LIVESTOCK HEALTH AND WELFARE

LONGMAN VETERINARY HEALTH SERIES

Forthcoming titles

The Health of Horses:
Edited by David G Powell & Stephen G Jackson

The Health of Poultry:
Edited by Mark Pattison

Small Ruminant Health:
Edited by Tony J Wilsmore & Peter J Goddard

Animal Breeding and Infertility:
Edited by Michael C Meredith

The Health of Dairy Cattle:
Edited by David G White

The Health of Pigs:
Edited by John R Hill & David W B Sainsbury

Food Hygiene:
Edited by Jeremy Hall

Nutrition and Animal Health:
Edited by John T Abrams

LIVESTOCK HEALTH AND WELFARE

Edited by
Roy Moss

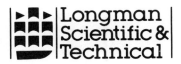

Longman Scientific & Technical,
Longman Group UK Ltd,
Longman House, Burnt Mill, Harlow,
Essex CM20 2JE, England
and Associated Companies throughout the world.

First published 1992

ISBN 0–582–060842

British Library Cataloguing in Publication Data
A catalogue record for this book is available from the British Library

Set by 3MM in 10/12½pt Plantin Roman.

Printed and Bound in Great Britain
at the Bath Press, Avon

CONTENTS

LIST OF CONTRIBUTORS

R Moss Esq., BVSc, MRCVS
Formerly Assistant Chief Veterinary Officer (GB)

I Ekesbo PhD, DVM, Dr.H.C.
Professor of Animal Hygiene, Swedish University of
Agricultural Science

A H Andrews BVetMed, PhD, MRCVS
Senior Lecturer in Farm Animal Medicine, Royal Veterinary
College, Hatfield

R Dantzer PhD, DVM
Directeur de Rechercher, Institut National de la Santé et de
la Recherche Médicale

M-C Salaün PhD
INRA Station de Rechercher Porcines

W H G Rees Esq., CB, MRCVS, OVSM
Formerly Chief Veterinary Officer (GB)

G Davies Esq., BVSc, Dip Bact, MRCVS
Head of Veterinary Intelligence and Resource Planning,
MAFF

R G Eddy Esq., BVetMed, FRCVS
Veterinary Surgeon, Somerset

A J F Webster MA, VetMB, PhD, MRCVS
Professor of Animal Husbandry, University of Bristol School
of Veterinary Science

H C Rowsell PhD, DVM
Executive Director, Canadian Council on Animal Care

W Sybesma
Director, Research Institute for Animal Husbandry, The Netherlands

LIST OF COLOUR PLATES (Pages 159–60)

FOREWORD

The interest shown by the general public in animal welfare issues is increasing and the moral status of animals has become an issue which is being widely debated in many parts of the world. Public opinion is divided on the ethics of livestock farming. Those who hold the view that, for the human population, food of animal origin is necessary for a balanced diet, appreciate that animal products must be marketed at affordable prices, but consumers are now demanding that the husbandry systems employed must give priority to the well-being of the animals. As many members of the community have scant knowledge of the realities of animal husbandry and food production a number of them look to members of the veterinary profession and other scientists responsible for advising farmers, to assure them that the welfare needs of the animals used for food production are receiving careful consideration.

Intensive farming systems using factory type buildings and production line methods are the ones most often criticized, but they cannot be condemned outright for they play a major part in the provision of cheap human foods. However, limits must be set on the lengths to which intensification methods can be allowed to proceed. There are commercial entrepreneurs who are developing farms into big businesses making sizeable profits, who do not consider the welfare of the animals their main objective.

Whatever system of husbandry is employed on an animal production unit, the standard of management is crucial to its successful operation. Good stockmanship demands that those in charge of the animals have a feeling for their needs and a knowledge of animal behaviour. Farms run on intensive lines, particularly those on which sophisticated machinery is used, need attendants who have special skills and it is important that they are given adequate training. It has been truly said that animal husbandry is a science which must be overlaid with tender loving care.

One clear aim of the book is to draw the attention of its readers to the basic facts that disease is a principal cause of suffering in animals and that the veterinary profession plays an important role in animal welfare by controlling and preventing outbreaks of disease. Because many overstocked intensive establishments do not provide healthy environments disease conditions can sweep through them. Advances in an understanding of the epidemiology of animal diseases have made it easier to prevent and control them and preventive medicine is now playing a larger part than ever before in animal production. Since several diseases of domestic animals are communicable to man, and some of these are of considerable public health significance, the subject is also of interest in human medicine.

The control of animal diseases by legislation has been in operation for centuries and, more recently, a substantial number of acts relating to animal welfare have been passed. The measures contained in some of these have been influenced by the views expressed by members of the general public. Such laws help to highlight the negative side of welfare by the avoidance of cruelty and disease, but more needs to be done to encourage a positive humane attitude to be adopted.

This book, which is a compilation of chapters written by authors who are recognized experts in their chosen fields, covers the subjects mentioned here as well as other related matters. Its value is enhanced because scientists from Europe and Canada have contributed, along with writers from Great Britain, to give a wide perspective to a theme which is of international importance. Although written primarily for members of the veterinary profession it contains information of value to all workers in the field of livestock husbandry. It meets the need for informed opinion by those advisers whose balanced views are valued by food consumers at a time when rapidly advancing technological methods are leading to a variety of developments in farming systems. Its effectiveness in achieving this aim is due to the scientific merit of the contributions and to the ease with which they can be read. It is to be hoped that the accumulated scientific and technical information it contains will be disseminated as widely as possible. All those concerned with the production of this work are to be congratulated on making such a valuable addition to the literature on the complex subject of livestock health and welfare.

J. O. L. King
May 1992

PREFACE

The need for this book became apparent after many years of discussion with colleagues both within and outside the veterinary profession on the concept of an holistic approach to the assessment of the status and maintenance of the well-being of farm livestock with regard to the particular environments and husbandry systems in which they are kept.

It is relatively easy for a veterinarian to make a careful clinical examination of an animal and its immediate companions and arrive at a preliminary diagnosis of its health status. Appropriate treatment, if required, will then bring about recovery, improvement or not, depending on the animal's original condition. However, complete recovery and maintenance of that recovery can only be achieved by ensuring that not only is the individual animal and its companions maintained in a fully healthy state but its surroundings, feeding and total environment contribute to the continued maintenance of that situation.

The concept of the holistic approach to the well-being of livestock is, however, only achievable through a partnership of the veterinary clinician with the pathologist, biochemist, nutritionist, ethologist, national and international regulatory authorities and many other disciplines and, of course, most importantly, the owner and the animal's attendants. Without such co-operation very little will be achieved in our efforts to continue to maintain all farm livestock in a satisfactory state of health and welfare.

The various chapters in this book deal with particular aspects of this co-operative approach, with the aim of providing a better understanding of the way in which judgements can be made on the status of the well-being of livestock and acceptable animal husbandry practices. How such judgements and acceptable practices are further translated into legislation and codes of practice is an important consequence, and a chapter is devoted to this aspect of the subject.

Valid judgements can, however, only be made in the light of available knowledge and the attitudes and perceptions of the public at any particular moment. Our knowledge of livestock and their reactions both physiologically and behaviourally to particular environments and husbandry practices continues to increase. However, interpretation of that knowledge does not always lead to agreement as to its significance in relation to an animal's well-being. Such disagreements can and do lead to confusion in the minds of both professional and lay people interested in livestock husbandry.

This book is written primarily for veterinary surgeons and veterinary students. It will also be of special interest to the livestock husbandry adviser, the livestock producer and attendant, to agricultural students in general and to the informed and interested layperson. It aims to dispel the confusion mentioned above and to draw together the various ways in which we are able not only to understand the welfare status of the animals with which we deal but also to deal with them in such a way that they are treated in accord with the fundamental requirements of the Council of Europe Convention on the Keeping of Animals for Farming Purposes, as expressed in Chapter I, Article 3 of that Convention, namely:

> Animals shall be housed and provided with food, water and care in a manner ... which having regard to their species and to their degree of development, adaptation and domestication ... is appropriate to their physiological and ethological needs in accordance with established experience and scientific knowledge.

It is hoped this book leads to a greater understanding of the complex relationship of the animal and the environment which man provides for it and the consequences of any part of that complex relationship. It is also a hope that this book will stimulate the reader to inquire further into the various aspects of the subject.

Roy Moss
October 1991

ACKNOWLEDGEMENTS

Without the enthusiastic support of all the contributors this book would not have been possible; to them my warmest thanks. In addition the constant encouragement of, and the advice solicited from and freely given by Dr David Sainsbury have been of inestimable value. I owe him a deep debt of gratitude.

Finally my thanks to all those, too numerous to name individually, who have been generous in the giving of advice and encouragement.

We are indebted to the following for permission to reproduce copyright material:

The author, Dr. M. Appleby for Fig. 4.5 (Appleby & Lawrence, 1987); the author, Dr. M. R. Baxter for Fig. 4.9 (Baxter & Schwaller, 1983); Birkhäuser Verlag AG for Tables 1.2 (Adler, 1974) & 1.3 (Simonsen, 1977); Blackwell Scientific Publications Ltd. for Figs 8.1, 8.4, 8.6 (Webster, 1987), 8.9 & 8.10 (Webster, 1984); the authors, M. J. Clarkson & W. B. Faull for Apps 7.13–7.19 (Clarkson & Faull, 1990); Elsevier Science Publishers BV for Fig. 4.1 (Done-Currie *et al.*, 1984), Tables 8.2 (Fuller, 1987) & 10.1 (Booman *et al.*, 1989); the author, D. Fraser for Fig. 4.3 (Fraser, 1987b) & part Table 4.4 (Fraser, 1987a & b); the author, J. M. Kelly for Apps 7.8 & 7.9 (Kelly *et al.*, 1988); Kluwer Academic Publishers for Fig. 4.11 (Baldwin, 1983); Kluwer Academic Publishers and the author, Prof. A. Oliverio for Fig. 3.2 (Oliverio, 1987); Longman Group UK Ltd. for Figs 8.2 & 8.3 (Webster, 1983); Ministry of Agriculture, Fisheries & Food/Agricultural Development & Advisory

Service for Figs 7.6 (MAFF, 1978), 7.7 (MAFF, 1982), Apps 7.1 (MAFF, 1984) & 7.2 (MAFF, 1979); National Sheep Association for Plates 5 & 6; the author, Dr. M. F. Seabrook for Table 4.7 (Seabrook, 1984 & 1987); Swedish National Board of Agriculture for Fig. 2.1; *Veterinary Clinics North America Food & Animal Practice* and the author, Prof. J. Breazile for Fig. 3.3 (Breazile, 1988); The Veterinary Record for Fig. 8.7 (Wathes *et al.*, 1983); The Veterinary Record and the author, M. R. Muirhead for Figs 7.1 (Muirhead, 1980), 7.8 (Muirhead, 1978), Tables 7.7, 7.8 (Muirhead, 1976) & 7.10–7.15 (Muirhead, 1980); the author, P. Zappavigna for Fig. 4.10 (Zappavigna, 1983).

Whilst every effort has been made to trace the owners of copyright material, in a few cases this has proved impossible and we take this opportunity to offer our apologies to any copyright holders whose rights we may have unwittingly infringed.

1 DEFINITION OF HEALTH AND WELFARE

R MOSS Esq., BVSc, MRCVS

Health and welfare—definitions
Animal welfare—the protagonists
Welfare codes of practice
Observational methods
Study of animal behaviour
Ethical considerations

In the United Kingdom on admission to membership of the Royal College of Veterinary Surgeons, the new member makes the following declarations:

> In as much as the privilege of Membership of the Royal College of Veterinary Surgeons is about to be conferred upon me I promise and solemnly declare that I will abide in all due loyalty to the Royal College of Veterinary Surgeons and will do all in my power to maintain and promote its interests.
>
> I further promise that I will pursue the work of my profession with uprightness of conduct and that my constant endeavour will be to ensure the welfare of animals committed to my care.

Having made these declarations the newly qualified veterinary surgeon is then admitted to the Register maintained by the Royal College under the terms of the Veterinary Surgeons Act 1966. This Act gives the veterinary profession in the United Kingdom a complete monopoly (with one or two minor exceptions) to practise the art and science of veterinary medicine. This right was not given to members of the veterinary profession for their own benefit but in order that members of the public and their animals are protected against incompetent unqualified practitioners.

As the *Guide to Professional Conduct* issued by the Royal College of Veterinary Surgeons in London points out, 'the second part of the declaration of a new member and the intentions of the legislature are therefore at one. The prime consideration is the welfare of animals entrusted to the veterinarian's care' (p. 6, Part I, para. 1.2: *Guide to Professional Conduct*, 1987).

Note there is no mention of the health of the animal. Yet the majority of the veterinary profession will think of themselves as being engaged in the day-to-day treatment, control and prevention of disease; in maintaining the health of the individual animal, the flock and the herd nationally and internationally.

Health and welfare—definitions

It is an interesting fact that health and welfare are treated by many people as separate subjects. Both are given the descriptive adjectives good and bad (poor). This is an attempt by the writer to indicate his or her declared (or even unstated) subjective or objective view of the holistic state of the animal they are describing in the particular circumstances of the time. Yet both the words 'health' and 'welfare' can be used in a description of the same condition. I think it will be agreed that an animal lacking correct nutrition will be in a state of both poor health and poor welfare. It will surely also be agreed that an animal affected by an infectious condition and showing clinical signs of that infection, e.g. a respiratory virus, can be considered to be in poor health. Yet it can also be argued that its welfare status may range from good to bad depending on the treatment and nursing it is receiving. With no treatment its welfare will be poor; but with acceptable treatment and nursing will not its welfare be good or at least satisfactory?

Many attempts have been, and continue to be, made to define both health and welfare. *Collins English Dictionary* 2nd edition defines *health* as 'the state of being bodily and mentally vigorous and free from disease'. The same source defines *disease* as 'any impairment of normal physiological function affecting all or part of an organism, esp. a specific pathological change caused by infection, stress [whatever that may mean], etc., producing characteristic symptoms'.

Welfare: health, happiness, prosperity and well-being in general.
Well-being: the condition of being contented, healthy or successful.

All of these definitions are helpful in any attempt to accurately define health and welfare. Yet none successfully succeeds in doing so. All the above definitions leave question marks. Duncan and Dawkins (1983) have written: 'The first and perhaps the biggest problem is one of definition. What do we mean by well-being or welfare or [and they introduce a new word] "suffering?"' What indeed do we mean?

Health

Dealing with health, Boddie (1946: 1) states 'the basis of the study of clinical methods must be a sound knowledge of anatomy, physiology and pathology as well as an intimate acquaintance with the appearance and behaviour of the animal in normal health.' Later on the same page he adds, 'only when he/she [the veterinarian] has become familiar with the normal animals that are his/her patients should the student turn his/her attention to the abnormal.' So a further concept is introduced: what is normal or, conversely, abnormal? The range of accepted normality will vary according to an observer's perceptions of it and can be very wide indeed.

The World Health Organization (WHO) definition of 'health' is also of interest here. 'A state of complete physical, mental and social well-being and not merely the absence of disease or infirmity . . . relative for each individual.'

Welfare

The Brambell Committee

Let us leave 'health' and turn to 'welfare', which has proved even more difficult to define in a way that is completely acceptable to all those interested in its definition. It is perhaps appropriate to first consider the *Report of the Technical Committee to Enquire into the Welfare of Animals Kept Under Intensive Livestock Husbandry Systems* (Brambell, 1965). This Committee, under the chairmanship of Professor F.W. Rogers Brambell, Head of the Zoology Department at the University College of North Wales, Bangor, was appointed by the Minister of Agriculture, Fisheries and Food, and the Secretary of State for Scotland, (at the end of June 1964). Its aims were 'to examine the conditions in which livestock are kept under systems of intensive husbandry and to advise whether standards ought to be set in the interests of their welfare, and if so what they should be.'

The report was published in December 1965. It is a seminal document (generally referred to as the 'Brambell Report') and contains much that is of importance and relevance to the scientific and ethical consideration of livestock health and welfare. The Committee wrote:

> Welfare is a wide term that embraces both the physical and mental well-being of the animal. Any attempt to evaluate welfare therefore must take into account the scientific evidence available concerning the feelings of animals that can be derived from their structure and functions and also from their behaviour. [chap. 4, para. 2.5]

The report also drew attention to the fact that, 'A principal cause of suffering in animals, as it is in men, is disease' (p. 11, para. 31). The report went on, 'we . . . accept the major importance of the disease risk in evaluating the welfare of an animal under any system of husbandry.' It is here implicit that absence of disease or disease risk is a plus factor towards good welfare.

The Report set out a number of principles on which the Committee based its judgements. They believed 'there are sound anatomical and physiological grounds for accepting that domestic animals and birds experience the same kind of sensations as we do' (para. 27). As noted above the Committee considered 'A principal cause of suffering in animals . . . is disease' (para. 31). The Committee was 'prepared to tolerate mutilation only where the overall advantage to the animal, its fellows, or the safety of man, is unmistakable' (para. 34). The Committee considered 'the degree to which behavioural urges of the animal are frustrated under the particular conditions of the confinement must be a major consideration in determining its acceptability or otherwise' (para. 36). They then set out one of the best known of their principles stating, 'an animal should at least have sufficient freedom of movement to be able without difficulty to turn round, groom itself, get up, lie down and stretch its limbs' (para. 37). The Committee considered a diet which 'should be such as to maintain it [the animal] in full health and vigour' was essential. 'Clearly . . .', the Committee said, 'an animal must be provided with adequate food and drink to prevent it suffering from hunger and thirst' (para. 39).

Farm Animal Welfare Council

Following the Report of the Brambell Committee the Government set up the Farm Animal Welfare Advisory Committee (FAWAC) which produced the first Codes of Recommendations (1968) for the Welfare of Livestock. In 1973 the FAWAC was replaced by the Farm Animal Welfare Council (FAWC), which was given the task of updating the Codes issued by its predecessor. The preface to each of the updated codes states:

> The basic requirements for the welfare of livestock are a husbandry system appropriate to the health and, so far as practicable, the behavioural needs of the animals and a high standard of stockmanship.

Later in the preface comes a list of provisions which it is suggested will fulfil the animals' basic needs:

- comfort and shelter
- readily accessible fresh water and a diet to maintain the animals in full health and vigour
- freedom of movement
- the company of other animals, particularly of like kind
- the opportunity to exercise most normal patterns of behaviour
- light during the hours of daylight, and lighting readily available to enable the animals to be inspected at any time
- flooring which neither harms the animals nor causes undue strain
- the prevention, or rapid diagnosis and treatment, of vice, injury, parasitic infestation and disease
- the avoidance of unnecessary mutilation

- emergency arrangements to cover outbreaks of fire, the breakdown of essential mechanical services and the disruption of supplies

It is interesting to note that the prevention and treatment of disease forms only one of the factors which will satisfy the welfare requirements of the animal and by implication prevent it suffering unnecessarily.

Council of Europe Convention

We have now been introduced to the word 'suffering' by both Duncan and Dawkins and the Brambell Committee. The former quote the latter report in which some examples of states of suffering are listed as fear, pain, frustration and exhaustion. Perhaps the Council of Europe Convention for the Protection of Animals kept for Farming Purposes (Council of Europe, 1976) will be of help in our attempt to seek acceptable definitions. Unfortunately, although the words health and welfare are mentioned in the Convention Document they are not defined. It is taken for granted that we understand their meaning in the context and purpose of the Convention which is as it states for the 'Protection' of animals. The Convention does however introduce a further concept, that of 'needs'. Art. 3 states:

> Animals shall be housed and provided with food, water and care in a manner in which—having regard to the species and to their degree of development, adaptation and domestication—is appropriate to their physiological and ethological needs in accordance with established experience and scientific knowledge.

The word 'needs' is also used in relation to space requirements in art. 4(2) and in art. 5, which deals with lighting, temperature, humidity, air circulation, ventilation and other environmental conditions.

Needs

There has been and will continue to be much discussion on what constitutes these needs, qualified as they are by the requirement that they be appropriate to the physiology and ethology of the particular species, having regard to their degree of development, adaptation and domestication.

Fortunately, we have been helped in our interpretation of the use of the word 'need' in the context of the Convention by Dawkins. She brilliantly makes use of the theory of consumer demand to achieve an understanding of the measurement of ethological need (Dawkins, 1983a). Her basic thesis is that there are ultimate and approximate needs which in the unnatural (Dr Dawkins' word) environment of the farm may become de-coupled. She believes that measuring the behavioural elasticity of demand under conditions where total time is restricted might therefore enable scientists to make an objective distinction between what animals regard as luxuries and what they regard as necessities.

We now have a number of words for which we seek an acceptable definition: health, welfare, suffering, need and one not yet mentioned and which, at least in legislation, predates all the others, cruelty. Each word will have a separate and particular meaning to all involved in livestock husbandry. Each person so involved will find themselves located at one or other position along the range of understanding of the meaning of health, welfare, suffering, need and cruelty. Most will occupy the middle ground but some quite legitimately will find themselves at one end or the other, appearing to be grossly out of step with the majority view. However, that majority view can and will change over time as evidenced by the changes in attitudes towards the keeping of farm animals during the past few decades.

Animal welfare—the protagonists

Who are the protagonists whose various viewpoints it is so important to understand?

First the livestock producer, who is in that business for profit. However, it also has to be said that in almost every case livestock producers do have a considerable concern for the health and welfare of the livestock under their charge. But profit must still remain of primary importance and to live with subclinical disease or even a low level of overt disease may not reduce that profit. In the world of livestock economics the prime consideration is the net profit per unit of capital invested. If the maintenance of satisfactory health and welfare means a lowering of profit, will the livestock producer be prepared to pursue the former, particularly as it may lead to reduced competitiveness in the market place?

The general public is the second of our protagonists, who in the majority of cases, are primarily concerned with the price and quality of the food they buy. However, some, and an increasing number, do wish to have a say in the sort of systems under which animals should be reared and fattened. A few committed animal welfarists believe animals should not be 'exploited' in any way. This section of the general public, which contains people with considerable expert knowledge of livestock farming practices, can and does have a considerable influence on our use of livestock for our own purposes. They continue to have an increasing importance in the consultative process adopted by governments, which politically have to balance all the, sometimes conflicting, interests of the general public. This process also takes into account what is, in the government's opinion, in the public interest, which is not necessarily the same as the interest of the public.

But how do the general public and government make judgements. Who is to provide the objective evidence for sound judgements to be made? This is the task of the scientist, and in particular the veterinary surgeon and the livestock husbandry specialist. But this task is not confined to the veterinary surgeon, scientist and husbandry specialist working in the research laboratory or on the experimental husbandry farms. The veterinary surgeon in general practice and the husbandry specialist working in the field have a very important part to play in the collection and evaluation of evidence on which governments will make judgements and take legislative action.

Welfare codes of practice

The 1970 Report

In September 1970 a report of the Farm Animal Welfare Advisory Committee (FAWAC) was published which set out the considerations that Committee members had taken into account in preparing the Codes and in their re-examination of disputed points (Farm Animal Welfare Advisory Committee, 1970). The report was addressed to the Minister of Agriculture and the Secretary of State for Scotland who had asked the Committee to allow its thinking on the content of the Codes to receive wider publicity than is generally normal for material prepared by a Ministerial Advisory Committee.

The Committee was chaired by Professor H.R. Hewer, and in his foreword to the Report he wrote of the two different approaches which were taken in formulating the contents of the first Codes of Practice. He labelled them, for convenience, the 'Ethical' and 'Scientific' approaches to seven key welfare issues; these are set out in the report at para. 12:

1. Adequate fresh air.
2. Food: sufficient and of a type to keep the animal in full health and vigour.
3. Fresh water readily accessible.
4. Avoidance of mutilations of benefit only to the farmer, or to which there are reasonable alternatives.

5. Freedom of movement (including the ability freely to turn round and exercise limbs).
6. Comfort of immediate environment (e.g. freedom from draughts, a bedded area).
7. Freedom to follow innate behaviour patterns except where its denial cannot reasonably be avoided.

(cf. preface of the present updated Codes of Recommendations (1968); see page 4).

Professor Hewer further stated that the first four would be unconditionally accepted under the 'scientific' approach (as well as the 'ethical') and the last three also, subject to other factors such as health and their validity in particular cases.

Chapter 1 of the Report then sets out first the 'Ethical Approach' to these welfare issues, and then the 'Scientific Approach'. In both approaches much emphasis is placed on 'stress' which, in relation to the ethical approach, is defined (para. 4) as 'an upset of homeostasis (a state of equilibrium in the living body with respect to various functions) which without intervention leads inevitably to death'. The point is made that a sharp distinction should be made between this definition and that (commonly accepted by the layman) of prolonged discomfort or pressure on life.

Para. 3 of the chapter contains the nub of the argument as to why both ethics and science must be used in combination when taking decisions on the suitability or not of animal husbandry practices. In para. 3 the report points out that it is widely agreed that there is insufficient scientific evidence on welfare issues, especially on animal behaviour and about the reaction of animals to imposed environments. Moreover, much of the practical experience is based only on assessments of the animals' ability to 'do well' in an economic sense. The paragraph continues:

> in this situation it is easy to fall back not on scientific evidence but on scientific opinion, which is by no means unanimous and which, like any other opinion, may be founded on subjective bias. Neither singly nor combined do the scientific and practical approaches provide an adequate basis for decisions on key welfare issues. They leave too much in doubt and they make too many assumptions. In particular, they place welfare needs second to considerations of productivity.

In dealing with the scientific approach a slightly different definition of 'stress' is considered (para. 14). The term is used to

> represent the total effect on the animal of its environment which, while it may lead normally only to a temporary state of imbalance, will, if pro-

longed or of a more severe nature, cause or lead to a departure from a state of health and well-being.

It is pointed out that within this definition it follows that health and well-being (which we have been trying to define) are indicators of the absence of this state of stress. Para. 14 of Chapter 1 finishes with the sentence: 'It remains to find out whether there is any measurable quality or function which can be used as a true criterion of health and welfare and of any deviation therefrom.'

Governments work through both legislation, which requires certain things to be done or not done (obligatory advice), and advice, which is not mandatory. The latter is generally expressed through codes of practice, which list a series of recommendations; if followed these should safeguard the welfare, health and needs of the animals for which they are concerned.

Content of Codes of Practice

All the Codes of Practice issued by the Government in Great Britain, which cover cattle, sheep, pigs, poultry (turkeys, domestic fowls and ducks), rabbits and deer, can be divided into four basic sections:

1. Housing, which includes the control of the ventilation and temperature of both climatic and totally controlled environment housing, lighting, mechanical equipment and services.
2. Space allowance for individual animals depending upon their species, age, sex and system of husbandry.
3. The provision of food and water, in both intensive and extensive systems.
4. Management, which includes the provision of isolation facilities, the loose housing of cattle and the housing of calves, farrowing quarters, sow quarters in piggeries, the tethering of sows, and the outside shelter of sows kept in extensive systems, the cleansing and disinfection of buildings, the facilities for handling cattle during routine tuberculin testing, vaccination, etc., and the provision of facilities to cover the risk of fire.

A similar course of action has been adopted by the Council of Europe Standing Committee for the Convention for the Protection of Animals kept for Farming Purposes. The Committee has already published a number of sets of recommendations, the first of which covered the laying hen and closely paralleled the contents of the Codes of Practice issued in Great Britain. These recommendations when adopted by those Member States of the Council of

Europe which have already ratified the convention, may be implemented either by legislation or administrative means.

Formulation of legislation

In the formulation of such legislation, the prime importance of the opinion of the scientist, and in particular the veterinary surgeon, has already been pointed out. These experts should, but do not always, seek objective evidence on which valid and meaningful decisions on the content of the legislation should be based. There can be a significant divergence of opinion between the pure behaviourist who believes in the simple 'mechanical' response of an animal to stimuli within its environment, and the ethologist who is more concerned with the wider implications of an animal's response to that environment through its perceptions and behaviour. Veterinarians are uniquely placed in this respect with their comprehensive understanding of both health and welfare. Most often they are the scientists who are called upon to observe the reaction of an animal to its environment in the working situation.

Table 1.1 sets out the basic animal/environment situation. On the left-hand side are the various individual (sometimes combined) environmental influences which are brought to play on an animal and its genetic blueprint throughout the whole of its life. That period of time is broken down on the right-hand side into the different periods of that life; these are self-explanatory.

The collection of information about the result of the interaction of environmental influences at various and often critical times in an animal's life is of prime importance to all involved in livestock production. It is in any particular case of great importance to the individual livestock farmer and his veterinary surgeon (nor should we forget its importance to the animal) when seeking to establish a diagnosis and advice on treatment. Some of the various clinical and laboratory methods that may be used in assessing the effect of environmental influences on individual animals will be discussed in subsequent chapters.

The collection of information is also of considerable importance to the livestock industry in general, and to the general public and government in their attempts to reach agreement on how livestock should be kept. In the case of those members of the Council of Europe who have ratified the Convention of the Keeping of Animals for Farming Purposes there is also the need to consider how that Convention and any recommendations agreed under it should be implemented.

Within Europe the other important legislative authority is the European Community. Directives have already been agreed and issued relating to the welfare of animals during transport and slaughter. Both these Directives have been based on Conventions formulated and agreed by *ad hoc* committees of the Council of Europe, which of course includes countries both inside and outside

Table 1.1 Environmental influences that may act on an animal at the various stages or events in its life

Environmental influences	Life stages/events
Feed	Pregnancy
Type	Parturition
Feeding method	Neonatal period
Ad lib	Rearing
Twice/thrice daily	Breeding
Natural/artificial	Fattening
Housing	Transport
Ventilation	Road
Forced/natural	Rail
Humidity control	Sea
Flooring	Air
Slats	
Solid floor	In markets
Drainage	
Bedding	At slaughter
Pen size and shape	
Single/group pen	
Family pen	
Tether/non-tether	
Handling facilities	
Disease	
Preventive medicine	
Routine testing	
Vaccination programmes	
Transport methods	
Land, sea, air	
On foot	
Construction	
Markets	
Methods	
Construction	
Slaughter	
Methods	
Construction	

the European Economic Community, which itself is a member of the Council of Europe as well as its constituent countries.

In 1989 the European Commission published for consultation draft regulations updating the present Directive on the transport of livestock. They also published draft regulations covering the keeping of pigs and calves up to the age of 6 months. All three drafts are based on the relevant recommendations produced by the Council of Europe.

There are a number of observational methods which have been, and continue to be used. Some are more applicable for use by the veterinarian in a clinical situation. Others are of more use for monitoring animals in the herd and in differing livestock systems. All will provide the veterinarian, and hence the livestock producer, with important information which should enable the veterinary surgeon to satisfy his primary requirement which, as previously noted in the oath taken by all veterinarians in the United Kingdom on becoming a member of the RCVS, is 'that my constant endeavour will be to ensure the welfare of animals committed to my care'.

Observational methods

All observational methods can provide all the protagonists in the welfare debate with information. Much of this will be of inestimable use in the search for acceptable livestock husbandry methods.

First, let us consider the information which can be obtained by an inspection of the individual animal and all facets of the environment to which it has been and is being subjected—a familiar situation to both the veterinarian in general practice and the State veterinarian in the field.

Professor G.F. Boddie in his book *Veterinary Diagnosis* (Boddie, 1946) sets out the method by which a clinical inspection should be undertaken. He writes first of a general inspection of, where necessary, both the individual or individuals concerned and then of the group or groups related to those individuals. The clinical examination of the individual follows; specifically, it must relate to a full examination of some or all of the following physiological systems:

1. Digestive system
2. Respiratory system
3. Circulatory system
4. Urinary system
5. Nervous system
6. Skin
7. Lymphatic system
8. Sense organs (eye, ear)
9. Genitalia and mammae
10. Locomotor system

Although in the vast majority of cases it will not be necessary to make an exhaustive examination of each and every system, all should have been considered during the first careful inspection of the animal. Only then will it be necessary for an examination to be carried out on one or more of the separate systems detailed above, the need to do so having been identified during the prior general inspection of the animal and its companions.

This detailed clinical inspection and examination of an individual animal plays an important part in any assessment of the welfare status of that animal. The Report of the United Kingdom House of Commons Agriculture Committee for the session 1979–80, sets out 'the principal nature of the abuses of animal welfare which veterinary staff' (State Veterinary Service personnel) 'have in mind when they make visits to farms.' Such visits will be undertaken either specifically in response to a report of a welfare problem, or during the routine welfare inspection of livestock holdings carried out by State Veterinary Officers in accordance with UK Government policy.

So the veterinary officer considers:

1. The general state of the animals' health.
2. The level of production standards; the veterinary officer must ask himself if the milk yield is acceptable taking into account all the factors concerned, or does it indicate a chronic disease, untreated, or an inadequate level of nutrition?
3. The presence or absence of disease, generally or specifically, and if present what action has or is being taken to resolve the problem?
4. The level of mortality; this will apply particularly to livestock kept in large groups in intensive conditions.
5. Signs of abnormal behaviour. Such behaviour has been divided into a number of categories in a report published by the European Commission (1983):

    (a) *Injurious behaviour*, including all those behaviours whose performance is detrimental for the actor and/or receptor.
    (b) *Stereotyped behaviours*, fixed in form and orientation, performed repetitively, no obvious function.
    (c) *Abnormal body movements* and/or locomotion (apart from those resulting from wounds, disease and so on).
    (d) *Redirected behaviours* performed in the absence of adequate substrate and/or those occurring with abnormally high frequency or intensity.
    (e) *Apathetic behaviours*, where the animal appears to be uninterested in what happens in its environment.

6. Evidence of pain or distress.
7. Disease control procedures exercised by the producer.
8. The necessity of any mutilations which may have been undertaken.

9. The stocking density; not just housed animals but to include those kept more or less permanently outside.
10. The care and skill with which means of restraint have been employed and their effect on the animals.
11. The appropriateness of the ambient temperature and humidity levels.
12. The adequacy of feeding and watering arrangements.
13. The quality of management in relation to the particular enterprise.

The Annex (ibid. House of Commons Agricultural Committee Session 1979–80) continues:

Veterinary Staff will also look at:
1. The presence or absence of an adequate supply of fresh water and wholesome food and its availability to the animals;
2. The adequacy and suitability of the accommodation and the suitability of the flooring;
3. The standard of maintenance of buildings, equipment and fittings;
4. The adequacy of alternative arrangements if essential equipment breaks down;
5. The adequacy of lighting arrangements.

The reader will have noticed here the introduction of two words which will almost certainly have somewhat different meanings to the various protagonists described earlier in this chapter: adequacy and suitability. Tethered sows on slats will be considered to be provided with both adequate and suitable accommodation and flooring by some producers and scientists but quite the opposite by many others, particularly those keenly interested in animal welfare. The Annex (ibid. House of Commons Agricultural Committee Session 1979–80) concludes:

> So many factors contribute to the welfare of animals that it is not always possible to say with any certainty in the present state of our knowledge, which factors or combination of factors contribute to its abuse. In very general terms, neglect, ill-health, disease, unnecessary pain or distress, poor stockmanship could separately or together cause abuses of animal welfare.

So here are two very detailed methods of inspection and examination of livestock which together should enable a veterinary surgeon to reach both specific and general conclusions as to the welfare status of a single animal or group of animals. Indeed, leaving aside detailed clinical inspection and examination, these methods should also enable livestock husbandry specialists, including livestock farmers, to do much the same thing.

Two further direct methods of assessing welfare status are of interest. But here we shall confine ourselves to the direct observation of the animal (or animals) and its reaction to the environment in which it is found.

Table 1.2 gives a basis for the evaluation of an animal's well-being proposed by Adler. Adler also suggested (Adler, 1974b) that such very objective clinical parameters as the levels of mortality and morbidity can be used to assess welfare. Are there any particular circumstances (or production systems) in which there are exceptionally high rates of mortality and/or morbidity? The last method has been suggested by Simonsen (1977). The list of factors considered important by him is given in Table 1.3.

The basis of selection from the above methods of assessment comprises:

1. Inspection of first the group (of animals) and second the individual or individuals.
2. A clinical examination of the individual.
3. An assessment of the environmental factors involved covering:
     (i) buildings, suitability, repair, ventilation;
    (ii) nutrition;
   (iii) production levels; and
   (iv) quality of management.

Study of animal behaviour

Up to now we have described observation and recording of the animal by an outside agency. What of the animal itself? What does it observe? Is it aware? Does it understand what is happening to it? Can it indeed suffer in the same way as a human being? Because an animal cannot describe its feelings verbally (and in any case even in human terms words are often inadequate to describe emotions) does not mean it cannot communicate. It does so by other forms of behaviour, which may include vocal communication using various sounds. Thus behavioural studies, the recording of an animal's response to a particular set of environmental circumstances, can provide much information on the mental, as well as the physical, state of the animal under observation. The response of an animal to a choice of environment may also help to provide an insight into an animal's mental and physical state. However, considerable care must be taken in the interpretation of such experimental results; both the choices presented to the animal may represent poor conditions, the one chosen being less aversive than the other.

Table 1.2 A basis for evaluating an animal's well-being (from Adler, 1974b)

SCIENTIFIC BASIS
Clinical parameters
    Mortality
    Morbidity
    Symptoms of health and well-being
Production parameters
    Growth
    Yield   } Protein metabolism
    Reproduction
Other parameters
    Behaviour data
    Physiological, endocrine data

ETHICAL BASIS
Rights of the animal as a living environment-conscious individual.

Table 1.3 Factors relevant to appraising an animal's well-being, as proposed by Simonsen (1977)

State of health
    Clinical evaluation
    Laboratory analysis
    Mutilations such as castration, beak-trimming, docking

Behaviour
    Registration of elements of behaviour within the categories:
        Normal
        Deviant
        Abnormal

Care-taking
    Registration of man hours per day per animal:
        (i) for ordinary management
        (ii) for special observation

Equipment
    Evaluation of quality and function, risks of functional disturbances

Duncan (1975) has described three types of research covering the investigation of the interaction of animals with the environment imposed upon them:

1. Research for welfare purposes, with very exact experimental protocols, controls and investigations into the physiological and biochemical reactions of the animals involved. In a paper presented at the first Danish

seminar on poultry welfare in egg laying cages Duncan (1978b) further subdivided the behavioural methods used in this specific welfare research into three:

(a) Step 1, look for unusual or inappropriate behaviour; Step 2, show independently that this is indicative of stress or reduced welfare.
(b) Step 1, subject birds experimentally to stressful situations such as deprivation, frustration or fright and observe their behaviour; Step 2, compare this behaviour to that which occurs under commercial conditions;
(c) Give birds a choice of environment and assume that they will choose in the best interest of their welfare. (The problem of interpretation of such choices has already been mentioned.)

2. Research with livestock for other purposes which may have welfare implications; by this is meant research into environment, housing, ventilation, nutrition and disease.
3. Operational research; this has been carried out, particularly in Sweden, and there would appear to be a vast untapped amount of information on what happens to livestock on farms, during transport and in slaughter houses, which can be used in conjunction with the results of research, for specific recommendations in relation to the keeping of animals under particular systems. This type of study will be more fully discussed in Chapter 2.

Operational research has a number of essential precursors:

(a) there must be clear-cut objectives;
(b) it must be very clear which observations are to be made and what use is to be made of them;
(c) the farm types must be clearly classified;
(d) it must be decided whether the farms are to be picked at random or specifically chosen;
(e) statistical evaluation to determine the extent of the studies required to make them statistically reliable and thus useful must be made;
(f) report forms must be designed;
(g) resources and costs must be considered.

However, this area would appear to be one of the most fruitful, since it involves observation of animals in practical situations, although in many cases the full scientific basis for definitive decisions is lacking. Even so, such studies will enable particular recommendations for the maintenance and perhaps improvement of animal health and welfare to be made.

Ethical considerations

Finally mention must be made of the need to consider the ethics of the animal/
human relationship in the use of animals for human profit. Recently, the word
'bioethics' has been used to describe what is really a synthesis of science and
philosophy. In fact it is arguable that animal welfare and bioethics are almost
synonymous. It is interesting to return to the report of the Brambell Committee (Brambell, 1965), in which can be found a number of statements and
recommendations that come close to being, if they are not exactly, bioethical
statements and judgements. In addition to those already quoted (p. 3) can be
added:

> 'there are sound anatomical and physiological grounds for accepting that
> domestic mammals and birds experience the same kind of sensations as
> we (humans) do . . .'; 'all farm animals . . . need companionship and are
> likely to suffer from solitary confinement.'

It is interesting here to note the similarity between these quotations (above
and p. 3) and the preface of the up-to-date Welfare Codes of Practice published
by the Ministry of Agriculture, Fisheries and Food in Great Britain following
advice from the Farm Animal Welfare Council (see p. 4). Also in the Preface
the Farm Animal Welfare Council makes very clear its attitude towards current methods of livestock husbandry. It states:

> 'Nearly all livestock husbandry systems impose restrictions on the stock
> and some of these can cause an unacceptable degree of discomfort or
> disease by preventing the animals from fulfilling their basic needs.'

The Farm Animal Welfare Council has also made clear its views in relation
to animal welfare and research. In June 1982 it stated in a MAFF Press Notice
that there should be no research into:

- adapting farm animals physiologically or anatomically to enable them to
  be used in more and more intensive systems unless there should be
  positive welfare advantages in doing so;
- the use of drugs to overcome disadvantages in husbandry systems otherwise unacceptable to animals.

By separating the consideration of health and welfare and dealing with them
as separate subjects, we confuse the issue of how are we to farm livestock
towards the end of the twentieth century. If we are to look for the production
of disease-free animals, and particularly animals which do transmit disease to
the human food chain, can we afford to consider livestock husbandry systems

which do not protect such disease-free status? Do we have to deprive an animal of some of its 'needs', which within the terms of Dawkins' argument might be considered as luxuries by the animals, to achieve that end? If we take the welfare status of an animal as an entity which must include an assessment of the health of the animal concerned then we can perhaps more easily take decisions on whether an animal is suffering unnecessarily. Such an assessment does, of course, accept that there will be occasions when an animal will suffer but with every effort being made to not only mitigate that suffering but to end it as soon as possible.

Each of the chapters which follow will develop a particular aspect of the holistic approach to the subject of health and welfare of farm livestock. The viewpoint will be first of all the needs and interests of the veterinary clinician in private practice and the veterinary surgeon in government service both in the field and in the higher levels of administration nationally and internationally. The livestock producer and livestock husbandry advisor will also find much of interest and practical application. However, the animals themselves remain central to the study and the effect on them of the way in which we deal with them for production and preventive medicine purposes will show whether our efforts to achieve satisfactory productivity and welfare are achievable.

2

MONITORING SYSTEMS USING CLINICAL, SUBCLINICAL AND BEHAVIOURAL RECORDS FOR IMPROVING HEALTH AND WELFARE

I. EKESBO PhD, DVM, Dr.H.C.

In all periods and in all cultures human beings seem to have given the highest priority in farm animal husbandry to efforts aimed at keeping their animals in good health and protecting them from disease. This in itself also involves certain guarantees for animals' welfare. Ultimately, however, animal welfare is and has always been dependent on the behaviour of the individual herdsman or woman. It is not unrealistic to say that the great majority of stockpersons of all earlier generations have fulfilled their responsibility for animal welfare.

If one discusses how to measure health and welfare and the influence on them of environmental and management factors, the two concepts health and welfare should first be defined.

The concept of health in the individual animal has been defined as 'harmony in functions between the organs and organ systems within the body, and harmony between the body and its environment' (Ekesbo 1983).

The concept of welfare is usually defined by indicating the needs which are to be met in order to provide for animal welfare. The Convention for Animal Protection of the Council of Europe (Council of Europe 1976) says that 'species-specific physiological, ethological, and health needs must be met'.

The expression 'animal husbandry' in what follows does not only mean the individual herd but also the individual animal and the individual farmer and stockperson.

Why the need for monitoring systems?

Interest in environmental protection, animal welfare and similar ethical questions has grown considerably in recent years, not only in young people but in all categories of people and professions in the Western democracies. Increased interest in the same issues is also evident in the former Communist countries of eastern Europe, following restoration of their democratic rights and freedoms.

Among farmers the situation is more complicated. During the 1950s and 1960s many farmers were very negative towards some of the new methods and systems introduced in animal husbandry. They regarded several aspects of these new methods as detrimental to the health and welfare of their animals, much as arable farmers reacted negatively towards intensive crop farming using monoculture and biocides.

However, two factors have been largely responsible for allaying farmers' doubts about intensive animal husbandry and the attendant risks of environmental pollution and bad animal welfare. One is the campaign of information, even propaganda, in favour of all new methods and techniques waged over the last 30 years. The other is the demand from society for greater efficiency in agriculture and its resultant economic advantages for the farmers. Most farmers have followed this advice and applied the intensive husbandry methods, despite their implications for animal health and welfare.

The situation has thus radically changed compared to the early 1960s. Many farmers have become strong defenders of cages and other confinement systems for poultry, sows, piglets or calves when animal health and welfare in such systems is questioned by consumers or by animal welfare organizations. Many farmers apparently feel that their own expertise is being questioned rather than the methods themselves.

However, among young farmers and especially on family farms there has in recent years been an increasing interest in more biological methods or environment-friendly systems in animal husbandry.

One apparent reason for this is the wish to reduce losses due to injuries and diseases caused by factors in the animals' environment (including management). Another appears to be a general uneasiness because of public criticism against what is regarded as factory farming. A third reason, and one which might often be forgotten, is the personal gratification of good animal husbandry and the sense of pride this creates for the stockperson. A further reason is that the traditional interest of farmers in environmental protection and animal welfare is again being asserted among farmers as a group. Experienced farmers realize that environmental protection and animal welfare are not incompatible with good economics. This means that many farmers, often of the new generation, are back in the same situation as their forebears in the late 1950s or the early 1960s. However, this generation often lacks the 'inherited' knowledge of the connection between husbandry and animal health and welfare. This generation demands scientifically based facts about these relationships.

Definition and measurement of farm animal health and welfare

Very simply, 'health' in the individual animal can also be negatively defined as 'absence of disease symptoms' (Ekesbo 1988). The individual animal is in that way characterized as either healthy or sick. This clinical diagnosis of health can be made more precise by observing the animal's behaviour in different situations, for instance observing the animal's feeding, resting or locomotion behaviour.

The behavioural observation can be supplemented with different chemical, physiological, microbiological, immunological and similar laboratory examinations of body fluids, body tissues and excretion products. An animal is thereby considered healthy if the obtained results are within the range of normal variation.

The health of a herd or any other animal population can be described by the frequencies of different diseases. But different definitions of diseases can be chosen. If clinical definition of a disease is chosen, it can be given in two different ways. The individual farmer can give the frequency of all diseases he is able to identify and register in his herd (Ekesbo 1966; Vilson 1973; Ekesbo et al. 1990). The method, when used correctly, has been shown adequate in giving results of great validity not only for the investigated animal, but also generally for all such animals. Analyses of such material have given a clear appreciation about the disease panorama in dairy cows (Ekesbo 1966). Furthermore, it has become possible with different degrees of certainty to stipulate risk factors for the most common individual diagnoses (Ekesbo 1966; Bäckström 1973; Lindqvist 1974). Such investigations have shown that udder disorders are the most common clinical diseases in dairy cows. For sows the MMA complex is shown to be the most common disorder.

Such information about the clinical frequency of single diseases is normally not available in official statistics. In most countries these are incomplete. In certain countries treatments performed by veterinarians are registered. These give a more accurate but still incomplete picture of the health condition in a herd or in a population, reliable only with respect to the few diseases always treated by a veterinarian. Consequently, the information regarding diseases that only seldom need veterinary treatment does not reflect their true occurrence.

Other sources of information are available for some specific diseases. For example, an estimation of the dairy cow mastitis situation can be obtained from milk cell counts, either from a single cow or from herd samples taken from the milk tank.

By recording the results from veterinary slaughter inspection, the health at slaughter can be determined for an animal, herd, species, region, population, etc. This is especially used for intensively bred calves and young stock, for fattening pigs and for poultry. If the animals are individually marked it is possible to obtain information on individual animals.

Knowledge of the connections between animal environment and animal health is of essential importance for all forms of animal husbandry. Only in this way can the cost/benefit analyses be made which make possible an economic comparison between different environments or different management methods. All such comparisons must of course avoid bias due to confounding factors. For instance, an evaluation of the impact of one or several animal environments on animal health cannot be based on health reports from the studied populations where some have been given medicine for prophylactic purposes and others have not.

In order to guarantee the accuracy of the analysis of animal health in a herd or in any animal population all factors affecting the frequency of each disease must be taken into consideration. Examples include age, breed, yield level and various environmental factors. Thus age is a risk factor for dystocia, hence for Holstein heifers the risk is about three times higher than for a Holstein cow at her second or third calving. Comparisons between herds or groups of animals therefore must take such risk factors into consideration. When comparing, for example, trampled teat incidence in groups of dairy cows housed in two different stall breadths the risk factors stall length and bedding material must be the same in the both groups. If not, stall length or presence or absence of straw might interfere with the results obtained. During recent years great progress has been made in defining such risk factors (e.g. Dohoo and Martin 1984; Bendixen et al. 1988b). Analyses of culling causes show that cows which have developed clinical mastitis are culled at a significantly lower age than cows without mastitis (Vilson 1976; Bendixen et al. 1988b).

For the objective measurement of the welfare of an animal or of a population several different parameters must be used (Ekesbo 1984, 1988).

The physical health of animals must be evaluated by a veterinarian specially experienced in the relationship between environment and animal health. The risk of bias due to confounding factors must be eliminated as much as possible, which requires profound knowledge of this type of epidemiology. This means that the experimental group and the control group must be similarly composed with regard to risk factors like age, breed, time of year, and season as well as environmental factors like the presence or absence of bedding, housing conditions, infection pressure, etc.

Furthermore, animal behaviour must also be studied and analysed, and the effects of different environmental factors evaluated. Here also the risk of bias due to confounding factors must be taken into consideration. Examples of bias are breed, age and environmental stimuli like straw, noise, etc. For ethological studies it is important to establish if the animals have had earlier experience of a comparable environment. Tied cows, for instance, often adopt special behaviour in getting up and lying down to tying devices, feeding barrier systems, stall lengths, etc. and do not change these behaviours when kept in other systems. Such experience can affect the animals' behaviour and thus cause false conclusions.

Close co-operation between qualified ethologists and veterinarians with experience in the field of environment–animal health interaction is most important in order to obtain scientifically reliable results when evaluating the different parameters.

To guarantee some degree of general validity for such studies they must be carried out under realistic circumstances, e.g. on animals in environments exposed to normal infection pressure. This means that studies have to be performed in commercial herds, which during such studies have to be divided into experimental and control groups under strict regulation of all environmental factors and taking bias from animal risk factors into consideration.

Measuring animal welfare thus always means measuring the animal's health, both physical and, as far as possible, mental.

Disease recording

Since the 1960s significant changes have occurred in dairy husbandry, with a definite trend toward larger herds, more intensive production systems and increased economic pressure to minimize the cost of production in order to remain profitable. Farmers as well as practising veterinarians are in need of more effective measures for herd health management with respect to control as well as prevention of disease.

During the 1960s and 1970s there appeared not only new techniques and new methods but also, if not new diseases, at least a changed disease panorama. The frequencies of environmentally evoked diseases increased considerably.

In recent years we have seen the introduction of new disease recording techniques as various research projects have sought a complete and accurate description of the disease situation in farm animals and have attempted to define risk factors for different diseases. Most studies have been carried out on cattle but there are also publications dealing with other species. Studies on cattle have been undertaken in France (e.g. Barnouin 1980; Faye et al. 1988), Holland (Grommers 1967), Sweden (Ekesbo 1966, 1988), Finland (Saloniemi 1980), USA and Canada (e.g. Dohoo and Martin 1984). On pigs studies have been performed in, for example, Sweden by Bäckström (1973) and Lindqvist (1974), and in Holland by Tielen (1974). In sheep work has been done by Ducrot et al. (1988), and in poultry by, for example, Svedberg (1976, 1988a). Also general approaches to the problem have been made in order to get functioning systems for health information from different geographical regions (e.g. Diesch 1988).

There have also been monitoring programmes for specific diseases: mastitis, retained placenta, dystokia (e.g. Saloniemi (1980; Dohoo and Martin 1984; Bendixen et al. 1986b).

Several practitioners in various countries use data processing for keeping records on cases and clients and some have developed their own programs for processing the material.

In Sweden a data processing system for mandatory reporting of veterinary diagnoses was gradually introduced province by province from 1970. This should enable the investigation of frequencies of cases which are treated or otherwise investigated by a veterinarian. It functions as follows. When the farmer calls his veterinarian the veterinarian fills in a special form on which the farmer's name, telephone number, the species of patient and, if one animal, the identity and the sex of the animal, plus a few words regarding its clinical history are recorded. If it is a telephone consultation the probable diagnosis, advice and possible drug prescriptions are noted. If it is a herd visit the veterinarian, after having investigated the animal(s), made the diagnosis, performed the treatment and prescribed any further treatment, completes the form and gives a copy to the farmer. The veterinarian keeps a copy for himself, and another copy is sent to the data processing unit. There is a fourth copy, which is always given to the farmer. This is to be used in case the animal has to be slaughtered or if it dies and is sent for postmortem examination. Part of this fourth copy can also be used if the veterinarian takes blood, milk or other samples for sending for laboratory investigation. The system has been mandatory for all veterinarians throughout Sweden since 1980. Once a year the veterinarian receives a summary of all reported cases in his practice. It is presented as the number of cases within each diagnosis. Farmers get annual information on a cow identity basis recording all disease consultations which have been performed on each cow by the veterinarian during the year. At present such a survey is available only for cows. For pigs, horses and other animals the farmer receives annually a list of all reported cases in his herd for each diagnosis but without mentioning the identity of the animal.

A problem with most monitoring programmes has been the absence of computer software able to process the field data, i.e. for making analyses and calculations. However, in recent years such software is beginning to be available (Frankena et al. 1990).

Example of a model for disease recording

Herd Sampling records

One model for dairy cows, which describes the herd health situation in most detail, was first developed in the early 1960s (Ekesbo 1966) and since then has been further elaborated (Ekesbo et al. 1991). The principal idea is that the farmer reports all diseases and injuries, and that information concerning housing and management of the herd as well as information about the identity, production, etc. of each herd member is made available.

The record of the occurrence of all diseases and injuries is obtained from the farmer or herd manager on a specially designed monthly report (Appendix 2.1). For each herd information regarding number of calvings, average number of cows per year and breed composition, and for each cow in the herd her identity, birth date, father, mother and similar genetic records, calving dates, production per lactation, sex of calf, etc. are obtained from the official Swedish dairy cow control organization. Each herd is visited and a description of its environment and management regime is recorded.

In the first version of this recording system (Ekesbo 1966) the identity of individual cows was not maintained. As there are breed differences in the occurrences of many diseases only purebred herds could fully utilize the results. The incidence of each disease per year was estimated relative to the number of calvings for diseases associated with parturition, and relative to the average number of cows for all other diseases. As a result of this study it was possible to obtain a good description of the panorama of diseases in the dairy cow population and to evaluate the role of several environmental factors, such as type of housing, grazing or zero-grazing, as risk factors in disease.

The experience gained from this study led to further development of the dairy cow disease recording method (Vilson 1976; Ekesbo et al. 1991). There are two components of the program: (a) the collection of data and (b) the utilization of data.

The farmer reports the identity of the cow for each disease or injury. On the monthly report, shown in Figure 2.1, is recorded the occurrence of every disease or injury, the cow affected, the date, and whether or not a veterinarian investigated the case. For several well-defined diseases and injuries categorized on the form, e.g. retained placenta, the farmer has simply to record their occurrence. For other diseases or injuries not included in the list, the farmer has to describe the signs and, when possible, the likely cause. For example, the farmer may report a hoof disease (No. 8 in Appendix 2.1) and indicate 'caused by slatted floor' or 'caused by interdigital infection according to the vet' or he may report other diseases (No. 13 in Appendix 2.1) and indicate 'metritis according to the vet' or 'diarrhoea caused by bad silage'. The aim behind this description of signs and possible aetiology is to avoid guessing at a diagnosis that may be unspecific and in some cases even false.

The reports are scrutinized and all diseases are coded. For example dystocia is coded as 001, mastitis as 020, trampled teat as 025, etc. For each group of diagnoses from No. 7 to No. 13, the appropriate diagnostic and associate disease code is determined on the basis of the description of the disease and signs provided by the farmer. Also results of laboratory tests, e.g. bacteriological milk investigations, are coded.

A disease file is subsequently created in the computer which includes herd and cow identification number, the disease code, the date and place where the disease occurred (e.g. at pasture or in the barn), cell counts, veterinary treatments, etc.

An environment file is created in the computer for each herd with a detailed description of the herd environment. It includes detailed information of how cows, calves and young stock are kept. For each herd detailed descriptions are recorded of relevant environmental and management factors including detailed characterization of the system as well as of the feeding regime and management. On a special form designed for data processing about 80 environmental and management factors are described. They comprise detailed descriptions of each barn or section of barn where dairy cows, heifers, calves or bull calves kept for beef are housed. These environmental factors include length, breadth and height of each animal room, details regarding manure handling, ventilation, watering and milking system, if urine drainage or not, length, breadth and surface type of stalls or cubicles, tying methods and type of manger or feeding gate. Management factors to be registered are type and approximate amount of bedding and feedstuffs used per animal per day. Also the day for letting the cows out to pasture in the spring as well as the day for housing them in the autumn are registered. Information is also gained regarding stockpersons—does the owner himself or herself, or an employee take care of the herd, and how is management for Saturday and Sunday organized, etc. Information about the herd environment can be recorded by specially educated technicians or by the veterinarian.

In a third file, the cow control file, detailed production and breeding information are gathered from the official dairy cow control organization for each herd and for each individual cow in participating herds. In this third file the information on individual cows regarding breed, age, calving dates and sex of calf born, annual production per cow and per herd, breeding information, etc. is stored.

Analysis of herd data

Once a year, or when the farmer or the veterinarian so wishes, collation and analysis of the disease reports are undertaken.

Computer programs have been developed to process the data and present them in a form that gives the veterinarian and the farmer a clear picture of the health of both single cows and the whole herd. The following information is presented once a year:

(a) All reported diseases and injuries in chronological order indicating date, cow identity, disease and if diagnosed by a veterinarian or not.
(b) All reported diseases distributed within the 13 groups (Appendix 2.1), per calendar month and indicating each affected cow.
(c) Each cow which was in the herd during all or part of the last 12 months in numerical order, indicating each reported disease and its date in chronological order. Cows without any reported remarks, i.e. cows healthy throughout the year, are noted. For culled cows the culling date and culling reason are indicated.
(d) Each cow in the herd in numerical order, indicating each reported disease since recording started in the herd. Also cows without any disease reports are indicated. For culled cows date of culling is indicated.

(e) The incidences within breed in the herd of all reported diseases distributed within the 13 groups during the 12 months of the last control year (in Sweden from 1 September to 31 August). The incidences (X) of diagnoses 1 to 4 are estimated according to the following formula:

$$X = \frac{I}{N-(\frac{W}{2})}$$

where I = the number of cases of the disease in question (i.e. number of cows affected by the disease and reported), N = number of cows which have calved, and W = number of cows not affected by the disease in question and which have either died at calving or been sold or slaughtered directly after calving. The incidences are presented as cumulative incidences.

The incidences (Y) of diagnoses 5 to 13 are estimated according to the following formula: $Y = I/(A+B+C)$, where I = the number of reported cases of the disease in question, A = the number of cows not affected by the disease in question which have been in the herd throughout the control year multiplied by 365, B = the total sum of the numbers of herd days for cows which have been in the herd less than a year and which were not affected by the disease, and C = the total sum of the numbers of days that each affected cow has been in the herd from the start of the control year until the day the disease occurred, for each disease. Y can also be presented as risk per 100 cow years, when Y must be multiplied by 36500. Instead of the control year any other period can be chosen. Thus comparisons between at-pasture and housed periods can be made.

(f) Incidences can be presented for more than the 13 groups shown in 2.1, with each group breaking down into subgroups; e.g. for diagnosis 13 there are about 40 subgroups.

(g) Each diagnosis can also be presented within age groups; this can be necessary for diseases where parity is a risk factor. The incidence of each diagnosis can also be presented within housing or pasture period or if it has happened inside or outside the cowshed.

Utilization of herd health data

The monitoring system described thus allows the assessment of the current herd health situation, the evaluation of the current health status of the herd relative to previous years or to other herds with similar or different environments, and the creation of a life health history for individual cows, sows, etc. The monitoring system will also identify animals or group of animals at risk for a particular disease based on the risk factors present in the herd in each time period evaluated.

The experiences gained from using this monitoring system indicate that it is possible to improve the farmer's knowledge of the health status of his herd as well of each cow in the herd. This is of great importance if disease incidence increases in the herd without any clear cause being established. This situation is not uncommon in modern animal husbandry. The results of analyses arising from this monitoring system are also of great value for decision making in culling and in the herd breeding programme.

Different sorts of compilations from such a monitoring system also give the farmer a much better basis for understanding connections between herd disease problems and environmental and management factors in the herd. Thus he can clearly see temporal connections between, for example, a cluster of reported trampled teats and a concurrence of animals in heat, which gives him the chance to take preventive measures, such as putting in stall partitions between each tied cow during such a period. Or he can see connections between changes in management, for instance the amount or type of bedding and udder or hoof health.

When a herd has been monitored for several years the programme's ability to discover temporal connections between variations in herd health and changes in environmental or management factors is much enhanced. Thereafter it has to be proved if the temporal connections are also causal.

It is not envisaged that this programme will be used by all farmers or veterinarians but rather by progressive farmers and veterinarians as a tool for designing a more effective herd health management programme and increasing their ability to control and prevent health-related problems. Tested in practice it has proved a reliable method for general use by progressive farmers and veterinarians acting together.

The data obtained through this disease recording system increase the possibilities for epidemiological studies aimed at identifying risk factors for diseases such as mastitis, trampled teats and parturient paresis (e.g. Bendixen et al. 1988a, 1988b; Oltenacu et al. 1988).

According to currently available literature no other programme so efficiently covers all diseases and injuries, both ones treated by a veterinarian and those diagnosed and treated by the farmer. With its software enabling collation and analysis, this programme offers a complete monitoring system for animal health. There is however one important provision: both farmer and veterinarian must be scrupulous and committed.

Relationship between animal environment and animal health and welfare

Monitoring systems using clinical or behavioural records enable elucidation of the relationship between the animal's environment and its health and welfare. Several investigations have shown that most major diseases in modern animal husbandry, including behaviour aberrations, are connected with factors in the animal's environment, including management, breeding or feeding, measures often designed to increase productivity. The following are examples of associations between diseases and environment.

1. Some diseases, e.g. parturient paresis and maybe also mastitis in dairy cattle, are positively correlated with the level of milk production (Bendixen et al. 1988a, 1988b).
2. The pecking directed to the cloaca region of mature chickens and egg-laying hens of high-producing hybrids has increased considerably and is a great problem in many flocks during the period from 16 to 30 weeks of age (Svedberg 1980).
3. Parallel to the increase in the growth rate of several breeds of pigs, poultry and cattle, skeleton disorders such as osteochondrosis (Reiland 1975; Poulos et al. 1978) have also increased. These disorders often cause serious clinical signs.
4. Changes of phenotype in some breeds, e.g. the Belgian Blue and Charolais beef cattle, have resulted in increased incidence of dystocia. More than 50% incidence of Caesareans is reported as the result of breeding for increased muscle mass, especially in the thigh region, of the newborn calf (Menissier and Foulley 1979).
5. It has been shown that zero-grazing (Dohoo and Martin 1984; Bendixen et al. 1986a, 1986b), minimal use or lack of bedding and slatted floors in the lying area (Ekesbo 1966) all increase the incidence of trampled teats and subsequent mastitis in dairy cows (Plate 2a). More than 40% mastitis is common in high-producing herds housed in unsuitable environments (Ekesbo 1966). A positive correlation has been shown between the use of so-called electric cow trainers and an increase in the incidence of subclinical mastitis (Bakken 1981).
6. Tail biting in pigs (Lindqvist 1974; van Putten 1979) and pecking in hens (Svedberg 1976) have also been shown to be associated with barren, monotonous environments.
7. Piglets weaned at 3–4 weeks and kept in cages or flat deck systems show a significantly higher incidence of abnormal behaviour. Such behaviours cause injuries, e.g. tail biting and ear biting (Algers 1984).

8. Manure gas poisoning is a disease problem associated with herds kept in houses with liquid manure handling systems (Bengtsson et al. 1967; Högsved and Holtenius 1968; Lindqvist 1974).

9. Foot disorders in cattle (Ekesbo 1966; Smedegaard 1982; Bee 1986; Colam-Ainsworth et al. 1989), pigs (Bäckström 1973) and poultry (Algers et al. 1984) have increased in herds or flocks where the animals are kept on unsuitable flooring.

10. Sows kept in stalls and crates, instead of loose in pens, show a higher morbidity. This is also true for their offspring (Bäckström 1973).

11. Hoof disease in tied cows seems to increase when short cut straw or sawdust is used as bedding instead of non-cut regular straw (Ekesbo 1966).

12. In specialized beef herds where the calves are purchased from different herds, the incidence of respiratory diseases is reported to exceed 75% (Miller et al. 1980). Respiratory disorders are a great problem in all herds of fattening pigs, beef calves and poultry flocks where an all in-all out system is not used. Respiratory disorders have also been reported from pig herds and turkey flocks because of dust problems (Collins and Algers 1984) created by a combination of too dry a climate, poor ventilation and unsuitable systems for feed distribution.

13. A total floorspace area of less than $0.7\,m^2$ per pig and air volumes of less than $3\,m^3$ per pig are shown to increase morbidity of fattening pigs (Lindqvist 1974).

The impact on livestock husbandry of good or bad health and welfare

It is easy to establish that poor animal health involves obvious losses for farmers—an extended breeding period means increased feed consumption, increased cost of labour and housing, etc. Economic assessments have been made of the cost of certain clinical diseases and also cost-benefit analyses with respect to changes in environment or management (Ekesbo 1973). Thus an average clinical mastitis case cost the farmer about £220 in 1986 (Clason and Everitt 1986).

The corollary of this is that good health conditions result in increased net cash for the farmer. As very few cost-benefit or similar economic analyses and studies have been performed it is difficult to assert with scientific objectivity that animal husbandry in environments which do not meet current health and welfare requirements will always incur an economic penalty for the farmer. But practical experience from many veterinarians and farmers indicates that this is the case. On the other hand there is a widespread belief that the effect of the animal environment can be judged simply from the animals' production. This method is both deceptive and inexact. The state of health, like production, is regulated by a host of different factors, many of which affect both. However, knowledge of these factors is too incomplete to allow definite conclusions regarding the state of health to be drawn from production data (Ekesbo 1966).

Consider the following example. Cow herd A kept in environment A produces an average of 8000 kg 4% milk. Cow herd B kept in a different environment B produces 7500 kg 4% milk. It is not possible to draw the conclusion that environment A is more suitable from the animal health and welfare point of view than B just from those production figures. An investigation of herd health might show that in herd A there are 20% trampled teats and 30% mastitis cases per year whereas in herd B there are 12% trampled teat cases and 18% mastitis. The investigation further shows that herd A has a very high intensity of veterinary treatments. Cows in herd A are regularly treated with antibiotic as soon as any trampled teat or mastitis case occurs, while in herd B only the mastitis cases are treated with antibiotic. It is further shown that herd A is fed a high proportion of concentrates whereas herd B only gets two-thirds of that amount per cow per year. The conclusion then must be that the difference in production between herds is mainly caused by the difference in feeding. The conclusion might also be drawn that there is a more detrimental effect on herd health from environment A than from environment B as there are higher incidences of trampled teats and mastitis in A than in B. It might also be concluded that both herds might increase their production with unchanged feeding regimes if they could change their environmental conditions so as to reduce the incidence of trampled teats and mastitis.

Attempts have been made to evaluate the role of the stockperson in animal welfare (Seabrook 1984). Such an evaluation meets the same difficulty as when one has to evaluate how different qualities in parents, teachers, etc. affect a child's mental health. However, there will be general agreement between experienced veterinarians that animal welfare in a herd depends to a high degree on the herd manager and his or her ability to establish a positive relationship with the animals.

When a positive relationship between herd manager and animals is absent, an extraordinarily important stimulus for the manager has been lost. This effect on the herdsman or woman, which has not been scientifically studied to date but which is empirically well known, should not be underestimated. There are reasons to assume that this effect on the keeper can increase his or her effectiveness, perhaps positively influence the keeper's health and in that way increase not only the pleasure derived from the work but also his or her productivity.

Scrutiny and approval of animal husbandry systems

Background and motives

Testing and approval of animal husbandry systems and of new techniques in animal husbandry have been regularly undertaken in Sweden since 1973, and in Switzerland since 1980.

New methods in animal husbandry that appeared during the last years of the 1950s caused mixed reactions among farmers and veterinary practitioners in Sweden. Some held that there was in certain instances a causal connection between these methods and decreases in hygiene standards and increases of some diseases. Demands for research into the effects on animal health of the new animal husbandry methods were made. Such research was deemed necessary in order to counter the new 'man-made' diseases.

In 1960 a research programme dealing with this problem was started for cattle and later also for swine and poultry. In 1966 it was proved that there is a clear connection between several environmental factors and the incidence or prevalence of different diseases in cattle (Ekesbo 1966) and later this was also shown for swine (Bäckström 1973; Lindqvist 1974) and poultry (Svedberg 1976, 1988a).

As soon as the first results of the research were published in the 1960s they were utilized in better adapting the new techniques to the health requirements of animals. This was achieved through courses for practising veterinarians and through information to farmers.

However, the new techniques introduced into animal husbandry were many, and some created new disease problems. Farmers were in a difficult situation. On one hand there was a great demand for efficient food production, which forced them to apply the new techniques, while on the other hand these techniques often appeared to cause animal health problems. The veterinarians protested against the way the new techniques were introduced as they found themselves having to increase their therapeutic measures against man-made diseases in the herds involved.

In this situation it was clear that veterinary medicine had to open a new frontier for combating these man-made diseases, i.e. identify the disease-evoking factors so they could be eliminated. For this purpose new knowledge in animal hygiene was necessary. In 1969 a two-week intensive course in animal hygiene was arranged for 48 specially selected veterinarians, two from each of the 24 provinces in Sweden. This was followed by one week's further education.

Animal hygiene is defined as 'The science regarding the influence on animal health and disease by factors in the animal environment and measures taken with such factors in order to promote health and to prevent disease'. The science thus encompasses the effects of factors such as buildings, pasture, waste and feed handling methods, climate, noise, light, dust and straw, in combination with microbiological factors or not. It also comprises the influence of the animal on the environment, e.g. soil and water pollution by intense distribution of liquid manure, and possible preventive measures against man-made diseases. It is thus one of the most important areas of preventive veterinary medicine and animal welfare.

The Swedish courses covered lectures in different aspects of animal hygiene, epidemiology and ethology, together with some instruction in building techniques, labour efficiency, economics, etc. The idea was that these veterinarians should be used as advisers by the technical sections at the regional agricultural boards. However, very limited interest was shown.

Ruth Harrison's book *Animal Machines* was published in 1964. It provoked reaction in Sweden, and marked the start of that country's animal welfare debate. In 1970 and 1971 the issue was debated in the Riksdag, the Swedish parliament. The Minister of Agriculture proposed that no farm animal buildings given state financial support should be built, or modernized, without having passed scrutiny of the plans by animal health experts. This approach was intended to 'design in' the animals' needs for good health and to eliminate poor design as regards animal health and welfare in connection with new building or the remodelling of animal houses.

This system became part of the animal welfare regulations from 1971 and was evaluated during 1972. In a statement following this evaluation, the Farmers Union found the system suitable for farm animal health and recommended that each farm should be given this scrutiny in connection with the modernization or construction of animal housing. This recommendation came into force from July 1973.

At the same time it was decided that all kinds of new technology identified as being a possible animal health and welfare risk should be tested or otherwise evaluated before it could be approved for general sale or use. In 1975 a special scientific section was created at the Department of Animal Hygiene, at the then Royal Veterinary College, for this evaluation.

The 1988 Swedish animal welfare laws and associated legislation contain new elements which are of interest when discussing monitoring systems. The main idea of the new law is that the environment and the management of farm animals must be adapted to the species-specific biological and health demands. One innovation is that animals must be protected not only against suffering but also against disease. Another is that scrutiny of building plans from the animal health and welfare point of view is now a formal part of the law, as is the scrutiny of new techniques or methods with possible animal health implications, before they are allowed onto the market. Before, this was only part of the animal welfare regulations.

The scrutiny system naturally places great demands on the knowledge of the veterinarians, specially trained and appointed for this task. After their training of two weeks they have to pass periodic courses of 2–3 days duration. There is a special scientific unit at the Swedish University of Agricultural Sciences, Department of Animal Hygiene to give these veterinarians further advice when necessary.

Scrutiny of animal housing design—the Swedish method

In practice the scrutiny is organized through the regional state veterinarians. They are able to co-operate with regional agricultural engineers and, if necessary, with other specialists when technical questions arise. A farmer who intends to construct or modernize his animal accommodation has to submit a special form where the planned animal environment and husbandry methods are briefly described with details of, for example, number, age distribution of animals, recruitment methods, solid or liquid manure handling, method of ventilation, length, breadth and height of the building, types of stanchions for tied cows or cubicles for loose cows, urine separation or not, etc.

When the scrutiny takes place an evaluation is made of possible health hazards, for instance whether the air volume per animal is adequate, whether there could be design modifications to diminish the risks of trampled teats and mastitis in cows, respiratory problems in horses, calves or pigs, diarrhoea in piglets or weaned pigs, navel-sucking in calves, and hoof or claw disorders in cattle, pigs or poultry. Thus if, for example, the air volume per pig in a pig fattening house is less than $3\,m^3$ per pig the farmer is advised that he must either increase the accommodation size or decrease the number of pigs kept in the accommodation. If in a new building for cows a farmer intends to make his stalls or cubicles 105 cm broad for Holstein cows he is told that he must make them not less than 120 cm broad and thus either increase the size of the shed or decrease the number of cows it contains. If it is a reconstruction of an existing shed, however, the farmer may be advised to increase the breadth from 105 to, say, 115 cm if greater modifications would be too costly or physically impractical. The reason for this is that in the latter case the two options are either no reconstruction and thus continuation of the existing but inadequate environment, or an improved environment, although one that is less than ideal.

The scrutiny is mostly done with a meeting between the veterinarian and the agricultural engineer. This is because each of the options that might have health advantages must be evaluated on its technical aspects. These scrutinies often involve visits to the farm, especially in remodelling cases, which are generally more complicated than new constructions. It is self-evident that the scrutiny must be done in close co-operation with the farmer, since the purpose is to protect his animals and himself from the drawbacks of disease and animal welfare problems.

Although formally this is an animal welfare procedure it also functions as an effective form of preventive veterinary medicine against environmentally evoked diseases.

Evaluations made by regional veterinary officers show that herds kept in housing which has been approved are distinctly healthier than herds housed in buildings constructed or modernized before this scrutiny procedure came into force.

Evaluation of new technology and new animal husbandry methods

Development of testing methods

Tests of new techniques from the animal health and welfare point of view are mandatory in three European countries, Sweden, Switzerland and the Netherlands.

New technology or new animal husbandry methods have been formally evaluated at the Department of Animal Hygiene at the Swedish Veterinary College since 1973. It was, however, already available on request in the early 1960s when 'The Ekesbo method' (Ekesbo 1984, 1988) was elaborated. The investigations are either carried out as full-scale studies or as model studies.

The basic principle followed at the Department of Animal Hygiene is to perform the evaluations in commercial herds, which are thus converted into experimental herds for the duration of the experiments. This means that a contract is drawn up between the Department and the owner of the farm stipulating, for example, that the management must follow a particular regime, which must not be changed, that no change in buildings must be made during the experimental period, etc.

The disadvantage of performing such investigations in commercial herds is that it puts very high demands on the scientists to control successfully all environmental and management factors. Experience since the 1960s, however, suggests that this is possible. The great advantage of performing the studies on commercial farms is that it is possible to use large groups of animals. This makes it possible to perform the studies under realistic conditions, for instance, with regards to infection pressure. Naturally great care has to be taken so that confounding factors, such as disease, do not distort the results. On the other hand some degree of infection pressure is a normal condition in most herds or flocks, be they broilers, dairy cows, calves, nursing sows or fattening pigs. Nonetheless, it is very important that the degree of infection pressure in the experimental herd is known and successfully controlled.

Example of testing a new husbandry method in Sweden

The advantage of full-scale studies may be illustrated by the following example (Algers et al. 1984). The task was to investigate if a new sort of cage for battery hens provided such an improved environment for the hens that it would be possible to keep five hens in it and still have enhanced effects on the hens compared with another commercially used cage containing four hens. When the experiment was planned the question was should the study be performed in a traditional experimental house specially designed for the study with about 100 hens in each group, or should the study be performed in a commercial flock where both systems were available for the study. The latter alternative was chosen and the experiment was conducted with two groups of about 20 000 hens in each, of which small groups of hens and cages were selected as experimental groups. The advantage was that the control and the experimental groups could be quite large, giving statistical reliability without great extra costs. Another important advantage is that the animals were exposed to all the factors which are present in a commercial group of animals of this size. It was also possible to create double control groups.

The principle of the Swedish system of evaluation

In the Swedish system the decision as to whether an investigation shall be undertaken is made by the regional veterinarian in connection with his scrutiny of the new building or remodelling project. He normally makes his decision after having taken advice from scientific experts in animal hygiene. It means that not only technical innovations purchased by firms will be tested but also innovations made by individual farmers. In the latter case the cost for evaluation is to a great extent met by state funds. When products intended for use by commercial firms are evaluated the cost of the evaluation has to be met by the firm which intends to purchase the device or system. The evaluation normally takes place on selected commercial farms, which for the testing period will be converted into research farms.

The principle of the Swiss system of evaluation

The Swiss system differs from the Swedish in the following way. Each technical system which is brought onto the market has to be scrutinized at one of the two research farms used for this purpose. The investigation cost is defrayed by the firm in question. Only commercially purchased technical devices are tested. If a farmer introduces a new device it will not be tested if the device is only used on his farm. For husbandry systems, like loose housing systems for egg laying hens, the testing on the research farm is supplemented with monitoring systems using clinical records from a limited number of commercial herds or flocks where the system is used for the testing period. If the system passes the scrutiny it is free to be marketed; otherwise it will not be allowed onto the market.

The principle of the Dutch system

The Dutch system is essentially a copy of the Swiss system, which means that all equipment put on the market for use on animal premises must be tested from the animal health and welfare point of view. The scrutiny of new equipment in Holland is due to be enforced by law after 1993.

Testing methods

Both the Swedish and Swiss evaluation methods follow the same principles. This means that each animal health and welfare evaluation of a new technical device or a new management system follows established scientific routines.

Here, as in all scientific investigations, the first prerequisite is careful experimental planning together with clearly and logically formulated questions and hypotheses. In principle, six methods or parameters can be used (Ekesbo 1984). Regular clinical investigation; records of *all* diseases and injuries, even trifling ones, by the herdsman; ethological investigation; recording of physiological parameters; slaughter records; and autopsy findings. The clinical investigations and the recording of diseases and injuries follow the principles described earlier in this chapter. However, the basic questions and hypotheses formulated in the testing, place in question how these six methods are used in detail. For instance, ethological studies connected with the evaluation of a new cow tie will focus on the cow's behaviour in getting up and laying down, and in feeding and resting. If a new management method involving the mixing of animals is to be studied it is natural to record competitive behaviour, especially if this is suspected of leading to attacks and injuries on conspecific animals. If the technique or method to be evaluated might influence parturition the ethological observations should cover an appropriate period both before and after parturition. Before starting evaluation each ethological observation to be recorded must be planned and defined in detail (Jensen et al. 1986).

Whether the evaluation is carried out in a commercial or experimental herd is determined by the hypotheses and questions asked. It must always be remembered that farm animals are exposed to infection pressure, which may be influenced by factors in the environment or management. According to experiences from Sweden (Ekesbo 1988) there are no disadvantages in performing such tests in commercial herds provided that the owner agrees to follow carefully the same management method throughout the evaluation.

Other factors to consider are the number of animals in the test, the time of year and the possible need for repetition of the study. The production must always be recorded as production levels may influence animal health.

Among other aspects to be considered are the composition of the control and experimental groups, including knowledge of the environment in which the animals were kept before they entered these groups. For instance, a cow's previous environment may influence her rising and lying down behaviour.

Systematic clinical investigation and ethological studies are the two parameters which give the most useful results. However, a general evaluation of all parameters used, as in all scientific investigations, must be performed.

Practical implications of animal housing scrutiny and the evaluation of new techniques

Examples of evaluated techniques and methods

During the last two decades evaluations have been performed of, for example, battery cages for pigs (Algers 1982a, 1982b), the number of egg-laying hens per cage (Algers et al. 1984), feeding barriers for cows (Hennichs and Plym-Forshell 1984), feeding systems for fattening pigs (Plym-Forshell 1986) and ultrasound devices for rodent control (Algers 1984). This evaluation process has often resulted in a technique being modified to better suit biological and health requirements. In a few cases it has resulted in new techniques not being introduced because of negative animal health and welfare consequences (Plate 3).

Implications for the farmer

These two procedures—the scrutiny of plans for remodelling or new building and the testing and evaluation of new techniques and methods—have been introduced to prevent 'man-made' diseases and so improve farm animal welfare. However, these two procedures do not replace sound management and other measures necessary for good animal husbandry. But they save the farmer a lot of effort that would otherwise be expended in counteracting environmental factors that negatively influence the animals' health. Thus these procedures aim at eliminating these negative health and welfare factors, enabling the farmer to concentrate on positive measures for farm animal health and welfare.

Even if the scrutiny of animal environments from the animal health and welfare point of view is beneficial for the individual farmer and his animals its influence on the consumer should not be underestimated. A production system that promotes the animals' good health and welfare is likely to find a more stable market for its products and run less risk of consumption decrease because of poor standards of husbandry. In the long term attitudes to animal welfare may be regarded as important as product prices by the livestock industry. But for farmers and others directly involved with animal husbandry, it is not only an economic but also an ethical issue. The importance c animals' welfare for job satisfaction and for the pride of the profession should not be underestimated.

Livestock health and welfare can influence consumer demand. People are more willing to buy products from animals which they believe to be healthy and treated well. Examples from countries such as Holland, Switzerland and Germany show that the introduction to the market of eggs from hens not kept in cages has been successful. From Sweden there are corresponding examples regarding pigs. Conversely, a 16% consumption decrease of broilers in 1987 was due to mass media reporting of contamination of birds by *Campylobacter* bacteria, interpreted as indicating poor animal husbandry in the broiler husbandry. Of course, such consumption decreases may be reversed by advertising campaigns, but in the long run such measures involve great risks if the advertising images do not agree with the realities.

Health and welfare oriented husbandry cuts drug use

The increase of 'man-made' diseases has led to a great increase in the use of drugs. Unfortunately drugs are often used routinely without any measures taken to eliminate the disease-provoking factor in the environment. In such cases drugs compensate for a bad environment or management. In 1986 following a request from the farmers' union the Swedish parliament banned the general use of antibiotics as feed additives. Antibiotics are now allowed only after veterinary examination for the treatment of sick animals. If environmental factors are shown to be aetiological these must first be corrected. The ban has significantly lowered the amount of antibiotics used in Sweden (Ståhle 1990; Figure 2.1).

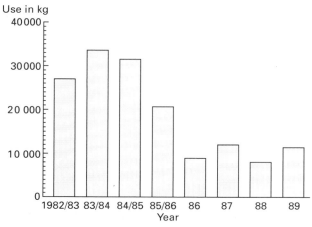

Figure 2.1 Use of antibiotics and chemotherapeuticals (excluding coccidiostats) in feed in Sweden 1982–89 (with kind permission of the Swedish National Board of Agriculture).

By using animal hygiene research results it is possible to create animal environments and management methods in which the animals show significantly less morbidity. As the cost of buildings, equipment and labour in such units need not necessarily be higher, when properly planned, and as the losses from disease are less than in normal commercial units, the profitability of the former can be better.

Husbandry systems are already available for keeping sows and piglets loose in straw-bedded pens with fully automated manure and feeding systems. Dry sows can be kept loose in groups with access to straw in the lying area. Cows loose housed with carefully designed bedded cubicles or tied in long stalls with bedding show less mastitis than cows loose or tied without bedding. Successful systems have been developed to replace cages for hens with different sorts of floor housing in environments that provide more stimuli.

Improving animal health in future? The role of man as a factor in the animal environment

Changing from a technology-based strategy to a biology-based strategy

Among the environmental factors which impact on the health of the farm animal the most important is man himself. We often discuss the effects of climate, manure or housing systems on farm animal health but often forget the effect of man.

In order to avoid diseases caused by the misapplication of technology, the strategy of animal husbandry must revert from being primarily technology-based to being primarily biology-based, where the technology is adapted to the animals' requirements for good health. This does not mean that technology should not be used. On the contrary, it means that it will be used but used in the right way.

Of course, the biology-based strategy requires biological knowledge. In order to fulfil this need for knowledge, three groups of people must be better educated in the ethology of farm animals—namely the farmers, the veterinarians and the animal husbandry advisors.

Improving the biological knowledge of farmers and others connected with animal husbandry

The problem is that the farmer of today, who is also the farmer of the future, needs more biological knowledge than he is currently given. Courses in the ethology of farm animals should be given at every agricultural teaching establishment. This is equally important at agricultural high school and agricultural colleges. Moreover, the ethology of farm animals should be a compulsory topic in all veterinary schools. Only in a few countries are courses in farm animal ethology included in the core curriculum of veterinary education. Scientific competence and experience in farm animal behaviour is a cornerstone in all clinical diagnosis. Such knowledge is more important for the veterinarian now than ever before because of changes in the animal environment on farms and their influence on animal health.

Only rarely are farm animal ethological courses compulsory in the education of farmers and agricultural advisors. Better ethological knowledge will mean that the most important factor in animal health, i.e. man, will be more of a good health promoter than a risk factor. The need for daily care would then be given more priority and the risk of substituting it with automatic devices would be diminished.

Such an educational programme must be based on good scientific research designed to investigate the connection between farm animal health, animal behaviour and the animal's environment, including management. Veterinarians must have knowledge of using monitoring systems based on clinical, subclinical and behavioural records. Such education must be derived from research within animal hygiene, including epidemiology, and applied ethology. If financial support is lacking for such research it may be necessary to change the current set of priorities and more weight given to the biological sector.

The role of the veterinarian and veterinary medicine in animal husbandry

Veterinary measures are urgently needed to reverse the trend of the last three decades, which have been characterized by an increase in farm animal diseases. By the application of available scientific knowledge it is already possible to improve livestock health with regard to several diseases associated with the group environment. Here, herd health monitoring systems have a central role to play.

In order to improve animal health in the future, animal diseases must be combated primarily by preventive measures aimed at eliminating the disease-evoking factors. This means that veterinarians must take an active part at the design stage in both animal housing and management. Such active veterinary involvement for combating environmentally evoked diseases has to be based on scientific knowledge of how different environments or environmental factors, including management, impact on animal health and welfare. Monitoring systems using clinical and behavioural records are a possible way to improve that knowledge.

It must become a ground rule that surgical or medical measures should be reserved for sick animals and should never be used as prophylaxis to compensate for inadequate breeding programmes or for inadequate environment, including management. Thus dystocia must be prevented by genetic measures. The progress in modern surgery and anaesthesia, which makes Caesarean section possible in farm practice, should not be used as an excuse for continuing to breed animals that are predisposed to the condition.

Similarly, tail biting and pecking must be prevented by correction of the environment, not by the general use of tail docking or beak trimming. Also, antibiotics in feed must not be used routinely in order to compensate for a bad environment.

Another important reason for increased disease problems in modern animal husbandry is the altered economic strategy. Traditional animal husbandry had a long-term view of the economy and followed a 'total' economic strategy, just as it had a total biological strategy based on holistic principles. In modern animal production the farmers are given advice by specialists and the result very often is a 'sectorial' economic strategy with a rather short-term view. As the costs for buildings, labour and feed are easier to estimate than the costs of diseases, the latter are often forgotten in the economic calculations and models.

Therefore it is necessary to obtain good veterinary research regarding the influence of different environment and management factors on the prevalence of diseases. The results of such animal hygiene research make it possible for veterinarians, together with agricultural economists, to analyse the costs for different diseases and also to make cost-benefit analyses of changes in breeding, environment and management. For instance, it is important for a farmer to know that alternative A for a planned dairy barn means a mastitis incidence risk of 30% and that alternative B means 15%. If the cost per mastitis case has been estimated, say about $500, he could more easily make his choice between A and B. In this way veterinary medicine can in future help the farmer to a more holistic and realistic assessment of his husbandry.

All this means that there must be changes in both undergraduate and postgraduate veterinary education with regard to knowledge of animal hygiene. Naturally, a prerequisite for such an education programme is an efficient and well-conducted programme of scientific research.

The role of animal welfare legislation

Traditional animal husbandry contained 'silent' ethical elements regarding the relationship between man and farm animal. Such guidelines, written or unwritten, will always be essential for animal husbandry. As the transfer of biologically based but unwritten husbandry traditions from generation to generation diminishes or even ceases altogether, the animal husbandry tradition for each species must be replaced by detailed guidelines in the form of national animal welfare laws and provisions designed to fulfil the same purpose. Results of monitoring systems using clinical and behavioural records are an important basis for animal welfare legislation.

Another reason for such guidelines is that the relationship between the farmer and his animals has been weakened, and in the large highly specialized herds and flocks it does not exist at all.

The provisions elaborated by the Council of Europe's Standing Committee on Farm Animal Welfare and based on the Council of Europe's Farm Animal Welfare Convention, ratified by 17 European nations in 1991, are a good start for such national provisions.

Practical implications of studies of the relationship between animal environment and health

Cattle

Dairy cows in many countries are still kept tied in short stalls with very little or no bedding. However, in some countries disease recording has shown the importance of soft bedding on the lying area and enough lying space. This has resulted in a change either to longer straw-bedded stalls or to loose housing with cubicles. In loose housing there is a growing problem with lameness caused by unsuitable floors (e.g. Colam-Ainsworth et al. 1989). Also, intensive feeding has caused a remarkable change in manure consistency: cows on intensive feeding regimes have a constant diarrhoea. This creates problems with dirty animals and especially dirty hoofs. Perpetually dirty hoofs leads to an increased risk of foot sores and foot rot in cattle.

Pigs

In most countries sows are kept in permanent confinement, usually in stalls or tied, in well-insulated houses without bedding. Considerable manual labour plus automatic dung cleaners and expensive ventilation systems are necessary as the climate must be well controlled.

As a result of clinical and behavioural records the system is changing in some countries. For example in the UK, Holland and Sweden farmers are starting to keep dry sows loose in groups of 15 or more, in rooms with plenty of bedding, often in uninsulated buildings where a reasonable climate can be obtained throughout the year without sophisticated ventilation systems. The boar is either loose in the group or kept in an adjacent pen.

Instead of investing in expensive climate-controlled sheds for early weaned piglets, the piglets stay with the sow in the farrowing pen until they are 5–7 weeks of age. Also, sows are no longer confined on perforated floors but housed loose in the pen with access to straw and the freedom to perform the functions of dunging, feeding and resting in different areas. The pen is about 5–6 m² and normally has an adjacent dunging alley with urine separation and automatic dung removal.

Sometimes the sow is kept in the farrowing pen with the piglets until weaning. Thereafter she is housed in groups of at least 15, often more, sows kept on either a totally bedded area or with access to a straw-bedded lying area. The piglets stay in the farrowing pen for at least two weeks after weaning before being put into pens for weaners.

Often, however, when the piglets are 2–3 weeks of age, the sows are moved with their piglets to group housing. As many as 12–16 sows with piglets may be kept together in one pen provided with plenty of straw. Piglets are given a separate feeding area, but can also feed with the sows. Feeding is arranged so that all sows can eat at the same time. The area per sow (and her piglets) is, as a rule, 8–10 m².

At 5–7 weeks the sows are normally taken to the dry sow section. The piglets stay in the same place until the age of 10–12 weeks, i.e. to a liveweight of about 25 kg, when they are transferred to the fattening unit or sold for fattening. The area per dry sow in group sow pens where all is bedded area is not less than 2.5 m² when 10–15 sows are kept together. When there is a separate bedded area (and a dunging area cleaned daily) the bedded area is normally not less than 1.3 m² per sow.

The principle when building new or remodelling pig housing is that, increasingly, the animals should determine such functions as manure disposal, heat control and climate control. For instance, in the summer the pigs will choose a suitable place for lying on the bedded area, when the doors and windows can be opened for ventilation; in the winter they may burrow into the straw bedding. Using an all in-all out system dung removal is undertaken with the cleaning between batches. Left to their own devices, the pigs always choose a dunging area which is quite limited and the rest of the bedded area stays clean. New straw bales are added once a week. Hence it follows that a system based on liquid manure handling is incompatible with a good animal environment.

Experience of the systems here described for dry sows and for sows and piglets indicates a reduced incidence of sow disorders related to farrowing and less diarrhoea in the piglets both before and after weaning.

For fattening pigs there are two main systems in Europe. In one the pigs are kept on a bedded area, with or without a separate dunging area which is cleaned daily or several times a week. Often this system is in a building where the pigs have access to the open air for at least part of the year.

Most pigs, however, are kept in closed buildings, sometimes on entirely slatted floors, or in pens with a solid concrete floor and a slatted floor in the dunging area. Fattening pig houses generally have no windows and often there is no straw or other material to provide stimulus for the animals. Tail docking is widely practised as tail biting is a problem. In some herds the lighting programme is set so that the animals are given light only at short intervals for feeding in order to prevent tail biting.

According to Sweden's 1988 animal welfare law tail docking of pigs is forbidden and pig houses without windows are not allowed. Moreover, straw or a similar material must be given daily to enable the pigs to fulfil their natural instincts.

In several European countries there is currently a trend to change fattening pig systems in the same direction as sows systems have been changing. In order to avoid some of the problems created by the barren environments in the fattening units, farmers have installed the pigs in so-called welcoming units before they enter the fattening pig unit. The welcoming unit is a pen where 40 to 100 pigs are kept in a group on a totally straw-bedded area for 3–6 weeks. If they are kept for 6 weeks the area is normally cleaned and bedded afresh after 3 weeks. This is to prevent the build-up of parasites in the manure—the life cycle for some parasites can make this possible after 3–4 weeks.

The interest in animal welfare among consumers has created a small market in Europe for farmers who keep their pigs in an environment even more adapted to the biological characteristics of the pig. Sows and piglets are kept in conditions described as 'without confinement'. There is more space per sow and always access to an outdoor area for the sows and mostly also for piglets. For fattening pigs there is access to both a bedded area and an outdoor area. Sometimes these farms have their own abbatoir in order to avoid the stress involved when pigs are sent to an outside slaughterhouse. The pork from these farms is specially labelled and sold for a higher price, often in a special display in the butcher's shop or butchery counter. However, the standards of humane production differ between European countries, and to achieve some sort of regulation of these standards, herd monitoring programmes using clinical and behavioural records are necessary.

Poultry

For laying hens there has been an interesting development in Switzerland (Oester and Fröhlich 1989; Matter 1989), where a ban on battery cages has created an increasing number of systems for loose housing of layers. It seems possible that the Swiss moves will be followed by other countries. Thus Sweden banned new installations of battery cages from 1988, with a total ban from the year 2000. Also in Sweden the development of loose housing systems aimed at improving poultry health and welfare has started (Algers and Viske 1990) and in this process monitoring systems using clinical, subclinical and behavioural records play an important role.

For broilers an interesting development has occurred during recent years in Sweden. In practically all countries salmonella has been a problem in broiler production. Investigations (Svedberg 1988b) have shown that the source is mainly the feed and that special precautions have to be taken in the feed factories. However, measures in the flock are also important. In Sweden, by restricting the number of birds per unit area it has been possible to decrease the morbidity and mortality in broilers, with implications for the quality of the product. Thus, up to the end of 1990 in Sweden, no case of salmonella in broilers had occurred in any flock where this programme had been carried out and which obtained its feed from factories where a special hygiene control programme (Svedberg 1988b) had been instituted.

THE HERD HEALTH
MONTHLY REPORT

HERD HEALTH MONTHLY REPORT

Owner:
Farm:

.... month 19....

	Housing	**Pasture**

1. Difficult calving

2. Retained afterbirth

3. Milk fever

4. Ketosis

5. Mastitis

6. Trampled teats

7. Other udder injuries ◆

8. Hoof diseases ◆

9. Foreknee/hock swelling ◆

10. Lameness ◆

11. Other traumatic injuries ◆

12. Loss of appetite ◆

13. Other diseases ◆

Other information of interest, please write on other side of this form.

MARK! All diseases or injuries which occur must be reported, not only diseases treated by your veterinary surgeon. For cases diagnosed by your veterinary surgeon please put a V in front of the cow number!

◆ If possible give cause on other side of this form.
D Date of disease. No. Cow identity number.

14. Young-stock diseases (if possible specify cause below):   No. cases . . . . . .
15. Calf diseases (if possible specify cause below):   No. cases . . . . . .
16. No. days with clear herd milk production decrease   No. days . . . . . .
    (if possible specify cause below)

17. Cows bought to herd.

18. No. normally slaughtered (culled) cows: . . . . (Specify date, cow no. and cause below).
19. No. emergency slaughtered cows: . . . . (Specify date, cow no. and cause below).
20. No. emergency slaughtered calves and young stock: . . . . . . (Specify date, cow no. and cause below).
21. Cows found dead (Specify date, cow no. and if possible cause below).
22. Young stock and calves found dead (Specify date, identity no. and if possible cause below).
21. Other information of interest, e.g. feed changes, change of herdsman and completion of above given records:

_____
_____
_____
_____
_____
_____
_____
_____
_____
_____
_____
_____
_____
_____
_____
_____
_____
_____
_____
_____
_____
_____
_____
_____

If milk sample(s) for mastitis test is(are) taken note here cow number and result of investigation:

_____
_____

3 OTHER CLINICAL DIAGNOSTIC METHODS
A H ANDREWS BVetMed, PhD, MRCVS

Stress and hormone release
Haematological examination
Standard biochemical tests
Other biochemical tests
Uses of normal biochemical testing
Other methods of health monitoring
Acknowledgements

For a long time it was hoped that physiological measurements would be able to objectively determine stress, well-being and unfitness. Such measurements involved monitoring the arousal of the sympathetic nervous system, the release of catecholamines from the adrenal medulla, increases in pituitary and adrenal activity as well as increases in levels of plasma corticosteroids (Selye 1950). Since that time, the ability to measure these parameters in experimental animals has become available. Thus it is possible to use small, permanently indwelling catheters for blood sample collection with the minimal disturbance to the animal. The amount of blood required for analyses is also very small. Moreover, the development of radioelectronic techniques for monitoring heart and brain activity has allowed physiological measurements to be made with the minimum of disturbance (Duncan and Filshie 1979). However, the results are difficult to interpret. It has to be remembered that these are normal physiological responses to allow the animal to adapt and cope with changes in its environment and circumstances. Stress is the rule, not the exception. Particularly in terms of changes in the normal daily life of the animal, it is difficult to decide if deviation is sufficient to produce suffering.

It is often easier physiologically to determine acute stress than other more long-term problems. While interpretation is difficult, measurement has become simpler. Improved developments often mean that in the assessment of alterations due to transport or handling, the choice of parameter can be made. This often depends on either the sensitivity of the analytical procedure or the ease with which it can be measured. The problem with such measurements is their involvement in welfare, i.e. the physical and mental well-being of the animals. In many cases the parameters used may have little relationship with welfare. The difficulty arises in the assessment of mental well-being or suffering. In many cases the physiological alterations which occur are influenced by the emotional state of the animal. Thus if a definition of suffering is taken to be an extensive arousal of the emotions (Brambell 1965) any behavioural indicator has to be evaluated in the context of the behaviour pattern of the animal and not divorced from it.

Certain relatively transitional emotional states such as anger, fear or frustration are accompanied by the activation of physiological signs by both the pituitary-adrenal axis and the sympathetic medullary system. This results in the instantaneous release of catecholamines and the slower release of glucocorticoids (Dantzer et al. 1983b). Evidence for this can be obtained by the measurement of concentrations of hormones in the plasma. Additionally, the degree of effect of these hormones on the target organs can be quantified. Thus, for example, they can be measured by the effect on plasma glucose and free fatty acid levels and the production of changes in lymphocyte and eosinophil numbers.

Long-term alterations in hormone levels and activities can be produced by the effects of the animal's environment on the range of behavioural responses and experiences allowed it.

The sympathetic adrenal medullary system is activated when there is a challenge of access to certain goal objects. Thus if access is restricted or prevented to perceived goals such as a mate, offspring, food, shelter or water, repeated attempts will be made to overcome the difficulty and regain or maintain control.

The pituitary-adrenal axis tends to be activated when there is little possibility of escape or control of the situation. Thus calves single-penned on slats will have a higher pituitary adrenal activity than those loose-housed in groups on straw (Dantzer et al. 1983a). This perhaps suggests that certain husbandry conditions which restrict the degree of control given to the animals will lead to increased pituitary and adrenal activity.

Stress and hormone release

Our ability to measure health, welfare and distress in animals is still in its infancy and is at present lamentably poor. In many cases to be effective it requires the continued monitoring of an animal to show any divergence from its own normal range of accepted values. In the population generally the variation is so great that animals outside the normal range are showing extreme abnormality rather than the more subtle alterations of the individual. Most of the biochemical indicators show a relationship between stress, pain and suffering. Their precise evaluation in pain or discomfort is more difficult. It is probably best that at present they are used for measurement in experimental situations rather than on the farm.

In many cases welfare has to be measured indirectly by quantifying any type of stress to which the animals are exposed, or by the diagnosis of disease considered to be stress- or welfare-induced, or by an increase in susceptibility to disease or by an adverse effect on production. We are unable to assess or quantify happiness of an animal. Stress is difficult to define but can be considered the non-specific response of the body to any demand made upon it (Selye 1973). The stressor agent may be pleasant or unpleasant but all produce the same biological stress response, which is non-specific and common to all types of exposure (Figure 3.1). There are two main parts of the environment to

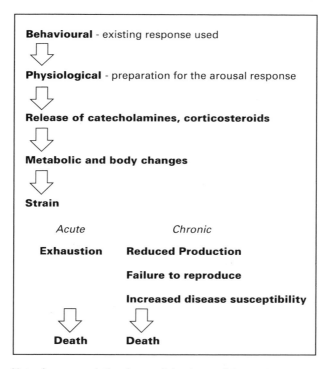

Note: Accommodation is possible at any of these stages

Figure 3.1 The progression of events caused by a stressor agent to which the animal does not accommodate.

which an animal can react. Firstly there are physical factors such as temperature, humidity, light and noise, and secondly social factors such as group size, available space, the dominance order within the group, etc.

Until recently, the two main systems involved in stress, namely the hypothalamic-pituitary-adrenocortical system and the sympathetic adrenomedullary system have been considered separately. However, there are several critical interactions between the systems and it has now been stated that the two systems should be considered together (Figure 3.2; Oliverio 1987).

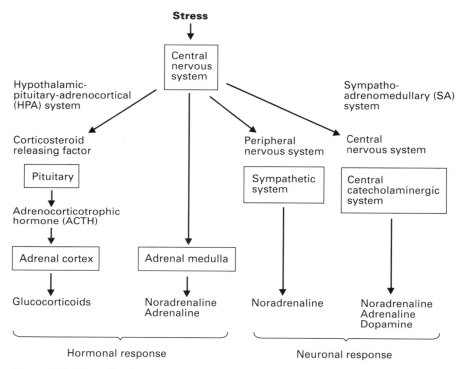

Figure 3.2 The activation by stress of the hypothalamic-pituitary-adrenocortical (HPA) and sympatho-adrenomedullary (SA) systems (after Oliverio 1987).

As previously stated, behaviour and physiological changes are the two indices of adaptation to stress most easily monitored. Thus when there is a change from the normal resulting in an arousal stimulus, behavioural responses are the first to be involved. These may be produced to deal with the changed circumstance, otherwise acclimatization and habituation may occur resulting in a satisfactory but slower adjustment. Thus physical stimuli on their own do not induce a stress reaction. It is only when the stimuli lead to an emotional response that a stress reaction occurs. Thus often gradual changes do not result in a reaction. However, if there is not a satisfactory response or a change is sudden, physiological alterations can come into play with the release of corticosteroids. When adjustment does not occur it can then, if not before, be supposed that there are welfare considerations. Such a failure to adjust can then lead to exhaustion or possibly reduced production.

The sympathetic adrenal medullary response tends to be activated when there is a challenge in the major areas of living such as food, water, shelter, mate or dependants (Dantzer et al. 1983b). This leads to repeated attempts to maintain control and there is continual arousal, increase in heart rate, blood pressure and peripheral vascular resistance. The neurohumoral response on the other hand is concerned with alterations experienced by the animal and how it is able to adapt and respond to these changes.

Adrenaline concentrations depend on different behavioural situations. Thus in bulls, rubbing, playful butting or avoiding disturbance produce a significant increase compared with standing, ruminating, walking, sniffing and licking (Schlichting et al. 1983).

Experimentally a less invasive approach to assessing brain function is by means of the so-called neuroendocrine window (Dantzer et al. 1983b). This is based on observations of the endocrine response following the use of pharmacological antagonists and agonists on the neurotransmitter being studied. Their use in farm animals is still not well elucidated (Gorewit 1981).

When a stimulus exceeds its normal level, either in terms of intensity or in the length of duration, it becomes a stressor. Thus the stimulus acts at a level above the capacity of the animal to readily cope and so requires the animal to put in 'effort'. This in turn can lead to a cascade of events which alter the physiological and behavioural patterns in the animal (Stephens 1980). Stressors and non-stressors result in the stimulation of the autonomic nervous system which at once releases adrenaline and noradrenaline from the adrenal medulla. This initiates the 'flight or fight' response and it is continued by release of other hormones which alter blood flow and respiratory function and begin an altered response to a new set of physiological priorities. The rise in these catecholamines causes an increase in blood glucose. The circulation is altered to increase the flow to the muscles and reduce it to the digestive system. Contraction of the spleen results in an increase in erythrocytes in the circulation, thereby increasing the oxygen-carrying capacity of the blood. The bronchioles dilate to allow a greater intake of oxygen. The pancreas is a mediator in the reaction by releasing glucagon. Glucagon may play an important role in increasing the metabolism of liver glycogen in mammals and in birds by increasing the circulating levels of free fatty acids from adipose tissues. Secretion of insulin is decreased.

Finally ACTH is released, which increases corticosteroid circulation and, in particular, cortisol to help counteract the stressor by combining the physiological modifications. This sequence of events is known as the general adaptation syndrome (GAS) (Selye 1946).

Subclinical disease

When animals are infected subclinically with disease, stresses of various sorts may result in the subclinical condition developing into clinical disease. This may be the result of reducing the natural defence mechanisms of the animal including leucocyte numbers and activity, interferon levels, etc.

Thus sheep suffering subclinical disease and then stressed by handling over a few days may break down with disease (Thurley 1977). A change in diet may precipitate problems or if this is coupled with a change in environmental temperature, may result in disease.

Immunocompetence also is affected by different types of stress leading to altered sensitivity to infectious disease (Kelley 1980).

Corticosteroids

Part of the stress response is the activation of the hypothalamus, pituitary and adrenal glands leading to the release of glucocorticoids. The main glucocorticoids are cortisol and corticosterone (see Figure 3.3), produced in the zona

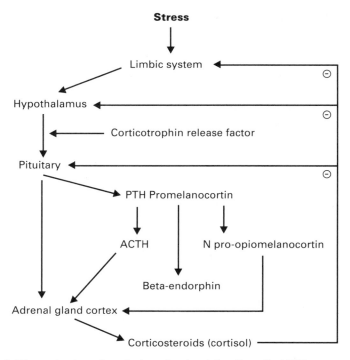

Figure 3.3 The activation of cortisol production (after Breazile 1988).

fasciculata. The neuroendocrine response to stress results in the release of endogenous corticosteroids. Cortisol has been found to be the major corticosteroid in many farm animals, including sheep (Bush and Ferguson 1953). It can be bound to plasma protein in some species; e.g. in man about 90% is bound (Bush 1957). Raised corticosteroid levels are an indicator of stress but they are also influenced by circadian rhythms, age and reproductive and emotional status. Corticosteroid levels tend to rise abruptly when ruminants and pigs are subjected to acute stress (Ladewig 1984). However, it is well demonstrated that, particularly in chronic distress, circulating corticosteroid levels are not always closely linked with the distress response. Thus often in chronic distress there are decreasing levels of circulating glucocorticoids due to a decrease in receptors on adrenohypophyseal corticotrophes to corticotrophin release factor.

The beneficial effects of glucocorticoid release are several. Glucocorticoids initiate great shifts in carbohydrate metabolism (Breazile 1988). The release of corticosteroids in distress leads to the diversion of glucose from muscle to the brain and other tissues, thereby maintaining essential metabolism. Energy stores are depleted and there is an increase in circulating energy substrates. Glucocorticoids are anti-inflammatory and immunosuppressive. Thus they act to reduce damage to cells and tissues as a result of their reduction in immune and inflammatory responses. A third effect is that glucocorticoids mediate the activity of adrenaline and other catecholamines on blood vessels and metabolic pathways.

Cortisol can be assayed by a competitive protein binding method (Bassett and Hinks 1969), which can be performed quickly and requires small samples. However, the method can be imprecise as other corticosteroids in the plasma may interfere with the evaluation (Farmer and Pierce 1974). A radioimmunoassay can also be used, which is more precise and sensitive (Dobson 1983) and requires less technician time. It involves measuring radioactivity following the preparation of a radiolabelled antibody to cortisol. This technique requires the purchase of expensive equipment as well as creating a possible radioactive hazard within the laboratory. Antibody to cortisol can be labelled with an enzyme and this enzyme can be measured by a calorimetric method. Salivary cortisol levels have been used in sheep and are relatively easy to collect and assess (Fell et al. 1985). Blood sampling equipment designed to reduce stress in animals being sampled is available.

A technique has been developed to measure cortisol in sheep plasma by modifying a kit used for measuring the hormone in human serum, where levels are considerably higher (Ford et al. 1990). The technique is non-invasive and produces a concentration of about 10% of that in plasma. It has, however, been found not to be so sensitive an indicator as plasma cortisol (Parrott et al. 1989).

Cow's milk contains cortisol at a concentration of 0.35–2.5 ng/ml (Bremel and Gangwer 1978; Schwlam and Tucker, 1978; Fox et al. 1981; Schutt and

Fell 1985) and is not dependent on the amount of milk present in the quarter. The plasma cortisol level is variable but a resting level of about 10.2 ng/ml can occur (Mayer and Lefcourt 1987). The mean plasma clearance rate in Jersey cows is 4.81 ± 0.487 ng/l plasma per minute. The mean cortisol secretion rate (= plasma clearance × mean critical plasma cortisol concentration) during lactation has been recorded as 26.4 ± 7.14 mg/ml (Paterson and Linzell 1974).

Effects on the animal

The action of cortisol on milk yield is variable. It would seem that injecting cortisol intravenously up to a dose of 100 μg has no effect on milk yield even if repeated (Mayer and Lefcourt 1987). This is equivalent to a plasma cortisol concentration of at least 31 μg/ml, 60 minutes after an intravenous injection.

Total plasma cortisol in cattle accustomed to handling and bleeding has been reported to be 25 mmol/l (Mitchell et al. 1988) and 33 ± 3 mmol/l (Herd 1989). Such values are unlikely to be obtained when cattle are not conditioned to handling and restraint. Consequently, high baseline values are often found, even in experimental work (Carter et al. 1983; Tennessen et al. 1984). It thus means that cortisol levels are difficult to interpret or evaluate when used to investigate the stressfulness of a situation on a single occasion. It must be remembered that rises not only occur because of blood sampling but can also result from the normal events of life. Thus elevated cortisol may occur during courtship, mating and active food consumption (Broom 1988).

Plasma cortisol levels in sheep can vary from 13 to 17 μg/ml when rested (Hargreaves and Hutson 1990). However, they tend to rise rapidly every time the sheep are exposed to sham shearing. The adrenal gland may show increased sensitivity after a series of sham shearings and electroimmobilizations. Similarly, herding cattle causes a rise in cortisol (Hattingh et al. 1989), while moving pigs into groups after being penned for five weeks on their own caused a short-lived cortisol rise (Barnett et al. 1981).

Cortisol response depends partly on previous experience of an environment. It is partly for this reason that attempts to show increased cortico-adrenal activity in intensively kept farm animals often produce conflicting or inconclusive results. Thus calves housed indoors on a slatted floor showed an increased response when placed in an outdoor pen with straw bedding compared to when they were returned to an indoor pen similar to their previous one. Calves reared outside showed a reverse relationship (Dantzer and Mormède 1985).

Cortisol levels in bulls tend to rise during lying down and for a period afterwards. This increase is greater in bulls loose-housed on slatted floors than on straw (Schlichting et al. 1983). Raised cortisol levels occur at stocking rates of 2 m^2/animal compared with 3 m^2/animal (Unshelm 1983). Moderate serum cortisol rises can occur when calves are transported or loaded or subjected to noise (Agnes et al. 1990). Transportation of goats for 2 hours results in higher plasma cortisol concentrations and for a longer duration than a 20-minute journey (Sanhouri et al. 1991). Baseline values tend to return one to two hours after the transport. The use of pentobarbitone sodium at 20 mg/kg BW can block stimulated as well as resting cortisol secretion (Sanhouri et al. 1991).

In pigs, measurements of total corticosteroid concentration, maximum corticosteroid binding capacity (MCBC) and free corticosteroid concentrations are determined in quantifying stress (Barnett et al. 1989). While corticosteroids have been used to measure stress, biological activity depends largely on the amount of unbound cortisol. Therefore to obtain accurate information on the significance of cortisol concentration it is suggested that other information is required, such as the concentration and affinity of binding proteins for cortisol in the plasma (Barnett et al. 1981). Thus in group-housed pigs, control corticosteroid concentrations were well below the maximum corticosteroid binding capacity (MCBC), with higher levels in the morning than the afternoon. However, in pigs penned individually the MCBC was lower and afternoon corticosteroid level was similar to the morning, suggesting a chronic stress response.

In egg-laying domestic fowl there is an increase in corticosteroid level, reaching a peak at ovipositioning. This rise is seen in hens in the presence or absence of a nesting box and the level of corticosteroid is slightly less as egg production proceeds. Stimuli such as handling, deprivation of food and water, heating and cooling increase corticosteroid levels. It is considered that a threshold level of 5–7 ng/ml exists but that quantitative evaluation does not appear to be well related to the level of stress (Beuving 1983).

Frustration can raise cortisol levels. Thus pigs trained to press a lever to obtain food will develop increased cortisol levels if they no longer receive food by pressing the lever (Dantzer et al. 1984). Animals with high pre-session plasma cortisol levels stopped pressing the pad quickly when no food was presented. Those with lower pre-session cortisol levels continued to press the pad despite the lack of food appearance.

ACTH

The direct criterion for assessing stress is considered by some to be the assay of adrenocorticotrophic hormone (ACTH). This stimulates steroidogenesis and the production of glucocorticoids. It is produced by the pituitary corticotrophes following stimulation by hypothalamic corticotrophin releasing factor (CRH), oxytocin and vasopressin. ACTH is formed from a prohormone called pro-opiomelanocortin (POMC), which also yields an N-terminal, 76-amino acid POMC peptide and beta-lipoprotein, which in turn produces several compounds including beta-endorphin (Breazile 1988). Thus stimulation of release of ACTH also causes secretion of N-POMC and beta-endorphin (Table 3.3). In chronic distress, ACTH release is less, due to reduced sensitivity of the pituitary cells.

The ACTH response to repeated stress stimuli is variable. It is thought this may be due to variations in the proportions of the main secretory stimulators such as corticosteroid releasing factor, oxytocin and vasopressin, as well as perhaps to other hormones and neurotransmitters which enter the adrenohypophysis via the hypothalamo-hypophyseal portal system. Influential factors present in the systemic circulation include angiotensin II, adrenaline, noradrenaline, vasoactive intestinal peptide (VIP) and cholecystokinin. Thus secondary stimulation of ACTH occurs in neurogenic or behavioural stress such as restraint or electrical shock when oxytocin secretion is increased but not vasopressin (Gibbs 1984).

ACTH inhibition is often seen when systemic stress is caused by hypotension or hypoglycaemia. However, basal glucocorticoid secretion can remain high in chronic distress such as social subordination. This is due to the reduction in sensitivity of brain receptors to corticosteroids resulting in an alteration of the glucocorticoid feedback system. In addition, there is diurnal variation in the ability of natural as well as synthetic corticosteroids to inhibit ACTH secretion.

Effects on the animal

In humans, the response to ACTH infusion increases following previous stimulation. This appears also to occur in farm animals. Thus there is an increased response to ACTH in lactating cows which have had to compete for several days for access to stalls (Friend et al. 1978).

The injection of ACTH into the cow can have an effect on milk yield dependent on the dose used and the route by which it is administered. The use of 200 IU ACTH subcutaneously had no effect on yield in Jersey cattle (Campbell et al. 1964). However, when a single or repeated injection of at least 200 IU ACTH is administered intramuscularly there is a severe drop (over 50%) in milk yield (Van der Kolk 1990b). This is equivalent to a plasma cortisol concentration of at least 31 ng/ml 60 minutes after intravenous injection. When the same cortisol rise is produced by an injection of cortisol this milk depression does not occur. It therefore suggests that the intramuscular injection of 200 IU ACTH is not having its milk depressant effect by production of cortisol alone.

Pigs placed in a new environment have a negative correlation between their blood plasma ACTH levels and locomotor activity (Mormède et al. 1984).

Administration of ACTH to pigs produces a higher behavioural activity following a fear signal.

Adrenaline and noradrenaline

Adrenaline (epinephrine) is a hormone produced in the adrenal medulla. Its main function is to regulate the sympathetic nervous system. Noradrenaline (norepinephrine) is a catecholamine stored in the chromaffin granules of the adrenal medulla. It acts as the neurotransmitter for most of the sympathetic prostaglandin neurones and also some of the tracts in the central nervous system. It also acts as a neurohormone and is primarily released following stimulation of the sympathetic system, particularly in cases of hypotension.

Adrenaline is released via stressors and causes increased blood pressure, with heart rate and cardiac output raised. It also increases mobilization of glycogen and the release of glucose from the liver. Noradrenaline also increases heart rate and raises blood pressure as well as causing vasoconstriction. In chronic distress there may be persistent secretion of adrenaline and noradrenaline with decreasing levels of plasma glucocorticoids. Both compounds can help stimulation of the secretion of the prohormone pro-opiomelanocortin (POMC).

Thus pigs placed in a new environment had a regular correlation between their adrenaline levels and locomotor activity (Mormède et al. 1984). Plasma adrenaline levels rise in calves exposed to noise, transportation or loading, although the noradrenaline concentrations did not change significantly in the same animals (Agnes et al. 1990).

Haematological examination

Leucocytes

The number of circulating leucocytes varies considerably according to many different factors, including the age and species of animal. Numbers tend to increase following inflammation, infection or certain forms of neoplasia. Numbers decline in certain debilitating conditions. Weaning results in a decrease in total leucocyte numbers while transport increases them. The white cell count in bovine early pregnancy is often reduced, possibly due to suppression by embryo-derived immunomodulating factors (Johnson et al. 1990). Generally speaking, although there are alterations in white cell numbers as the result of stress affecting cortisol levels, the changes are only an indirect indication of the problem and often are not quantitatively related to the stress.

Neutrophils

These are found in the circulation or in capillary beds or the bone marrow. A sudden increase in demand results in mobilization of the bone marrow pool.

Neutrophilia occurs in several ways. There can be a movement of cells from the inactive capillary beds—the marginal area—following stress or exercise or use of adrenaline. Acute corticosteroid release results in a decreased migration of neutrophils from the blood vessels and increased mobilization from the bone marrow pool. There is a suppressive activity of neutrophils with elevated cortisol levels. In chronic steroid conditions, e.g. athletic training, there is increased neutrophil production. Rises also occur in response to infection.

Neutropenia can result from an increase in neutrophil destruction, for example in autoimmune disease. The movement of neutrophils into the inactive capillary bed (marginal bed), as occurs following endotoxin shock, also results in neutropenia. It can also happen where there is an increased demand for neutrophils without any compensating inflow from the bone marrow; this has been observed in cattle. Decreased bone marrow production can be due to bone marrow suppression along with anaemia and thrombocytopenia.

Monocytes

These are found in bone marrow. Increased monocyte levels occur in chronic disease, particularly chronic inflammatory conditions, often characterized by suppuration and necrosis. Monocytopenia has been reported in cattle and horses following an acute corticosteroid response. Monocyte levels tend to be reduced in calves after weaning (Phillips et al. 1989).

In infections monocytes produce the cytokine interleukin-1, which stimulates the release of ACTH via either the brain or the adrenohypophyseal corticotrophes. Macrophages in the tissues also have this property.

Basophils

Basophils are produced in the bone marrow, and occur more often in horses than ruminants. Basophilia is seen in hypothyroidism and in hypersensitivity involving an antigen or allergen. There are so few circulating basophils that basophilia is effectively undetectable.

Lymphocytes

These are concerned with humoral antibody formation and cell-mediated immunity. They circulate in the blood and lymph and are also found in the lymph nodes, spleen and gut-associated lymphoid tissue. Numbers decrease with age of the animal and this is particularly so in horses. Increases otherwise tend to be associated with neutrophilia. Lymphopenia usually reflects a reduction in lymphopoiesis. Abnormal reductions can occur when corticosteroid release occurs, e.g. stress. Acute viral infections can also cause a reduction, as can neoplasia.

Activated lymphocytes produce the cytokine interleukin-1 which can stimulate the release of ACTH.

Eosinophils

Eosinophils are found in the bone marrow. Eosinophilia occurs in diseases affecting tissues containing many mast cells, e.g. skin, lungs, gastrointestinal tract and uterus. Tissue damage causes mast cells to degranulate and release histamine which results in the release of eosinophils from the bone marrow into the general circulation.

Eosinopenia occurs with adrenaline or corticosteroids. They thus reduce in chronic stress often a result of, for example, prolonged training of horses. In acute stress there is increased catecholamine secretion whereas more chronic problems increase corticosteroid secretion. Levels tend to decrease in calves at weaning and transit (Phillips, et al. 1989).

Neutrophil:Lymphocyte ratio

Circulating leucocyte alterations have been noted following adrenocortical activity and stress. As glucocorticoid concentrations increase, lymphocyte and eosinophil numbers tend to decrease while the number of polymorphonuclear leucocytes increases. This results in a rise in neutrophils in most domestic species and heterophils in birds (Sayers, 1950). Thus in pigs there is a rise in neutrophils and a decrease in lymphocytes and eosinophils following marketing (Clemens et al. 1986) and, castration and electric shock (Ellersieck et al. 1979). The N:L ratio has been shown to reflect plasma cortisol levels following the feeding of dietary cortisol (Widowski et al. 1989). In chickens the heterophil:lymphocyte ratio is related directly to the number of stressors received by chicks (McFarlane and Curtis, 1989). The H:L ratio is a more reliable indicator than corticosterone, heterophil or lymphocyte concentration on its own (Gross & Siegel, 1983).

Polycythaemia

The haematocrit or packed cell volume is the volume of erythrocytes in the blood and is measured by centrifugation. Activation of the sympathetic nervous system can be measured by the haematocrit value.

This is an abnormally high packed cell volume (PCV). There are two forms: relative and absolute polycythaemia. Relative polycythaemia is an increase in PCV without a rise in the red cells and red cell-producing tissues. This is seen in dehydration or following splenic contraction which occurs after excitement, apprehension or fright. This is particularly common in the horse. Absolute polycythaemia is where there is an increase in PCV due to an increase in the red cells and red cell-producing tissues. This is uncommon and usually follows an abnormality in the cardiovascular, respiratory or endocrine systems. It can follow excess continued cortisol production.

Anaemia or oligocythaemia

As overhydration is unlikely to occur naturally in animals, all cases of anaemia are absolute and can be divided by aetiology into haemorrhagic, haemolytic and aplastic or hypoplastic. Acute haemorrhagic anaemia is usually the result of trauma or, rarely in large animals, warfarin poisoning. Chronic haemolytic anaemia usually involves the alimentary tract, urinary tract or blood-sucking parasites. Acute haemolytic anaemia can be due to infections such as babesiosis and bacillary haemoglobinuria, or due to toxicosis, for example chronic copper poisoning or acute brassica poisoning, or to antibody/antigen reactions. Chronic haemolytic anaemia again can be due to infections, toxins or antibody/antigen reactions as well as congenital conditions such as porphyria.

Hypoplastic or aplastic anaemia and chronic hypoplasia can be nutritional due to starvation, protein deficiency, mineral deficiency such as cobalt or copper, or vitamin deficiency such as vitamin B_{12}, folic acid, thiamin, niacin or hypoplastic or aplastic anaemia. There can also be depression due to chronic renal disease, hormonal disorders or debilitating disease such as *Trichostrongylus* infections. True aplasia is unusual and very serious, often due to irradiation, bracken poisoning, oestrogens or other drugs.

Fibrinogen

A less direct assessment of stress can be obtained by determination of plasma fibrinogen (Factor I). It is a soluble plasma glycoprotein consisting of six polypeptide chains, produced by liver parenchymal cells and is a precursor of thrombin. Fibrinogen is part of the body's defence mechanism against injury and disease. It can migrate into the extravascular space to contain or localize an invasive disease process or following injury. Inflammatory responses are often accompanied by an increase in circulating plasma fibrinogen levels. Increased levels of fibrinogen are dependent on ACTH, although the effects appear to be extra-adrenal (Seligsohn et al. 1973). Assembly and transport of calves often leads to an increase in concentration.

Some use has been made of the ratio of plasma protein to fibrinogen (PP:F). This provides a useful method of investigating the actual amount of fibrinogen increase over plasma proteins particularly in conditions where dehydration occurs. A normal ratio of PP:F is about 13:1 in cattle (Prathaban and Gnana-prakasam 1990) and 14.7:1 in buffaloes (Prathaban and Nagarajan 1984). A PP:F ratio of 10:1 in cows indicates a marked increase in fibrinogen (Schalm et al. 1975).

Fibrinogen can be measured by collecting blood in EDTA and centrifuga-tion. The fibrinogen is precipitated with sodium sulphate and incubation. The mixture is centrifuged, the precipitate washed with sodium hydroxide and the quantity determined by the Biuret method. The Biuret method can also be used for determining total plasma protein.

Cattle of different types tend to have variable fibrinogen responses, thus *Bos indicus* calves have higher levels (Phillips et al. 1989) at weaning, assembly and transport than *Bos taurus* (Phillips et al. 1989).

Standard biochemical tests

Plasma proteins

The total protein is usually measured by the Biuret method although refracto-metry can be used for a rapid result. Plasma proteins include:

Albumin
Globulins (immunoglobulins and other proteins)
Enzymes
Transfer proteins
Protein hormones
Clotting factors

Increased concentrations are usually due to:

1. A reduction in extracellular fluid, e.g. dehydration; this results in similar relative increases in both albumin and globulin.

2. Chronic diseases and those resulting in an immune reaction, thereby increasing gamma globulins.

Decreased concentrations occur due to:

1. An increase in extracellular fluid.
2. Excessive protein loss—usually albumin is primarily lost. This can be due to haemorrhage, protein-losing enteropathy or renal protein loss.
3. Decreased protein synthesis. Often this is due to dietary deficiency, malabsorption or liver failure.

Albumin

This is usually determined because measurement is quicker than for globulins, although the BCG dye binding albumin method tends to be erratic on occasion (Kerr 1989). Albumin is produced in the liver and so it is affected by liver disorders, malabsorption, protein-losing enteropathies or protein deficiency. Elevated levels occur in dehydration, shock and haemoconcentration.

Globulin

This is usually derived by measuring total plasma protein and albumin levels and then subtracting them. Elevated levels occur in acute and chronic disease. Decreased levels occur in malnutrition and lack of passive absorption of globulins in young animals.

Immunoglobulins

These can be measured by various methods but the zinc sulphate turbidity test (ZST) does provide a useful measure of immunoglobulins. The immunoglobulins are divided into alpha, beta and gamma fractions, which is accomplished using electrophoresis.

Urea

This is the nitrogenous waste product of the breakdown of amino acids. Urea is produced in the liver and transported to the kidneys in the plasma.

Increased levels can be due to a rise in plasma urea concentrations, or increased breakdown of poor quality dietary protein which is deaminated in the absence of the essential amino acids, carbohydrate deficiency, poor renal perfusion or renal failure, urethral obstruction or ruptured bladder. Decreased renal blood flow occurs in dehydration, adrenal insufficiency and shock and so can be an indirect non-specific indicator of adaptation problems.

A decrease occurs with marginal or low dietary protein levels. It can arise from a failure of the urea cycle to convert ammonia to urea, as occurs in liver failure or nephrosis not complicated by renal insufficiency.

Creatinine

This is a nitrogenous waste product and is a breakdown product of creatine, derived mainly by the irreversible non-enzymatic degradation of creatine phosphate in the muscles. It is unaffected by the diet or by liver or urea cycle metabolism. An increase in creatinine often does indicate renal failure, urinary tract obstruction or impairment of renal function.

Ammonia

This is produced from amino acid catabolism or nitrogen excretion before urea formation. If the urea cycle fails it leads to a build-up of ammonia. Problems are uncommon in farm animals. However, an increase is likely if there are errors in urea cycle metabolism, patent ductus arteriosus leading to a porto-caval shunt or in the end-stage of liver failure.

Selenium/vitamin E

Deficiencies of selenium and vitamin E can suppress components of the immune system (Boyne and Arthur 1979; Eskew et al. 1985). Conversely selenium and vitamin E supplementation can enhance the humoral immune response (Spallholz et al. 1975; Peplowski et al. 1980). Resistance to disease or improved animal health have followed the use of vitamin E and selenium supplementation (Teige et al. 1982; Smith et al. 1985). Enhanced serum antibody responses to *Pasteurella haemolytica* vaccination have occurred with the combination of selenium and vitamin E (Droke and Loerch 1989).

Performance and health status of cattle in the feedlot environment may not be improved by selenium and vitamin E supplementation, particularly if disease levels are low (Droke and Loerch 1989).

Glucose

Normal brain function is dependent on adequate glucose concentrations. Glucose is absorbed from the gut and when not required it is stored in the liver and muscles as glycogen. This is broken down when required and once exhausted, lipolysis or eventually proteinolysis occurs. Thus raised glucose values have been observed in tied calves at the start of the fattening period. This is not due to nutrition but is the result of enhanced catabolism thereby tending to reduce weight gain. This state is probably mediated by both the hypothalamic pituitary adrenocortical system and the sympathetic adrenomedullary system.

Increases in glucose levels occur following a high carbohydrate meal, after sudden exercise, severe or acute stress, corticosteroid activity, treatment with glucose-containing fluids or diabetes mellitus. Stress due to pain, restraint of intractable animals or transportation leads to a rise due to glucocorticoids but, more importantly, adrenaline. Thus blood glucose levels increased in goats at least half-an-hour after the start of a journey and over 30 minutes after plasma cortisol levels rose. They remained high 90–150 minutes after the end of the journey and 1 to 2 hours after cortisol values decreased. Pentobarbitone sodium administration at 20 mg/kg body weight 30 minutes into the journey reduced glucose elevation (Sanhouri et al. 1991).

Decreases normally arise through acetonaemia or, although highly unlikely, could be due to insulin-induced hypoglycaemia, adrenal insufficiency and occasionally with hepatic insufficiency.

Beta-hydroxybutyrate

When energy is deficient and there is a lack of glycolytic products, ketosis develops, and ketone bodies, including beta-hydroxybutyrate, achieve significant concentrations in the blood. An increase in beta-hydroxybutyrate is usually the result of absolute carbohydrate deficiency.

Bilirubin

This is a by-product of haem breakdown:

			+ Albumin	Conjugated with glucoronic acid ↓		
Haem	→	Bilirubin	→ Plasma	→ Liver	→	Bile
			Indirect bilirubin	Direct bilirubin		
			Water insoluble	Water soluble		

Increased plasma bilirubin occurs in several conditions, including fasting hyperbilirubinaemia, which is seen in horses, intravascular haemolysis, liver failure and obstructive biliary disease.

Cholesterol

This can be measured but is of little value in large animals.

Triglycerides

Fat is stored as triglycerides in the fat reserves. When required they are broken down by lipases and esterases within the fat store itself. This releases into the plasma free fatty acids and glycerol. Triglyceride is measured by breakdown with lipase and esterase, producing total glycerol, which is measured. Free glycerol can be determined by assaying without the use of the lipolytic enzymes.

High triglyceride levels occur in diabetes mellitus, hypothyroidism, renal failure, nephrotic syndrome, pancreatitis and equine hyperlipidaemia.

Creatine kinase (CK) Creatine phosphokinase (CPK)

There are three isoenzyme types (K being present as a dimer, i.e. it has two subunit groups, M and B). This produces CKMM (skeletal muscle), CKMB (cardiac muscle) and CKBB (brain). A rise in CK is seen in damaged muscle due to exertion, surgery, deficiencies, catabolism, hypothyroidism and cerebrocortical necrosis.

Lactate dehydrogenase (LDH or DH)

LDH is one of the largest protein molecules in the body and is involved in glycolytic conversion of pyruvate to lactate and vice versa in gluconeogenesis. Pyruvate is reduced by nicotinamide adenine dinucleotide (NADH) in a reaction catalysed by LDH. LDH has four subunits or protomers (i.e. it is a tetramer and the subunits are in two forms, H and L, producing five isoenzymes—HHHH (LDH1), HHHL (LDH2), HHLL (LDH3), HLLL (LDH4) and LLLL (LDH5)).

LDH1, also known as HHHH and hydroxybutyrate dehydrogenase (HBDH or HBD), is associated with kidney, erythrocyte and primarily cardiac muscle. LDH2, LDH3 and LDH4 are associated with muscle and lung, while LDH5 is associated with the liver. LDH tends to have a long half-life and also often produces retrospective information. It can be used to determine muscle damage and as it is released for several hours it may be useful in indicating stress.

Gamma glutamyl transferase (γGT; GGT)

This indicates long term damage to the liver.

Sorbitol dehydrogenase (SDH)

SDH is often used as an indication of hepatic damage in horses and ruminants. It is an indication of acute liver damage and as it has a short half life it will fall rapidly once any insult to the organ is removed.

Glutamate dehydrogenase (GLDH, GDH, GMD)

This is often used in ruminants as an indicator of acute hepatic damage.

Aspartate aminotransferase (AST, previously SGOT)

AST is widely found in tissues including the liver, skeletal muscle, heart muscle and erythrocytes. Therefore it is not an indicator of specific organ damage, but is used to suggest muscle or liver damage.

Alanine aminotransferase (ALT, previously SGPT)

This is considered to be of limited use in diagnosis in large animals, although it is primarily a muscle enzyme.

Alkaline phosphatase (ALP)

ALP is found in the skeleton as well as liver and intestinal wall. The normal range tends to be variable particularly in horses and is higher in young animals. Raised values can indicate bone disorders and liver problem.

Non esterified fatty acids (NEFA)

These are now often used to indicate ketosis in ruminants.

Sodium

Usually sodium is present in excess and is regulated by excretion via the kidney and the gut. It is concerned with water balance. An increase in sodium levels is unusual but can result from fluid deprivation, dehydration, central nervous system trauma or disease. It has also been seen in hyperadrenocorticism with hyperaldosteronism or corticosteroid excess. Decrease occurs in kidney failure as the renal tubules do not reabsorb sodium, in adrenal insufficiency, some acute or chronic disorders, and intestinal obstruction.

Potassium

This is generally found within cells and is concerned with electrolyte and water balance, although less so than sodium. Increases in potassium are unusual and generally small. They can occur in kidney failure, particularly with acute pyelonephritis or adrenal insufficiency. Decreased potassium levels occur in diarrhoea, malabsorption syndrome, unusual renal loss, inadequate potassium intake or an abnormal redistribution between the extracellular and intracellular fluid.

The horse tends to develop notably low plasma potassium levels without any harmful effects. This occurs when sodium excretion is elevated, for instance when eating hay or with profuse sweating following prolonged exercise (Kerr 1989).

Chloride

The concentration of chloride anions in the blood is affected by the other main anion, bicarbonate. Under normal conditions, plasma chloride tends to follow the same changes as sodium. Changes in chloride and other electrolyte concentrations in mastitic milk have prompted observations of changes in its electrical conductivity. These can be measured by electronic devices in the milking parlour allowing early detection of mastitis.

High plasma chloride concentration is often present in acidosis and where there is increased plasma sodium concentration, dehydration or renal insufficiency.

Low plasma chloride concentration occurs where there is alkalosis or low plasma sodium concentrations. It can also occur in colic, particularly where there is obstruction high in the gastrointestinal tract allowing fluid to pool in the stomach and upper small intestine. Plasma levels in horses can fall markedly when excited or frightened. Low levels can also be seen in hyperadrenocorticism, where there is chronic loss of potassium ions.

Total carbon dioxide

This is the only measure of acid/base status which does not require a special procedure to collect blood for analysis. Most of the CO_2 in the plasma is in the form of bicarbonate and this measurement can be useful in acid–base balance disturbances due to metabolic problems but not those due to respiratory problems.

Calcium

Plasma calcium circulates in both the bound and unbound forms in almost equal proportions. An increase in circulating calcium levels occurs noticeably in hyperparathyroidism, which is uncommon, or due to the over-treatment of parturient paresis. Decreased levels can occur with parturient paresis in cattle and hypocalcaemia in sheep, and are a sign of chronic renal failure and hypoalbuminaemia. They can also occur in prolonged reduction in feed intake, malabsorption, hypoproteinaemia and vitamin D deficiency.

Phosphate

This is a major component of bone as well as being involved in many metabolic pathways. Plasma concentrations tend to be controlled by parathyroid hormone. Increased levels of phosphate in farm animals may often be due to diet and high levels may occur in the pig with no clinical signs. They occasionally occur in chronic renal failure of farm animals. A decrease in plasma phosphate may be seen in post-parturient haemoglobinuria or downer cow. It can also occur following vitamin D deficiency, malabsorption syndrome, starvation, cachexia or renal tubular defects.

Magnesium

High levels of magnesium in plasma are unusual but may occur in conjunction with other abnormalities, such as acute renal failure. Hypomagnesaemia is common in ruminants, usually resulting from dietary magnesium deficiency, but it can also arise following diarrhoea, hepatic insufficiency or excessive renal loss.

Copper

Problems usually arise in ruminants. Copper poisoning can occur with haemolytic anaemia. However, serum copper levels tend to increase in weaned suckler calves following market transit stress and bovine respiratory disease

(Orr et al. 1990). A decrease in blood copper levels is most commonly seen in ruminants. In some cases there are signs of deficiency. However, on occasions animals can show no abnormalities but have low circulating copper levels. Injection of copper in some of these cases results in an increase in weight gain, showing it to be a copper-responsive condition.

Cobalt

In simple stomached animals cobalt is used as vitamin B_{12}. In ruminants cobalt can be converted to vitamin B_{12} and so a deficiency of cobalt is possible.

Zinc

Deficiency of zinc can result in skin lesions, lameness and fertility problems. Recently it has been found that in weaned suckler calves serum zinc levels decreased following market transit, stress and bovine respiratory disease. While part of the reduction could be attributed to a lowered feed intake, serum zinc still decreased after infection with infectious bovine rhinotracheitis even when feed intake was held constant (Orr et al. 1990).

Other biochemical tests

Interferon

A diminished ability to resist disease has welfare implications, and interferon production may be one method of quantifying this. It can be produced by activated lymphocytes and has an action on the adrenal cortex similar to ACTH, being able to stimulate secretion of glucocorticoids. In some instances this can increase the normal distress response.

Interferon can be assayed by measuring antiviral activity in serum by use of a conventional cytopathic effect inhibition bioassay (Ojo-Amaize et al. 1981). This is compared with a laboratory standard of known interferon concentration. Interferon can also be examined by neutralization assay.

The test has been used to indicate the susceptibility of pigs to viral infections after transport (Artursson et al. 1989). The ability of peripheral blood mononuclear leucocytes to produce interferon after stimulation with virus and their ability to multiply in response to the presence of a T-cell mitogen also give an indication of susceptibility to stress or ability to counteract disease.

Growth hormone

Growth hormones are synthesized in somatotrophes, a subclass of pituitary acidophilic cells. Catecholamines such as noradrenaline and dopamine modulate the secretion of growth hormone resulting in an increased release.

Changes in growth hormone levels can arise following stress (pain, apprehension, cold and surgery). It also increases following exercise, anorexia or severe hypoglycaemia. The stress responses may be mediated by catecholamines acting on the hypothalamus. Thus although plasma GH has been found to rise in pigs following stress and exercise, which in itself is at times a stressor (Machlin et al. 1968), physical stress did not have an effect on GH values in market weight pigs (Weiss et al. 1970). Porcine growth hormone can be assayed by a double antibody procedure.

It appears that a rise is more likely when there is physical restraint and handling rather than from a subcutaneous injection (Robert et al. 1989).

Prolactin

Prolactin is secreted from the pituitary and is concerned with the initiation and maintenance of lactation. Catecholamines such as noradrenaline and dopamine modulate the secretion of prolactin by reducing release.

Rises in prolactin concentration have been reported following acute stress in ruminants (De Silva et al. 1986). Serum concentration of prolactin can be quantified using a homologous double antibody radioimmunoassay procedure. However, prolactin levels in pigs do not always alter. A rise in prolactin in pigs is more likely following physical restraint and handling than from a subcutaneous injection (Robert et al. 1989).

Uses of normal biochemical testing

Metabolic profile

This test was designed for dairy cows. Although its use has been questioned on economic and interpretative grounds, it can form a useful guide for economic milk production if used on a regular basis. Originally it was hoped that the use of biochemical parameters might be able to indicate imbalances or the optimum relationship between input in terms of food and output in the context of milk, fertility, pregnancy and weight gain. The test can be of some use up to a point when interpreted in relation to the feed inputs and changes in condition and milk production. However, the wide range of normal values and the variation in alteration of some biochemical parameters—some of which only represent the immediate situation (i.e. magnesium, glucose), others which only show long-term changes (e.g. albumin) and yet others which show very limited alteration (e.g. calcium)—make for difficulties. However, the more often testing is performed in a herd, particularly when involving individual animals, the more useful it can be. Problems of assessment and cost have led to the production of mini-profiles (Blowey, 1975).

Originally the caption 'metabolic profile' involved estimation of various parameters in seven high-yielding cows, seven medium-producing cows and seven dry cows. The analyses undertaken were for serum inorganic phosphate, calcium, magnesium, potassium, sodium, total serum protein, albumin and globulin, blood urea nitrogen, blood glucose, packed cell volume and haemoglobin. Occasionally plasma non-esterified free fatty acids, serum copper and iron were quantified. The mini-profile involves sampling about six cows around peak lactation—e.g. at 4–10 weeks. This usually includes testing for blood glucose, serum urea nitrogen and albumin. Some laboratories prefer the use of beta-hydroxybutyrate rather than glucose to test for energy deficiencies. This is because it is more stable than glucose and has a reverse relationship to blood glucose.

Horse fitness tests

Horses can be used for racing, hunting and endurance trials. The performance of such animals is partly dependent on their conformation, genetic make-up and physiological adaptability. However, it also depends on the fitness of the animal. The horse is more adapted than other species to conserve and utilize oxygen, and the changes that occur are dependent on the type of exercise to which the horse is exposed.

Trotting

This results in an increased osmolarity of the plasma mainly due to a rise in sodium and lactate levels. There are also rises in blood potassium, calcium and magnesium but not chloride. The plasma phosphate level tends to decrease.

High levels of creatinine, urea and lactic acid also occur in the blood and the last two remain high for over an hour.

Cantering

This does not usually result in elevated blood lactate or uric acid levels.

Galloping

Horses develop an increased osmolarity of the plasma primarily due to sodium and lactate levels. There are also rises in blood potassium, calcium and magnesium but not chloride. Thus the changes are similar to those in trotting although they tend to return to normal after about an hour. Plasma phosphate levels tend to decrease. During training the serum creatinine, haemoglobin and haematocrit levels increase.

Long-distance races

While blood sodium and bicarbonate levels remain the same, there is a rise in potassium and a fall in calcium. In these races there is a very marked increase in blood lactate levels. There are also rises in blood free fatty acids, glucose and glycerol. Glucagon levels tend to show a marked rise and cortisol levels increase. However, uric acid, creatinine, urea, albumin and creatine phosphokinase levels increase.

Endurance rides

These are not races but involve completing courses of 80 to 150 km in one or two days. While participating, the animals show a rise in blood phosphate and plasma free fatty acid and glycerol levels. In many cases there is an initial rise in blood glucose, possibly due to excitement, followed by a decrease as liver glycogen becomes depleted with prolonged exercise. There is a fall in plasma sodium, potassium, calcium, magnesium and chloride. Falls in calcium and magnesium occur towards the middle of the ride whereas those of sodium and potassium occur at the end. These losses are mainly via sweat. Some rise also occurs in blood lactate, lactate dehydrogenase and creatine phosphokinase. The degree of haemoconcentration and increased plasma protein levels depend in part on the weather and are quickly corrected at the end of the ride. In some studies, disqualified horses showed higher packed cell volumes and total protein concentrations at the finish than horses successfully completing the ride

(Sloet van Oldruitenbourgh-Oosterbaan et al. 1991). Acidosis is not a feature of the rides because of compensation.

Fitness assessment

It has proved difficult to assess fitness or predict performance by biochemical or haematological testing. However, it is probable that performance will be poor when in the resting animal there are high levels of aspartate transferase (AST), alanine transferase (ALT), alkaline phosphatase, gamma glutamyl transferase (YGT), alkaline phosphatase (SAP), creatine phosphokinase (CK) or lactate dehydrogenase (LDH). Training does reduce blood lactate levels.

Jumping horses

As with other horse events, wide variations in parameters occur between individuals. However, following exercise there has been found to be an increase in sodium, calcium, blood plasma protein, lactate dehydrogenase and blood glucose (Art et al. 1990). It is suggested that in jumping trials, because of the conditions and variations in courses, the post-exercise value of each horse should be compared with the others under the same conditions and not to mean values.

Three-day eventing

This competition involves cross-country, show jumping and dressage. The types of changes in parameters are similar to a combination of the alterations seen in racing and endurance rides. The most obvious changes tend to be seen after the cross-country event (Rose et al. 1980).

Other methods of health monitoring

Temperature monitoring

Temperature has long been used as a measure of health. All homeothermic animals have two thermal regions. The first, approximately measured rectally, is the stable inner core and represents about two-thirds of the body mass. The other is the outer shell which is of variable temperature and acts as the protective barrier in contact with the environment. Infrared energy is produced and emitted by all animals and the amount emitted depends on the animal's absolute temperature plus the degree to which the animal emits energy, i.e. the emissivity. As the emissivity of animal skin approaches unity measurements of infrared energy can be converted directly into temperature (Palmer 1981) by a portable infrared thermometer. This gives a method of studying animals in health and disease. It has the advantage of being non-invasive.

An interrogator transponder system consisting of a Doppler radar transmitter/receiver and a small transponder unit placed either on or in the animal can be used. The addition of a circuit to the transponder allows the accurate recording of body temperature and early disease detection. When the animal is stressed, blood is redistributed from the skin and splanchnic areas into the muscle masses. As a result, the subdermal temperature falls and can be recorded by the interrogator/transponder or infrared systems. The systems can help in the determination of disease resistance and heat tolerance in different breeds and species (Seawright 1976).

Milk temperature can be used to detect oestrus and mastitis.

Endorphins

Plasma beta-endorphin concentrations can be measured by means of a radioimmuno assay. Endorphins tend to be released in response to stressful stimuli. Work on sheep has shown levels to increase following shearing, electroimmobilization, handling, transport and slaughter. Endorphins have also been used to assess effects on pigs at and prior to stunning (Anil et al. 1990).

Automatic weighing

In many production systems it is necessary to weigh the animals. This involves restraining and weighing all or a sample of animals to obtain the information. Poultry have been weighed using an automatic weigh sampling device consisting of a strain-gauged perch linked to a microcomputer (Turner et al. 1984). Weights are recorded by computer which can identify and eliminate false data.

Remote observation

The use of a closed-circuit television and video system can be helpful in ascertaining disease problems and normal or abnormal behaviour such as parturition and oestrus. It is probable that imaging systems will experimentally be able to identify the behaviour of animals and edit the video film accordingly.

Cows can be fitted with a harness incorporating a plastic plate fitting under the tail. When the tail is raised horizontally for a prolonged period of 2–3 minutes it produces a signal which is transferred to a control box, thus initiating an alarm. This can be used to determine calving.

Electroencephalograph

This has been used to assess sleep and waking patterns in farm animals in an attempt to determine the acceptability of changes in their environment. It involves the implantation of electrodes. In work undertaken to assess activity the animals also had electrodes present in the eye and neck muscles. These were linked with an electro-oculogram and electromyelogram. Different stages could be recognized from the awake state, the relaxed state, slow-wave sleep stage and paradoxical sleep stages (Ladewig and Ellendorff 1983). Pigs kept in an open pen with straw and then in a farrowing crate with a slatted floor showed no significant change in their sleep-awake response but during their awake phase rooting was a prominent activity when straw was present. However, this could be due to previous experience with slatted floors.

Environmental sensors

Air quality sensors to detect pathogens have yet to be developed. Ammonia sensors have been used but are not yet reliable due to humidity and temperature imbalances (Ross and Daley 1988).

Acknowledgements

The author has drawn heavily on the experience of others and particularly that of a former colleague, Dr M G Kerr. Much of the laboratory test interpretation is based on her thoughts as outlined in *Veterinary Laboratory Medicine: Clinical Biochemistry and Haematology* (Kerr 1989). Roger Ewbank was generous enough to discuss his thoughts and comment on the manuscript.

COLLECTION OF DIAGNOSTIC SAMPLES

It goes without saying that for good laboratory investigation the right samples must be taken by appropriate means and stored and transported in a suitable fashion. No laboratory test can act as a substitute for clinical examination and interpretation. It is an aid to diagnosis and must always be interpreted in that light. In many instances, where several animals are ill, a group of those which are sick should be tested. In some instances it is also useful to obtain samples from those animals in the group which are apparently well. This can act as a means of contrasting various parameters between the sick and healthy animals, or it may show that others have subclinical infection and are therefore likely to succumb at a later date.

It is always best to contact the laboratory undertaking the testing to find what measures they require for sampling in terms of amount, anticoagulants, separation, containers to be used, labelling, history, etc. Blood sampling usually involves the use of EDTA for haematological investigation and fibrinogen determination. Biochemical tests usually require plasma obtained with the use of the anticoagulant heparin. However, oxalate-fluoride anticoagulant is used for determination of glucose as it will stop the activity of enzymes. Clotted samples are used to obtain antibody titres as well as for metabolites and alkaline phosphatase. Ideally, in all cases, the serum or plasma should be separated from the erythrocytes before packaging and transport. This reduces the possibility of haemolysis during transit as well as preventing possible alteration in values due to exchange of enzymes and minerals between the cells and plasma or serum (Allen 1991). However, in many cases a travel time of 48 hours will not significantly alter the result. In some samples, such as when testing for glutathione peroxidase, it is necessary to provide red cells as the enzyme is present within them. In such cases a packed cell volume also has to be estimated. When packaging samples for transport, the appropriate postal regulations must be observed.

COMMON TEST FINDINGS FOR CONDITIONS OF LIVESTOCK

Please note that these levels are generalizations and should only be used as a guide for interpretation. In practice, considerable variation will occur according to the stage at which the problem is investigated, its severity, its specific cause, the species and the individual involved. The clinical examination of the animal is paramount when interpreting the results.

Key:
* Acute
** Chronic
*** Excessive
† Horses
‡ Cattle (ruminants)

Problem	Blood Tests	Other Tests
Abomasal torsion	Cl $\downarrow$ H $\uparrow$ HCO_3 $\downarrow$ K $\downarrow$ Na = Protein (total) $\uparrow$	Urine pH $\downarrow$
Acidosis (metabolic)	Cl $\uparrow$ H $\uparrow$ K $\uparrow$ HCO_3 $\downarrow$ pCO_2 $\downarrow$ pH $\downarrow$	Urine pH $\downarrow$
Alkalosis (metabolic)	Cl $\downarrow$ H $\downarrow$ HCO_3 $\uparrow$ K $\downarrow$ Na = pCO_2 $\uparrow$ pH $\uparrow$	

Problem	Blood Tests	Other Tests
Anaemia (haemolytic)	AST ↑ Bilirubin (indirect) ↑ Bilirubin (total) ↑ LDH ↑ Globulin ↑ ** Protein ↓ * ↑ ** PCV ↓	Urine haemoglobin ↑
Anorexia	Bilirubin (indirect) ↑ † Bilirubin (total) ↑ † Ca ↓ ‡ Mg ↓	
Anorexia (prolonged)	Albumin ↓ Ca ↓ ‡ K ↓ Mg ↓ P ↓ Total Protein ↓ Lymphocytes ↓	
Ascites	Cl ↓ Na ↓	
Cardiac muscle problems	AST ↑ CK ↑ LDH ↑	
Congestive heart failure	H ↓ HCO_3 ↓ Creatinine ↑ pCO_2 ↓ pH ↑ Urea ↑	
Dehydration	Albumin ↑ Cl ↑ Globulin ↑ K ↓ Na ↑ Protein (total) ↑ Urea ↑ PCV ↑	
Downer cow	AST ↑ CK ↑ LDH ↑ Urea ↑	
Endurance exercise	Ca ↓ Cl ↓ CK ↑ *** Creatinine ↑ *** Glucose ↑ then ↓	

Problem	Blood Tests	Other Tests
Endurance exercise (*cont.*)	H ↓ ★★★ HCO₃ ↑ ★★★ K ↓ LDH ↑ ★★★ Mg ↓ Na ↓ P ↑ pCO₂ ↑ ★★★ pH ↑ ★★★ Protein (total) ↑ Urea ↑ PCV ↑	
Enteritis	Cl ↓ Fibrinogen ↑ H ↑ ★ HCO₃ ↓ ★ K ↓ Na ↓ pCO₂ ↓ ★ pH ↓ ★ Protein (total) ↑ Erythrocytes ↑ PCV ↑ Neutrophils ↑	Urine pH ↓
Excitement	Cl ↓ ★ Glucose ↑ H ↓ HCO₃ ↓ pCO₂ ↓ pH ↑ Lymphocytes ↑ Neutrophils ↑	
Exercise	Ca ↑ Glucose ↑ H ↑ HCO₃ ↓ K ↑ Mg ↑ Na ↑ P ↓ pCO₂ ↓ pH ↓ Urea ↑ Lymphocytes ↑ Neutrophils ↑	Urine pH ↓
Exhaustion	Cl ↓ Na = Urea ↑	

Problem	Blood Tests	Other Tests
Fear	Cl ↓ ★ H ↓ HCO$_3$ ↓ pCO$_2$ ↓ pH ↑	
Haemorrhage	Cl ↓ Na ↓ Protein (total) ↓ PCV ↓	
Hyperglycaemia	Cl ↓ Glucose ↑ Na ↓	
Hyperlipidaemia	Cl ↓ Na ↓	
Hypocalcaemia (Lactation tetany in horse, lambing sickness in ewe, parturient paresis)	Ca ↓ P ↓ ‡	
Hypomagnesaemia (cattle, sheep)	Ca ↓ (often) Mg ↓	
Ketosis	Glucose ↓ Ketones ↑ Urea ↑	Urine pH ↓
Kidney problems	Albumin ↓ Ca ↑ ★★ Ca ↓ ★ Creatinine ↑ K ↑ Mg ↓ Na ↓ P ↑ ★ P ↓ ★★ Protein (total) ↓ Urea ↑	Urine: Casts ↑ Cells ↑ Protein ↑ SG ↓ Culture Biopsy
Liver problems	Albumin ↓ ★★ AP ↑ AST ↑ Bilirubin (direct) ↑ Bilirubin (indirect) ↑ Bilirubin (total) ↑ Fibrinogen ↑ YGT ↑ LDH ↑ Mg ↓ Protein (total) ↓ ★★ SDH ↑ Urea ↓	Urine: Bilirubin ↑ pH ↓ SG ↓ BSP clearance ↑ Biopsy

Problem	Blood Tests	Other Tests
Malignant hyperthermia	AST ↑ Ca ↓ CK ↑ LDH ↑	
Malignant oedema	AST ↑ CK ↑ LDH ↑	
Pain	H ↓ HCO$_3$ ↓ pCO$_2$ ↓ pH ↑	
Peritonitis	Cl ↓ Fibrinogen ↑ Globulin ↑ H ↑ HCO$_3$ ↓ K ↓ Na ↓ pH ↓ pCO$_2$ ↓ Protein (total) ↑ ‡ ↓ ★ Lymphocytes ↓ Neutrophils ↑ ★ ↓ diffuse	Urine pH ↓
Pregnancy toxaemia	AP ↑ AST ↑ Glucose ↓ H ↑ HCO$_3$ ↓ LDH ↑ pCO$_2$ ↓ pH ↓ Protein (total) ↑	Urine pH ↓
Protein-losing enteropathy	PCV ↑ Protein (total) = or ↓	
Respiratory infection	Fibrinogen ↑ Globulin ↑ ★★ H ↑ HCO$_3$ ↑ pCO$_2$ ↑ pH ↓ Lymphocytes ↓ ★ ↑ ★★ Neutrophils ↑	
Shock (endotoxic)	Albumin ↑ Glucose ↓ Protein (total) ↑ Urea ↑ Erythrocytes ↑ PCV ↑	

Problem	Blood Tests	Other Tests
Skeletal muscle problems	AST ↑ CK ↑ GSPx ↓ LDH ↑ Urea ↑	Urine: Myoglobin ↑ Biopsy
Stress	Glucose ↑ Lymphocytes ↓ Neutrophils ↑	
Sweating (excessive)	Cl ↓ H ↓ HCO_3 ↑ K ↓ Na ↓ pCO_2 ↑ pH ↑ Neutrophils ↓	
Toxaemia (acute)	Ca ↓ Protein (total) ↑	
Transport	H ↓ HCO_3 ↓ pCO_2 ↓ pH ↑	
Vagal indigestion	Cl ↓ K ↓ Na = Protein Total) ↑	
Volvulus	K ↓ Na ↓	
Water deprivation	Cl ↑ Na ↑ PCV ↑	Urine SG ↑

BEHAVIOUR, STRESS AND DISEASE

R DANTZER PhD, DVM and M-C SALAÜN PhD

Domestication and behaviour
Behaviour—methods of study and mechanisms
Abnormal behaviour
Stress and behaviour
Discomfort
Conclusions

Nutrition, reproduction and health have long been the main disciplines of interest in the field of animal sciences. Behavioural studies were carried out only in relation to these disciplines. The aim was to optimize those behavioural patterns that positively contribute to productivity (e.g., food intake, reproductive behaviour) and to get rid of those behavioural patterns that were perceived as counterproductive (e.g., exploratory behaviour and social activities).

Attitudes have changed drastically in the last two decades. Confronted with an increased incidence of environment-related diseases, veterinarians were the first professionals in the 1960s to claim that the intensification process in animal husbandry had gone too far and that it was necessary to improve the quality of the environment in which animals are housed. The response was a boom in sales of health products and feed additives! It took 10 more years to see the emergence of an authentic interest in the behaviour of farm animals, mainly under the pressure of welfarists concerned with the issues of pain and suffering possibly engendered by housing conditions and management practices in intensive husbandry. Since that time, an impressive amount of knowledge about farm animal behaviour has accumulated.

Drawing from this literature, the present chapter aims at showing how the consideration of behaviour of farm animals can actually help to optimize the environmental conditions under which they are kept and to decrease in this way the risk of disease.

Domestication and behaviour

In the course of evolution, animals have adapted to certain habitats in which survival is optimal. The process of natural selection favours those animals which are the best adapted to their ecological niche and this adaptation is expressed in morphological as well as functional characteristics. In case the environment changes to less favourable conditions, animals try actively to reduce the impact of the adverse situation on their organism and if they are not successful, they leave to find more suitable surroundings.

Domestication has taken place via a selection on the ability of animals to tolerate the presence of human beings in their immediate environment. Since no active selection has been practised on other behavioural traits, there has been no major change in the species-specific behavioural repertoire of farm animals. Differences between domestic and wild populations are the result of quantitative changes in the threshold at which a response can be elicited rather than the expression of qualitative changes in behaviour (Price 1984). An example is nest-building in sows. This behaviour is still present in the repertoire of modern breeds of pigs but its full expression requires a higher than normal level of stimulation. The fact that the potential for a full expression of the species-specific behavioural repertoire has not been fundamentally altered is evident from the successful survival of feral chicken, pigs, cattle, sheep, horses and goats.

Genotypic adaptation occurs at the population level over many generations. However, this is a slow process and its role in adjusting the behaviour and physiology of farm animals to confinement remains unclear (Ricker et al. 1987). Tennessen (1989) argued that the most effective adaptation of farm animals to confinement is at the phenotypic level. Early experience tunes physiological, behavioural and emotional responses and in this way allows animals to cope with their environment. In spite of a long history of domestication, farm animals are not fully able to adapt to any type of production system. When environmental pressure on the organism is excessive, adaptive processes break down and functional disorders may appear. The recognition of these disorders requires a good knowledge of normal behaviour.

Behaviour—methods of study and mechanisms

Methods of study

In the biological sciences, the study of behaviour is dominated by two main approaches, ethology and experimental psychology. Ethologists usually are interested in the way behaviour, like other morphological and physiological characteristics of the organism, contributes to individual survival. Field observations are a key feature of this approach since by definition the adaptive nature of a given behaviour can only be deduced from the econiche in which it has evolved. In contrast, experimental psychologists study intermediate processes, such as learning and motivation, to understand how the brain processes information from the external and internal environments. This is usually done by confining animals to laboratories and studying arbitrary behavioural patterns under strictly controlled conditions, for example requiring animals to press a lever in order to obtain a food reward, as a measure of feeding behaviour.

In animal science, this distinction is somewhat blurred. At a descriptive level, the behaviour of farm animals is studied in the commercial environment they are provided with and the comparison between different environments, including more natural ones, allows an assessment of the extent to which the expression of certain behavioural patterns is constrained. To study mechanisms, more standardized conditions are necessary and this is usually achieved by reducing the environment to the minimal features that are sufficient for the animal to express the behaviour under investigation. This domain of research is termed 'applied ethology' or 'applied behavioural science'.

Description of behaviour

An important step in the description of behaviour is the identification of the different behavioural patterns that form the repertoire of a given species. Ethograms are full catalogues of the basic species-specific behaviours, including communication patterns (Table 4.1). This qualitative description is usually

Table 4.1 Main behaviours composing the behavioural repertoire of farm animals

Maintenance	Reproductive
Ingestive behaviour	Oestrous behaviour
Exploratory behaviour	Sexual responsiveness
Body care	Mating behaviour
Association and social behaviour	Parturient behaviour
Territoriality	Nursing
Rest and sleep	
Social communication	

accompanied by a quantitative description in which time serves as the basic unit. Time budgets define mean time spent in main activities (Figure 4.1). The part played by a given behaviour in the time budget of an animal cannot, however, be used as a measure of the biological importance of this behaviour.

Ethograms and time budgets represent static descriptions of behaviour at a macroscopic level. Each behaviour is actually composed of a number of el-

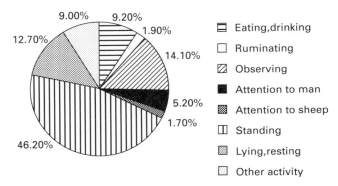

Figure 4.1 Time budget of sheep housed indoors during a 10-hour period in daytime (adapted from Done-Currie et al. 1984).

ementary behavioural patterns that have characteristic relationships with each other and serve different functions. These basic behavioural units need to be defined in objective terms and quantified by their frequency, duration and time of occurrence in relation to others (sequential analysis). Agonistic interactions in sows, for example, include mutual investigation, threat, avoidance and elements of physical aggression such as head-to-head, bites directed towards the ears, neck and shoulders of the opponent, shoulder-to-shoulder opposition, perpendicular attacks, chasing and submissive posture (Jensen 1982) (Figure 4.2).

The problem with this description at a microscopic level is that it mixes postural and functional labels. Ideally, function should be the outcome of description rather than part of it. In research on aggression, basic aggressive strategies have actually been defined in terms of (1) targets for attack by the offender and (2) protective postures adopted by the opponent. In pigs, the strategy of the fighter is to charge the opponent in a perpendicular way in order to bite its ears, face or neck. In order to prevent this and because of the relative lack of body flexibility that characterizes pig morphology, the opponent faces the attacker and moves laterally towards him. This results in a typical shoulder-to-shoulder apposition posture that the fighter tries to break by turning away and coming in perpendicularly. However, his opponent maintains apposition so that both pigs circle together in this posture. This fighting pattern may last several minutes but it is interrupted by pauses during which the two animals stand panting shoulder to shoulder before resuming the battle. The loser eventually turns away, squeals, runs or takes refuge in a corner and presents its hind quarters (a non-target site for biting) to the victor. The way these behaviours are organized and the variation from this fighting pattern have been described in juvenile pigs (McGlone 1985b). The importance of target areas for attacks is demonstrated by the decreased incidence of fighting observed in pigs regrouped in pens equipped with 'hide' areas in which

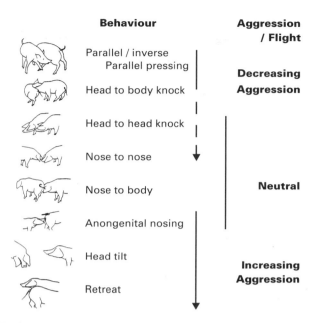

| Behaviour | Aggression / Flight |

Figure 4.2 Typical patterns of agonistic interactions in group-housed dry sows (adapted from Jensen 1980, 1982).

animals can position their head and neck (McGlone and Curtis 1985). In spite of the usefulness of this description, there are still some methodological problems related to the difficulty of identifying threat and submission postures (McGlone 1986).

The identification of the different functional categories of a given behaviour is a necessary step for the study of mechanisms. In the case of aggression, for example, it is obvious from the preceding discussion that this behaviour cannot be treated as an entity and that it is necessary to dissociate offence from defence. 'Anti-aggressive' drugs such as anxiolytics do not act in the same manner on these two categories, since defensive behaviour is attenuated by diazepam at doses which increase offensive behaviour. In terms of hormonal mechanisms, offensive behaviour depends on circulating androgens whereas defensive behaviour is modulated by glucocorticoids.

Another example is female sexual behaviour, which includes three different components: proceptivity, i.e. active attempts by the female to contact with the male; attractivity, i.e. features that attract the male; and receptivity, i.e. acceptance of the male (Leshner 1978). In primates, these distinct components have been shown to be mediated by different hormonal mechanisms. Attractivity is dependent mainly on peripheral influences of oestrogens on vaginal mucosa. Proceptivity is mediated by androgens elaborated by the adrenal cortex. The hormonal mechanisms involved in receptivity are still elusive.

Another useful way of describing behaviour is to take into account its temporal dimension, by distinguishing preconsummatory (or appetitive), consummatory and postconsummatory components (Table 4.2). The appetitive sequence brings the subject in contact with the target. In natural conditions, typical appetitive behaviours such as the search for food or the quest for a sexual partner occupy an important part in the time budget. In confinement, animals are only allowed to express consummatory behaviours and not the appropriate appetitive behaviours. The physiological processes that are implicated in the consummatory step are often controlled by the many sensory-motor reafferences that result from the expression of the corresponding appetitive behaviour. In addition, the duration of the sequence of consummatory behaviour is normally a function of the availability of the natural object toward which it is directed, and the satiety mechanisms that bring an end to the sequence are tuned to its normal temporal course. When food is directly supplied in a highly concentrated form, the total bulk of nutrient is ingested within a few minutes. In such conditions, the normal sequence of eating behaviour, which involves rooting in pigs, pecking and ground scratching in poultry, and chewing and licking in cattle, cannot be carried out at full length. When animals are kept on slatted floors without bedding, these activities are often redirected toward penmates (see the next section of abnormal behaviours).

Mechanisms of behaviour

If they are given the opportunity to do so, most pregnant sows will engage in nest-building on the last days preceding parturition. This behaviour is displayed not only by animals living in the wild but also by animals that have been housed in confinement before being moved outdoors. In this latter case, nests that are built by naive animals have all the necessary qualities to offer full thermal protection to piglets (Stolba and Wood-Gush 1984). Components of nest-building, in the form of pawing and attempts to gather material, also can be observed in confined sows, suggesting the predominant role of internal versus external factors in the determination of this behaviour. The physiological mechanisms underlying nest-building can be studied in several ways, from the identification of the environmental stimuli which are necessary for its development and execution, to the investigation of the role of changes in the sow's internal state mediated by hormones.

External and internal stimuli represent what behaviourists call proximal factors, i.e. factors which are directly responsible for the behaviour under study and antecedent to its expression. Ultimate factors represent another set of factors which correspond to the final aim of the behaviour under study. In the case of maternal behaviour, for example, it could be speculated that sows

Table 4.2 Preconsummatory (appetitive), consummatory and postconsummatory components of a few behavioural activities

Behaviour	Preconsummatory	Consummatory	Postconsummatory
Feeding	Food search	Ingestion	Grooming Resting
Body care	Scratching	Dustbathing Wallowing	Shaking
Sexual behaviour	Courtship	Mating	Grooming Resting
Agonistic behaviour	Approach Threat	Fight	Escape Flight
Farrowing Laying	Nesting	Parturition Oviposition	Grooming Resting

are building nests because they are foreseeing their progeny's thermal needs. Although this appears very unlikely, we are still inclined to propose ultimate factors as explanations for some categories of behaviour. In the case of the establishment of dominance orders, for example, animals have been claimed to fight in order to set up priority of access to future resources in case they become scarce. If this is so, growing pigs should fight more when food is restricted than when it is abundant. However, food availability was found to have no influence on the incidence of fighting in piglets brought together after weaning (McGlone 1986). Aggressive interactions are actually triggered by the identification of conspecifics as strangers on the basis of their olfactory stimulus characteristics. This discussion should not lead to the conclusion that behaviour can only be explained by it proximal factors or that animals do not develop expectations about goal objects. Ultimate factors determine the survival value of behaviour and are therefore important in a phylogenetic perspective.

Behaviour of farm animal species cannot be understood without reference to their sensory-perceptual world. In pigs, olfaction is dominant over vision. Olfactory stimuli emanating from one animal and perceived by another induce behavioural and endocrine changes in the recipient animal. Such signals, known as pheromones, have been identified in pigs, and include 3-alpha-hydroxy 5-alpha-16-en androgen metabolite found in the submaxillary gland of boars. Removal of this gland decreases the sexual response of the sow to the operated male and reduces the male's own libido (Perry et al. 1980). Another metabolite, 5-alpha-androst-16-en-3-one (androstenone) is responsible for boar taint and is elaborated by preputial glands. It facilitates the immobility reaction in oestrous sows. Olfactory stimuli also play a role in aggression. Androstenone decreased the duration of offensive and submissive behaviour in piglets

(McGlone 1985a). In addition, urine collected from ACTH-treated pigs and sprayed in the air during late fight increased submissiveness (McGlone 1985b). Pigs are able to recognize other animals belonging to the same social group and to differentiate them from animals belonging to a different social group. The main sources of odour are from the orbital and suborbital scent glands, the carpal glands and the apocrine sweat glands which are numerous on the upper neck and the back. Lipid secretions from these glands could be degraded by the skin microflora into a complex mixture of branched and unbranched short-chain fatty acids. The composition of these mixtures would depend both upon the characteristics of the individual pigs and the microclimate of its pen, which could explain why pigs are able not only to identify other animals from the same group but also to recognize individuals from social groups other than their own.

There are close interactions between olfaction and internal states. Ewes, for example, normally display a strong aversion to amniotic fluids, which disappears and is replaced by a marked attraction at time of parturition (Levy and Poindron, 1987). This change in olfactory preferences is brought about by the rise in oestrogens that precedes parturition. It leads the female to lick its newborn lamb instead of attacking it. By licking this social object, the ewe forms in her brain an olfactory template of it, which is subsequently used as a reference point to enable her to distinguish her lamb from alien lambs. The formation of this olfactory memory is made possible by the neural action of oxytocin on brain structures sensitized by oestradiol (Kendrick et al. 1987). After birth, the ewe's perception of her lamb gradually evolves to include visual and olfactory cues which, after a few days, become sufficient for recognition.

In birds, vision is the predominant sensory modality. The size of the comb, a morphological feature that is dependent of circulating androgens, is the main stimulus for triggering aggressive behaviour in cocks. Birds learn to know each other by visual inspection and the mere presence of other birds, without the ability to physically interact, is sufficient to reduce fighting when animals are regrouped (Zayan et al. 1983).

Information from the external and internal environment is ultimately integrated in the brain. The way this information is processed and leads to changes in behaviour is the object of intense research by neuroscientists. However, this research is mainly carried out on laboratory animals and the corresponding knowledge is rarely available in farm animals.

Abnormal behaviour

Behavioural plasticity of farm animals allows them to adapt to environmental conditions very different from those they originally evolved in. However, there is a limit to adaptability beyond which disorders appear in the form of disturbed behavioural patterns. The distinction between normal and disturbed behaviour is a gradual one. It is important to dissociate environment-induced behavioural disorders from primary or secondary neurological disorders since the symptomatology can be the same. Behavioural disorders are characterized by a diminished responsiveness to exteroceptive stimuli, unusual forms of conduct, unsound bodily movements, reduced or exaggerated activity and behavioural patterns considered as abnormal. Abnormal behaviour is defined as a persistent undesirable action which is displayed by a minority of the population, is not due to any obvious neurological lesion and is not restricted to the situation that originally elicited it.

At the level of the Commission of the European Communities, a group of experts has set up a list of abnormal behaviours that are observed in farm animals and that are considered as indicators or signals of a maladjustment between animals and their environment (Wiepkema et al. 1983) (Table 4.3). These behaviour patterns are very heterogeneous because of differences in causation, function and methods of evaluation. The most common abnormal behaviours recognized by experts are excessive oral activities such as tail biting in pigs, feather pecking in hens, cannibalism in both species, tongue rolling or urine drinking in group-housed veal calves and wool pulling in sheep. Another important category of abnormal behaviour includes stereotyped activities like pacing in laying hens, tongue playing in veal calves and bar biting in tethered sows.

Abnormal oral activities

Abnormal oral activities involve components of the feeding and food gathering repertoire. They express the inability to carry out in a normal way the species-specific food intake sequence. In intensive husbandry, food is provided once or twice a day, in a processed form rich in energy and low in roughage. There is therefore little need for the animal to seek and masticate the food and time devoted to eating is dramatically reduced in comparison to natural conditions. Because of the lack of appropriate stimuli in the surroundings, the strong need to peck, root or graze is redirected towards social congeners. Typical examples are feather pecking in hens and tail biting in pigs (Plate 4).

The behaviours have been attributed to a bewildering variety of environ-

Table 4.3 Behavioural abnormalities in farm animals

Categories[1]	Performers	Housing[2]
1. Injurious behaviours		
Tail biting/cannibalism	Fattening pigs	Modern, unbedded
Tail/ears biting	Piglets	,,
Sucking penmates	,,	,,
Coat licking	Veal calves	Crates
Sucking penmates	,,	Group housing
Urine sucking	,,	,,
Feather pecking/cannibalism	Laying hens	Battery cages
	,,	Floor housing
Feather pecking/cannibalism	Broilers	Floor housing
2. Stereotyped behaviours		
Bar biting	Tethered sows	Modern, unbedded
Sham chewing	,,	,,
Weaving	,,	,,
Sham chewing	Fattening pigs	,,
Tongue playing	Veal calves	Crates
,,	,,	Group housing
,,	Dairy cattle	All systems
,,	Fattening bulls	Group housing
Stereotyped pacing	Laying hens	Battery cages
3. Abnormal body movements		
Abnormal lying down or standing up	Cattle	Slatted floor housing
4. Redirected behaviours		
Licking	Veal calves	Crates
Sham ruminating	,,	,,
Sham dustbathing	Laying hens	Battery cages
Leaning	Dairy cattle	Cubicle system
Dog sitting	,,	,,
Milk-sucking	,,	Various systems
Wood gnawing	Fattening bulls	Slatted floor
Mouthing prepuce	,,	,,
Mouthing coat	,,	,,
Hysteria	Laying hens	Floor housing
5. Apathetic behaviour		
Motionless sitting on hind quarters	Tethered sows	Modern, unbedded
,,	Fattening pigs	,,

[1] The categories are not mutually exclusive.
[2] The mentioned housing system indicates in which conditions the behaviour can be observed, but it does not mean that the housing system as such is always the cause of abnormal behaviour.

mental factors such as crowding, impoverished environment, poor ventilation, uncomfortable temperature, disease and boredom (Table 4.4). Nutritional factors like monotonous diet and dietary deficiency have also been claimed to play an important role since they would result in the appearance of a specific appetite for nutrients present in feather or blood of conspecifics (Hughes 1982; Fraser 1987a, 1987b). Abnormal oral activities usually start with recreational chewing or pecking parts of a conspecific's body, exhibited by a few animals (primary biters or peckers). At this stage, environmental factors still play a major role, by modulating the frequency of redirected chewing and pecking and therefore the likelihood of accidental injury (Figure 4.3). Nutritional factors are likely to take over after the appearance of injuries. The 'injury' stage is characterized by a generalization of behaviour, the habit spreading to other individuals in the group by visual communication (Blackshaw 1981; Hughes 1982).

It is well known that only a few animals in a pen indulge in feather pecking or tail biting. Fraser (1987a) observed large inter-individual variation in the degree of chewing behaviour and attraction toward blood. This certainly explains why most of the biting is done by certain penmates while others experiencing the same environment and diet do not bite at all. These characteristics are partly under genetic control, as shown by the occurrence of familial differences in the proportion of peckers and pecked hens and a relatively high heritability for this trait (0.56). Therefore it should be theoretically possible to control this behavioural disorder by selecting lines in which the proportion of primary peckers is low.

Abnormal oral activities can also reflect more general management problems. For example, early weaned piglets raised in battery cages show a higher frequency of belly nosing of penmates than those housed in a maternity pen with bedding (Fraser 1987). Similar behaviour has been observed in veal calves removed from their mother immediately after birth. As the need for suckling does not significantly decrease before five weeks of age, calves kept in groups tend to redirect this behaviour toward the navel and penis of other animals (Van Putten and Elshof 1982).

The elaboration upon these few examples of abnormal oral activities should not be taken as evidence that this issue has already been solved. The exact causes which are responsible for the development and maintenance of these behavioural disorders remain mostly unknown and, in particular, the interaction between external and internal factors has not yet been worked out.

Stereotypies

Stereotypies are repetitive actions that are fixed in form and orientation and serve no obvious function. The apparent lack of function of these activities

Table 4.4 Factors reported to promote abnormal oral activities (from Sambraus 1985; Fraser 1987a, 1987b)

Overlarge group size
High stocking density
Unregulated feeding
Dietary deficiency
Specific appetite for nutrient present in feather, blood
Not enough feeding space for all animals
Malfunctioning drinking equipment
Parasite infection
High noise level in the barn
Too high level of noxious gases (CO_2, NH_3, H_2S)
High humidity
High temperature
Draughts
Excitation
Boredom

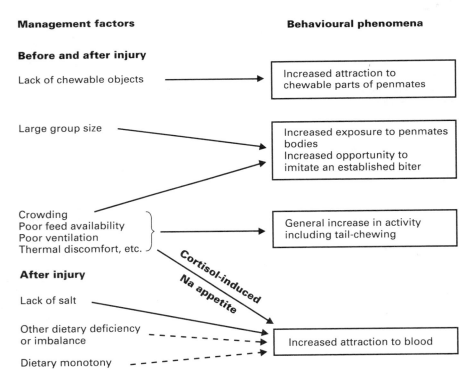

Figure 4.3 Proposed model suggesting how management factors may influence behavioural phenomena favouring tail biting. The more speculative relationships are shown with broken lines (adapted from Fraser 1987b).

differentiates them from other repetitive movements that are often found in the behavioural repertoire of many animal species, such as body grooming and displays.

Because they interfere less with production than abnormal oral activities, stereotypies have been relatively neglected in animal production. In the last decade, this situation has changed because of concern about welfare issues in intensive husbandry and the belief that stereotypies are both signs of inadequate environmental design and indicators of mental suffering (Kiley-Worthington 1977; Dawkins 1980; Broom 1983).

The term 'stereotypy' refers to repetitive sequences of activities that consist of a few fixed elements carried out at a higher than normal rate and occurring in nearly the same order in successive cycles. Behavioural elements may differ from individual to individual. For example, stereotypies in stalled sows usually involve chewing and licking activities directed toward objects in the immediate environment or executed in the absence of such objects (vacuum activities or sham chewing and licking). However, the number of behavioural elements and the way they succeed each other vary between individuals. In a typical case, a sow will pick up a chain placed in front of her and chew it from the bottom to the top; she will then drop the chain and root it down, before displaying sham chewing while attempting to pick up the chain again. The whole sequence is then repeated, endlessly. Another animal placed in the same conditions will alternate between bar licking, trough licking, sham licking and sham chewing (Cronin 1985). In veal calves kept individually in boxes and bucket fed with milk replacers without any roughage, biting and licking of parts of the crate dominate during the first 10 weeks of life and are replaced later by self-directed activities such as tongue playing (De Wilt 1985; Wiepkema et al. 1987).

The development of stereotypies is characterized by a progressive narrowing of behavioural diversity. While sows living is semi-natural conditions exhibit more than 100 different behavioural patterns, this range decreases to a little more than 30 in sows housed in stalls (Stolba et al. 1983). Stereotypies themselves include less than ten different patterns, with a mean number of three to four acts per individual (Cronin and Wiepkema 1984). The final elements which form the basis of the stereotypy are not arbitrary but depend on the predominant behaviours in the eliciting situation. For example, stereotypies which are displayed before feeding in stalled sows are built upon elements of redirected activities consecutive to thwarted attempts to reach the food trolley (Rushen 1984).

In tethered sows, stereotypies develop in four distinct stages following tethering: (1) escape attempts lasting on average 45 minutes; (2) a phase of stuporous inactivity which lasts about one day; (3) a progressive reappearance of outward-directed activities (16 days) that form the background on which (4) basic stereotypies develop (Cronin 1985) (Figure 4.4). This gradual emergence of stereotypies is also apparent when animals of different parities are con-

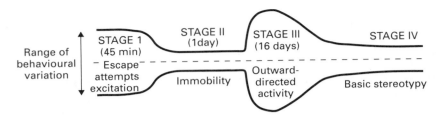

Figure 4.4 Development of stereotypes in second-parity sows tethered for the first time. The vertical axis represents the range of behavioural variation and the horizontal axis time (from Dantzer 1986).

sidered (Stolba et al. 1983; Cariolet and Dantzer 1984). Parity 1 is characterized by frequent and long-lasting periods of drowsiness. In parities 2 and 3, the levels of locomotion and investigative activities rise significantly, and some individuals may already display a high frequency of stereotyped behaviours. These behaviours increase in frequency and duration over successive parities. In addition, patterns of stereotyped behaviour show qualitative changes with increasing parities; self-directed patterns (e.g. sham chewing, head weaving) tend to replace environment-directed stereotypies (e.g. bar or chain biting) (Stolba et al. 1983).

Stereotypies usually develop in situations characterized by restriction of movement (limited space or tethering) and by lack of exteroceptive stimulation. Frustration and (or) conflict also has been demonstrated to induce stereotyped activities. Hungry hens exposed to food that they could see but not eat displayed escape movements that developed into stereotyped pacing within a few sessions (Duncan and Wood-Gush 1972). Similar stereotypies have been reported in laying hens in the absence of a suitable nest site (Brantas 1980). The thwarting of food motivation appears to be an important factor in the development of stereotypies. Stereotyped activities are common in horses and sheep fed concentrate diets (Willard et al. 1977; Done-Currie et al. 1984; Mardsen and Wood-Gush 1986). In tethered sows housed in gestation stalls, there is a positive relationship between the frequency of stereotypies and the degree of food restriction, with a threshold around 2 kg per sow per day (Rushen 1985; Appleby and Lawrence 1987) (Figure 4.5). Pigeons which develop spot-pecking while maintained at 80% of their free-feeding body weight stopped stereotyping within one day of free-feeding (Palya and Zacny 1980). In a similar way, stereotyped chain chewing induced by an intermittent distribution of food to food-restricted pigs was greatly reduced when pigs were fed before the test (Dantzer and Mormède 1983a).

Social factors represent another contributory component in the genesis of stereotypies. Naive pigeons developed stereotypies at a higher rate when placed in visual contact with other birds displaying stereotypies than when placed with non-stereotyping birds (Palya and Zacny 1980). The stereotypies

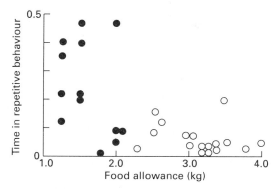

Figure 4.5 Relationship between proportion of observations spent in stereotypies and daily food allowance in individual gilts. Solid circles represent gilts kept on low food levels whereas open circles represent gilts kept on high food levels (adapted from Appleby and Lawrence 1987).

that developed by imitation were true stereotypies because they did not disappear when adjacent birds stopped displaying stereotypies. It is likely that the same contagion phenomenon occurs in groups of sows.

Most speculation on the neural basis of stereotyped behaviour has been built upon pharmocological data showing the psychostimulant drugs such as amphetamine induced stereotypies in laboratory animals (Lyon and Robbins 1975), in farm animals (Sharman and Stephens 1974; Fry et al. 1981) and in birds (Deviche 1985). There is good evidence to suggest that performance of stereotyped behaviour depends on brain dopamine systems involved in the control of movement and that the intervention of these systems is modulated by other neurotransmitters, particularly endogenous opiates. This last conclusion is based on experiments showing that stress activates endogenous opiates (Dantzer et al. 1986) and that blockage of opiate receptors decreases the frequency of developing stereotypies but not well-established ones (Cronin 1985).

Because of the putative role of endorphins in reward processes, the effects of blockade of opioid receptors on stereotypies have been interpreted to suggest that the performance of stereotypic behaviour results in the release of endogenous opiates which reduce the negative emotions experienced by the sow and allow her to adapt to her condition. Since these endogenous opiates are addictive, like morphine, the sow would become at the same time addicted to this behaviour. More traditional explanations of stereotypies focus on their compensatory function or their de-arousal properties. In the first case, the eliciting situation causes a low arousal level that the animals find aversive; they therefore actively seek means of increasing arousal and, because of the lack of exteroceptive stimulation, the only way to do so is to perform behaviour which involves richly innervated parts of the body (e.g. mouth). In the second case, the environment is supposed to elicit a state of hyperarousal that needs to be dissipated by alternative activities or requires the animals to engage in distracting activities. From what is known currently about the mechanisms of stereotypies and their neural basis, it appears more reasonable to conclude that stereotypies do not serve any obvious function besides being the expression of activation engendered by the environment (Dantzer 1986). Behavioural responses energized by this activation depend on the stimuli available and the disposition of the animal. They do not gain strength because of any rewarding properties but simply because of the positive feedback of sensory stimulation engendered by these motor acts on the neural systems that control them and the progressive sensitization of these repeatedly activated neural systems. Because of the high inter-individual variation in the likelihood of developing stereotypic behaviour even in the more unfavourable conditions (e.g. Wiepkema 1987), stereotypies must be viewed as the outcome of neuronal functional abnormalities that occur in certain predisposed individuals. The best way to prevent such disorders is to provide the animals with appropriate stimuli which can take the form of adjunct objects such as straw or toys (e.g. Fraser 1975; Grandin et al. 1987).

Sickness behaviour

Animals that are ill with infectious disease are typically described as lethargic and apathetic. They are reluctant to move and do not show much interest in normal activities, including food and water intake and interactions with other animals. They develop rough hair coats. This picture of a lethargic, depressed, anorexic and febrile individual is well known by veterinarians since it is the recognition of these signs by the animals' owner which usually motivates consultation. The first task the veterinarian is confronted with is to separate those non specific signs of sickness from the specific ones, in order to diagnose what disease the animals are suffering from. For these reasons, there has been little interest in the investigation of the mechanisms responsible for the behaviour of sick animals.

Some recent research on the biological basis of the fever syndrome has actually opened new perspectives on the mechanisms of sickness behaviour and its adaptive value.

The febrile process is triggered by products released from accessory immune cells, including macrophages and monocytes. In contact with specific components of the cell wall of pathogens, activated cells release endogenous pyrogens which act both in the local microenvironment to stimulate immune mechanisms, and at a distance to coordinate a whole set of metabolic and neural responses to infection. The exact nature of endogenous pyrogens has been recently elucidated. The main endogenous pyrogens are represented by interleukin–1, interleukin–6 and tumour necrosis factor. Fever is due to a central action of these factors on the anterior hypothalamus. Other neural activities of endogenous pyrogens include pituitary-adrenal activation, by a stimulation of the secretion of hypothalamic corticotrophin-releasing factor (Besedovsky et al. 1986; Berkenbosch et al. 1987; Sapolsky et al. 1987), sleepiness (Krueger et al. 1984), anorexia (McCarthy et al. 1985, 1986), general malaise (Tazi et al. 1988), decreased activity (Otterness et al. 1988) and reduced interest in social activities (Crestani 1990). The cellular and molecular mechanisms underlying these effects are the subject of an intense research effort.

Although the development of antipyretics has led to the systematic treatment of fever signs, fever is actually an evolutionary mechanism which is very effective in combating viral and bacterial infections (Kluger 1979). The febrile response is due to an increase in the themoregulatory set point so that animals feel cold at normal temperatures. This results in a decrease in heat losses and an increase in heat production, of which the main effector is shivering. The resulting hyperthermia stimulates the activity of the immune system and decreases the viability of pathogens. In addition, sequestration of blood iron and zinc decreases the availability of these oligo-elements for the growth and multiplication of pathogens. As argued by Hart (1988), the behaviour of sick animals is not a maladaptive response nor the effect of debilitation, but rather an organized, evolved, behavioural strategy that potentiates the role of fever by conserving energy and protecting the sick individuals from external dangers.

Stress and behaviour

Stress is usually conceived of as an excessive demand over the animal's adaptive abilities. Since Selye's original contribution (Selye 1936), stress has been recognized as a main component of everyday life. Everybody knows about stress, even if nobody knows what it means exactly. In livestock production, stress is used to describe both the conditions which lead to production losses and diseases (e.g. transport stress, weaning stress, nutrition stress) and the resulting pathology (e.g. the acute stress syndrome in pigs). The term stress is used not only for labelling but also for explaining (if animals die or develop pale, soft and exudative meat, it is because they are stressed). It is only a small step from there to conclude that they need 'anti-stress' drugs to palliate their exquisite sensitivity to stress!

The reality behind this mythical concept of stress has been worked out to some extent in farm animals (Dantzer and Mormède 1983b). In animal sciences, the positions about stress have oscillated between two extremes: one pointing out decreased defence mechanisms due to genetic selection for intensive production and environmental pressure which favours anabolism over catabolism; the other attributing the troubles to over-responsiveness of hormonal systems involved in adaptation. These two extreme views are the outcome of a tradition of physiologically oriented research which has concentrated on the pituitary-adrenal axis and peripheral effects of stress hormones, without being able to decide whether the observed hormonal reactions were adaptive or maladaptive. In addition, the popularity of the stress concept has long obscured the fact that there was a gap between the initial formulation of Selye's stress theory, which had mainly been elaborated on the basis of anatomo-pathological findings, and the results of modern biochemical methods of hormonal assays. As a typical example, the three phases of the stress reaction (alarm, resistance and exhaustion) have no obvious equivalent in terms of changes in plasma corticosteroid levels. Moreover, exhaustion never occurs in real life. The only point of convergence between Selye's theorization and the result of hormonal measurements is the occurrence of an enhanced pituitary-adrenal activity following exposure to a wide variety of stressors. This response is so constant that it has become the operational definition of stress in physiologically oriented research.

In order to understand what stress is about, it has been necessary to adopt a different perspective emphasizing the fact that living organisms adapt to their environment by integrated responses which depend on reciprocal interactions between behaviour and hormones.

Relations between hormonal and behavioural responses to stress

Classical hormonal responses to stress involve the sympathetic adrenal medullary system—the emergence reaction, as defined by Cannon (1935)—and the pituitary-adrenal system—the general adaptation syndrome, as defined by Selye (1936). Psychological stimuli are as effective as physical stimuli in activating both hormonal systems. In pigs, for example, short-term exposure to a novel environment is sufficient to increase plasma cortisol levels to values comparable to those reached after an injection of ACTH. Moreover, the intensity of the cortisol response is a function of the degree of novelty experienced by the animals. Calves housed in strawed pens responded with higher cortisol levels when introduced to a novel pen with a slatted floor than when exposed to an enclosure with straw. The reverse trend was observed in calves raised in slatted pens (Figure 4.6).

Frustration and conflict are also very effective in inducing pituitary-adrenal activation. Pigs trained to work for food by pressing a panel with their snout responded to the frustration produced by the interruption of food delivery by a large increase in circulating cortisol levels and this increase was a positive

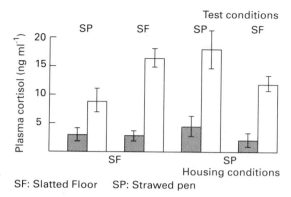

Figure 4.6 Plasma cortisol response to different degrees of novelty in veal calves usually housed in strawed pens (SP) or slatted floor pens (SF) (from Dantzer et al. 1983c).

function of their tendency to continue pressing the panel in spite of the lack of reward.

When confronted with a threat, all individuals do not respond in the same way. Some individuals rapidly master the situation. Others pay little attention to it. Still others try hard to cope with the problem but with little success and rapidly enter a state of passivity and resignation. There are therefore many coping strategies for the same problem. An important question in face of so many different strategies is how to evaluate their relative effectiveness and adaptive value. This is usually done by reference to the outcome with respect to the original problem (i.e. is the problem materially solved?), or on ethical grounds (i.e. is the behaviour acceptable in regard to current ethics?). On biological grounds, the effectiveness of a given behavioural attitude can be appreciated on the basis of its physiological consequences rather than on the way it is expressed. In other terms, coping can be defined as any process the individual interposes between the aggression and himself in order to decrease physiological activation. This concept has been substantiated by work on laboratory animals, showing that the critical factors are represented by the ability to predict and control the occurrence of external events.

In a typical experiment, rats were exposed to painful electric shocks with or without the possibility to put an end to this stimulus (Weiss 1972). Rats which could control electric shocks by turning a wheel with their forepaws developed less gastric ulceration than rats exposed to the same intensity and frequency of shocks but without being able to modify their occurrence.

There is an impressive amount of evidence to show that the pattern of hormonal response to stress depends not on the physical characteristics of the stressor, but on the perceptual experience of the subject and the behaviour he engages in (Figure 4.7). The sympathetic adrenal medullary system is acti-

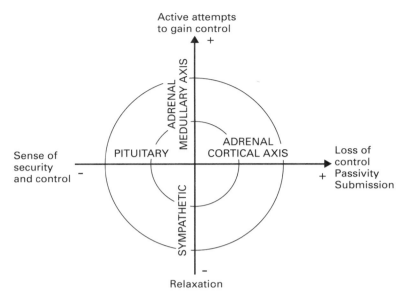

Figure 4.7 Model of the neuroendocrine substrates of the emotional reaction to environmental stimulation. A sympathetic adrenal-medullary effort/relaxation axis is contrasted with a pituitary-adrenal-cortical loss of control/security axis in a two-dimensional space. The normal neuroendocrine activity of the population under study corresponds to the intersection of the two axes and the circles to the normal range of variation of hormonal activities (from Dantzer et al. 1983c).

vated when the power to control access to goal objects such as food, water, shelter, mate and dependants is challenged and leads to repeated attempts to maintain control. This response is associated with continued arousal and increase in heart rate, blood pressure and peripheral resistance. In contrast, the reverse trend, i.e. deactivation of the sympathetic adrenal medullary system, is achieved during the relaxation state that accompanies grooming and attachment behaviour. The pituitary-adrenal system is maximally activated under conditions of uncertainty, when coping attempts are thwarted and potentially disastrous threats are perceived which cannot be escaped or controlled. The subjects then tend to withdraw from their environment and protect themselves. In contrast, low pituitary-adrenal activity is associated with feelings of security and control.

The interactions between behaviour and hormones are not unidirectional from behaviour to hormones. The individual's hormonal state at the time it enters the situation modulates the neural activity involved in the perception of the impinging stimuli via the general metabolic rate, the functional state of sensory receptors and effectors and action on neural activity. As a typical example, pigs treated with ACTH or a synthetic corticosteroid, dexamethasone, responded to a fear signal (a tone paired with electric shocks) as if they were more fearful than without hormonal treatment (Mormède and Dantzer 1978).

All these notions can be incorporated in a model of hormone–behaviour interactions in response to aversive situations (Figure 4.8). This model is important because it points out that the study of the physiological correlates of adaptation is meaningless if, at the same time, behavioural reactions are not assessed. This model also incorporates the notion that in many cases the success of adaptation depends on the opportunity for the animal to express the appropriate behavioural response. If animals are exposed to a cold draught, they normally alter their position and seek shelter. However, if they cannot move away, they have to increase their heat production and decrease their heat losses in order to adjust to the draught. In other words, the basic adaptive response is behavioural and the neuroendocrine changes which take place are crucially dependent on the behavioural strategy adopted by the subject.

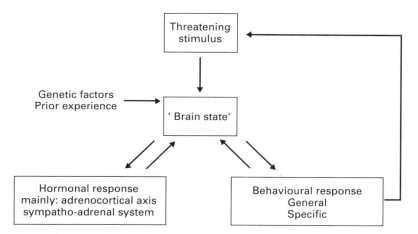

Figure 4.8 Model of the relationship between environmental threatening stimuli and bodily responses. The responses which are initiated by the central nervous system depend on the 'brain state' at the time of stimulus perception. The behavioural response is given a specific quality which corresponds to two main modes of responding, either active (e.g. flight or fight) or passive (e.g. withdrawal, immobility or freezing). Peripherally released hormones depend on the behavioural attitude and they feed back to the brain to modulate the acquisition and retention of the behavioural response (from Dantzer and Mormède 1983b).

Practical implications for the assessment of adaptive abilities

There would be little or no need for further research in the field of animal welfare if it was sufficient to simultaneously record behavioural and neuroendocrine responses of animals to their environment in order to assess their possible state of stress. The main problem is still the choice of the exact criteria to be used and the way the results can be interpreted.

In the case of well-identified acute stressors, the selection of a suitable measure of stress is relatively easy since most physiological and hormonal indicators reflect the operation of the stress factors under study. As a typical example heart rate was observed to increase two-fold when pigs had to walk up a 30° ramp in order to reach the upper level of a two-deck lorry whereas it increased by only 40% when the ramp was lowered to 15° (Van Putten 1982).

In cases of chronic stressors, the situation is less straightforward. The sensitivity of stress indicators can be increased by submitting animals to a standardized challenge in order to assess their behavioural and physiological reactivities, instead of measuring only baseline values. The so-called open-field test, which consists of placing animals into a new environment in order to assess their ambulatory activity, vocalizations and changes in plasma hormones, is commonly used for that purpose. There is still some controversy, however, about the exact meaning of the variables measured in this test. By analogy with rodents, for which the test was initially developed, it has been postulated that it provides measurements of fear. Since rats and mice normally live in burrows and are inclined to avoid predators by staying motionless when they cannot escape, a high level of fear is usually associated in these species with a low level of ambulation. However, in ungulates in which the usual defence reaction is more likely to be running than freezing, an excessive ambulation may be due more to repeated attempts to find a way out and rejoin penmates than to low emotionality. In spite of these problems, the open-field test is a useful technique for assessing differences between animals in the way they react to novelty.

Another possibility is to assess learning abilities in different tasks motivated by reward or punishment. In this case, it is better to select tasks which allow determination of the relative strength of the active and passive coping strategies that animals tend to adopt in face of incoming dangers.

The sensitivity of endocrine investigation techniques for long-term studies can be enhanced by recourse to dynamic tests such as the ACTH stimulation test and the dexamethasone test for the pituitary-adrenal axis (Dantzer et al. 1983c; Mormède et al. 1983; Meunier-Salaün et al. 1987). Other useful indicators include measures for immunocompetence, especially when they are relevant to the pathological state that is supposed to be influenced by the stress factors under study (e.g. proliferative response of pulmonary lymphocytes to non-specific mitogens, in transported calves prone to the shipping fever syndrome; cf. Dantzer and Kelley (1989) for a recent review).

Discomfort

Although a common approach to welfare is to look for ways of eliminating sources of stress and suffering, there are more direct ways of ensuring well-being. Positive approaches to welfare are based on the consideration of the so-called 'behavioural' needs of farm animals. This terminology, which has been incorporated in the European legislation on farm animal welfare, is based on the postulate that any constraint on the expression of basic species-specific behavioural patterns results in undue suffering. Instead of arguing about the exact definition of suffering and the degree of awareness and subjective experience accessible to farm animals (Griffin 1976; Dawkins 1980, 1990; Singer 1990), a more pragmatic approach consists of tailoring housing conditions and management procedures to the way animals are behaving. Several techniques are available for doing so, ranging from ergonomics to studies of preferences.

Ergonomics

Animals can be considered as workers who have to comply with the requirements of producing meat, eggs or milk in an environment designed to optimize productivity. The ergonomic approach aims at optimizing the design of the working environment by taking into account both the workers' characteristics and the nature of the work to be accomplished.

The availability of sufficient space for ordinary activities is the first requirement for animals which have to live in confinement. A quick glance at accepted norms in intensive husbandry shows that the minimum amount of space is 250–500 cm^2/kg metabolic weight (a measure of body surface, which is calculated by elevating body weight to the power 0.66). This norm corresponds to the surface area occupied by animals which are standing or lying in sterno-abdominal recumbency.

On the basis of body dimensions, allometric equations have been defined to compute minimum static space requirements for growing pigs (Petherick and Baxter 1981; Curtis et al. 1989) and cattle (Boxberger 1983) and relate them to the commercial unit in intensive husbandry, i.e. body weight (Table 4.5). In the case of growing pigs, it is interesting to note that decreases in performance are observed only when the allocated space is lower than the minimal area necessary for pigs to lie on their sternum and abdomen.

Although the determination of static space requirements is a good starting point, it is obviously insufficient for describing the normal space requirements. Animals do not stay standing or lying, they move from one position to the other and, in addition, they make use of the space available to engage in a

Table 4.5 Estimation of minimum space requirements in pigs

Production situation	Space requirement[1]	Reference
Sow (tethered)	Standing up and lying down (mm) Length $= 384\,W^{0.33}$ Width $= 126\,W^{0.34}$ Height $= 177\,W^{0.29}$	Baxter and Schwaller 1983
Piglets } (group) Growing pigs	Resting area $= 0.034\,W^{0.67}$ Total area $= 0.05\,W^{0.67}$ Feeding length $= 1.1 \times 0.61\,W^{0.33}$	Pertherick and Baxter 1981 Baxter 1989

[1] W = body weight in kg; length, width, height expressed in mm/pig; space area expressed in m²/pig.

number of activities more or less useful to the production system they are part of. In sows, the sequence of movements that are involved in lying down and standing up (Figure 4.9) cannot be expressed in a normal way if there is no additional space both in front of the animal and laterally to it. On this basis, two-thirds of the stalls that are commercially available in the UK were recognized as imposing constraints on the execution of basic movements of sows (Baxter and Schwaller 1983). What it means is that sows are obliged to alter their normal way of moving from one position to the other and, by doing so, they increase the degree of stress imposed on their joints. This can lead to pain in the short term but also to an increased risk of arthritis in the long term, associated with a reluctance to move and, therefore, problems with micturition and drinking. In addition the risk of self-inflicted injuries increases, especially on the teats when the sow brings her hind legs under her belly before raising her bottom (De Koning 1984). From these considerations, it is easy to understand why lameness, urinary problems and the metritis-mastitis-agalactia syndrome can become a significant problem in stalled sows.

Another important area is the design of troughs and other livestock equipment. A compromise has to be found between the ease with which the trough can be cleaned by the stockman and the prevention of food wasting by the animal itself. In order to solve this problem, the best approach is to consider the way the animal moves its head and collects food (Figure 4.10) instead of relying on empirical designs which too often turn out to be totally inadequate! Innovative designs have come out of recent work by animal behaviourists (Wierenga 1983; Baxter 1984; Phillips et al. 1987; McFarlane et al. 1988). For example, in dairy units, a sufficient walking area for connecting the different elements of a cubicle system is a key feature for the functionality of such a system (Wierenga 1983).

The question of the optimal space necessary for maintenance activities such as feeding, drinking, elimination, body care and interaction with conspecifics

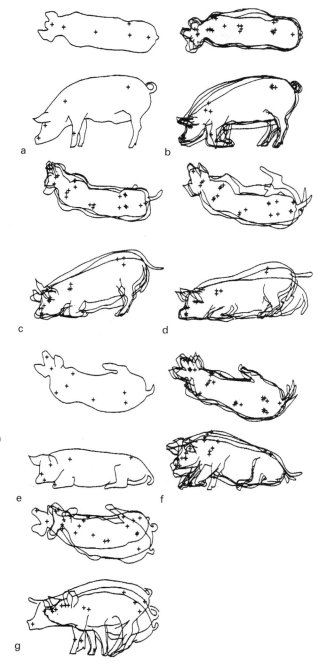

a b c d e f g

Figure 4.9 Stages of movement in lying down (a–d) and standing up (e–g) in sows. Drawings were made from frame-by-frame analysis of video recordings of free-moving sows (adapted from Baxter and Schwaller 1983).

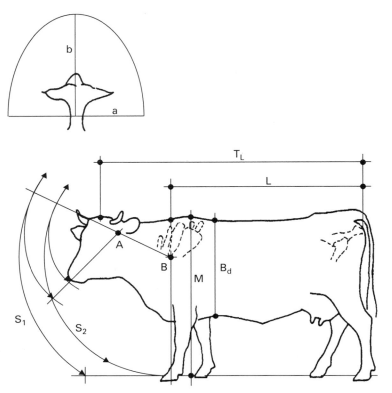

Figure 4.10 Movements of cattle during feeding. S_1 and S_2 represent cow's reach with and without the tongue protruded (adapted from Nygaard and Oybwad 1969). (Reprinted by Zappavigna 1983.)

is still far from being solved, because of the lack of sufficient data on the way these activities are carried out in the natural repertoire of the species under consideration. In growing pigs, for example, there is empirical evidence to suggest that the relative locations of the feeder and the drinking nipple are very important in determining the way the resting and dunging areas are actually used by the animals (Buré 1987). Although this empirical knowledge is likely to be shared by experienced pig farmers, there is no rationale for making a sound choice of one design over others.

Comparative studies

Ideally, the key to understanding what constraints are imposed upon the expression of species-specific behaviour patterns by artificial environments would be to have a full description of behaviour in natural environments. However, the definition of what is a natural environment is far from being easy and an alternative strategy is to study the behaviour of farm animals in semi-natural enclosures, with sources of food easily accessible and no predator. The work by Stolba and Wood-Gush (1984) is a good example of what can be done to determine key features for the release of species-specific behavioural patterns and to incorporate them in the design of an environment more adapted to production requirements.

Preference studies

Based on the postulate that if given the choice between several alternatives, animals select the one which is the best suited to their needs, techniques for assessing preferences have been introduced in applied behavioural science. These techniques allow the assessment of both qualitative aspects (e.g. do animals prefer light over darkness?) and quantitative aspects (e.g. how import-ant is the preference for light in comparison to other stimuli?) of behavioural needs (Duncan 1978a; Dawkins 1980, 1990) (Figure 4.11). It is obvious that

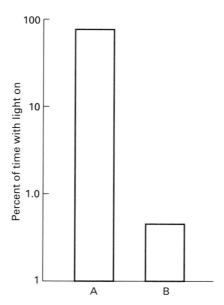

Figure 4.11 Percentage of time with light on when pigs are put in a cage in which they can turn the light on or off by inserting their snout in either of two slots (A); in which the time the light is on is related to the time their snout is inserted in the slot (B). Note that when the light is cheap (A) the light is on for a longer time than when it is costly (B) (adapted from Baldwin, 1983).

taking into account the animal's point of view by directly asking it what it prefers is better than relying on anthropomorphism to decide what is good and what is bad for the animal. For example, a series of studies on preferences of piglets for the different flat deck floors that are commercially available in Western Germany revealed that some floors were clearly avoided and some were clearly preferred, with many falling in between (Marx and Schuster 1980, 1982). These findings have clear implications in terms of thermal comfort.

The interpretation of choice tests is not always that easy. For example, pigs work very hard for turning on heat lamps when they are put in the cold in a climatic chamber environment. But if they are exposed to the same temperature outdoors, they prefer to root the ground instead of staying in the hut where the heating equipment has been set up (Baldwin 1983). In addition, preferences are based on short-term needs and this can be detrimental to long-term needs. Despite these limitations, preference tests represent valuable tools for investigating the subjective feelings of animals.

Alternative systems

Modern livestock production mixes up empirical design with sophisticated control equipment. There is no reason for pens to have a rectangular or square shape apart from the conformity with our own representation of harmony and order. This arbitrary nature of the design of pens can be easily generalized to other aspects of housing and management.

Due to the big surge of interest in the welfare of farm animals, alternative systems are currently the object of much interest from both professional and political authorities. One of the most advanced projects is the get-away cage system as an alternative to battery cages for hens (Wegner 1983). It is characterized by a larger size and the provision of perches at different vertical levels, laying nests and areas for dust-bathing. In still another system, the aviary system, hens use the three dimensional space of a building, which is equipped with roots, nests and dust-bathing areas. All these systems have advantages and disadvantages, in terms of behavioural needs and economics, and more research is needed to improve the efficiency of such systems. Pigs also have benefited from this interest in alternative systems, with designs ranging from the duplex studio (Fraser et al. 1986) to the structured familial pen (Stolba and Wood–Gush 1984).

Although such alternative systems represent a radical departure from traditional designs, more limited improvements to the present designs are also possible, ranging from the use of pen partitions with hides to enable pigs to protect their head and shoulders from the bites and blows of opponents (McGlone and Curtis 1985), to the introduction of operant conditioning systems for control by animals of their own environment (Balsbaugh and

Curtis 1979; Nehring 1981; Edwards and Riley 1986; Morrison et al. 1986; Hunter et al. 1988).

Although it is clear that there is much potential for improving the way animals are kept, the sole consideration of the animals' point of view is unlikely to be the solution since another important actor in the system, i.e. the stockperson has to be taken into account.

The human–animal relationship

Modern livestock production requires that the stockperson enters and imposes upon the perceived physical, social and cognitive environment of the animal. The size of present-day livestock units and the recourse to automation enable only brief contact between animals and stockpersons, with little opportunity for individual recognition of animals. The stockperson is more often part of the environmental and physical constraints to which animals are exposed than a caregiver. The way animals react to him or her is likely to be influenced by both their previous experience of contact with humans and the particular conditions under which interactions take place. This topic has been the subject of some recent research, especially in pigs and dairy cows (Hemsworth and Barnett 1987; Metz 1987; Seabrook 1990). Two main approaches have been used, with emphasis on the side of the animal or on the side of the stockperson.

As a typical example of the first approach, pigs were submitted to handling treatments which lasted for a few minutes per week and consisted of stroking the animal when it approached the caregiver (pleasant treatment), discouraging contacts by giving painful electric shocks to the pigs on approach of the caregiver (unpleasant treatment) or limiting contact apart from that received during the routine husbandry practices (control treatment) (Hemsworth et al. 1981a, 1981b, 1986a, 1986b, 1986c, 1987, 1989). The unpleasant treatment group displayed increased withdrawal and avoidance of human beings, a retarded growth rate and higher corticosteroid concentrations at rest and in presence of the caregiver (Table 4.6). Reproductive performance was also adversely affected since boars submitted to the unpleasant treatment were unable to display a fully coordinated mating response and had smaller testicles whereas gilts tended to reach puberty later. In addition, avoidance and withdrawal behaviour of the sow toward human beings were negatively associated with the number of piglets born per sow and per year.

An important aspect of the human-animal relationship is the determination of the optimal period for exposure to human beings during development. Human contact limited to the developmental period during which social bonding occurs is very effective in improving later handling characteristics (Boissy and Bouissou 1988).

On the side of the caregiver, there has been some work on the stimulus

Table 4.6 Effects of aversive handling on behaviour and zootechnical performance of pigs

Variable	Experiments
Fear level: Higher time to interact with experimenter in a standard test	Hemsworth et al. 1981a, 1986b, 1987 Gonyou et al. 1986 Dryden and Seabrook 1986 Pearce et al. 1989
Reproductive behaviour: Increased age for a full coordinated mating response by boars	Hemsworth et al. 1986c
Adrenal activity: Higher corticosteroids levels Increased size of the adrenal cortex	Hemsworth et al. 1986c, 1987 Gonyou et al. 1986
Performance: Decreased growth rate	Hemsworth et al. 1981b, 1987 Gonyou et al. 1986
Lower pregnancy rate of gilts Smaller testicle size	Hemsworth et al. 1986c

aspects which are perceived and responded to by the animals (e.g. voice, smell, gaze, general attitude) (Hemsworth et al. 1986a, 1989) as well as the intrinsic qualities which are necessary for good stockmanship (Seabrook 1984, 1987) (Table 4.7).

Table 4.7 Critical factors for the development of a good relationship between stockperson and animals (from Seabrook 1984, 1987)

Factor in the relationship	Action of the stockperson
Competence: Technical knowledge related to experience	Interest and motivation to use technical information
Confidence, consistency	Security and consistency of management procedures
Consideration: Observations of animals	Effective development of perceptuals skills: ability to detect changes from the normal pattern of animals and environment Provision of positive stimuli
Communication: Physical contact Social communication	Stroking, scratching and patting Use of voice and social gestures

Conclusions

Health and welfare cannot be assessed without recourse to objective indicators. From the preceding sections, it is clear that we are not short of behavioural and physiological indicators, But the crucial question is what these indicators are supposed to indicate. This task is made even more complex by the lack of agreement about exact definitions of suffering and welfare in animal production.

Instead of spending time in sterile discussions about the meaning of such concepts, we are advocating a more pragmatic approach to these issues. There is sufficient evidence to accept the fact that at least some elements of awareness and consciousness exist in farm animals. It is difficult, however, to argue more precisely on the kinds of mental experience which are occurring in different animals housed in different ways (e.g. is the well-fed and sheltered battery-cage bird suffering more than the pigeon scratching for a living in the city?). The major problem we are faced with is not the recognition of negative emotions or suffering but an agreement on the maximal amount of constraint which can be put on an organism without unacceptable loss of its physical and mental integrity. The basis for such a decision is a full understanding of the behaviour of farm animals. For a long time we have known more about the behaviour of exotic species than that of the animal species which are used as livestock for our own well-being. This situation has fortunately changed during recent years, but much more remains to be done.

5 LEGISLATION FOR HEALTH

W H G REES Esq., CB, BSc, MRCVS, DVSM and
G DAVIES Esq., BVSc, Dip Bact., MRCVS

The background

Agriculture is an industry like any other and it might be thought that the health and welfare of farm lifestock were matters for the stockowner alone. However, governments have long recognized that they have a part to play in controlling disease and more recently they have also come to take some responsibility for the welfare of farm animals in the national herds and flocks.

The responsibility for disease stemmed from the need, in the 19th century, to safeguard the supply of food to the burgeoning populations of the industrial revolution. The authorities of the time also came to realize, as the processes of disease transmission were unravelled by scientific research, that the task of controlling potentially devastating disease was not within the command of the individual stockowner; there has to be some form of public control. This requirement for controls, particularly controls on the movement of livestock, underlies much of the legislation in the animal health field.

Why do governments intervene?

For the purposes of enacting legislation, or more particularly for determining whether governments should intervene, livestock diseases can be divided into three groups:

(a) Diseases which the stockowner can control alone—mastitis, parasitic gastroenteritis (PGE) and liver fluke are examples of disease that the farmer can control by his own individual efforts. Success will depend on his ability to use modern techniques including preventative measures (vaccination, controlled grazing) or treatments (antibiotics, parasiticides).

(b) Diseases which the stockowner cannot control by his own unaided efforts—obvious examples are foot-and-mouth disease (FMD), which in temperate climates is spread from herd to herd by the wind, and swine fever or contagious bovine pleuropneumonia (CBPP), which are usually spread by the movement of animals that are part of the livestock trade.

(c) Zoonotic infections and other conditions where control gives little direct benefit to the stockowner; the benefit accrues to public health. This group of diseases includes salmonellosis in poultry and Q fever, which cause little economic loss to the industry but can give rise to diseases in human beings either through contact with livestock or through consuming animal products. In recent years this category has expanded to include residues in meat or milk and animal welfare has also come to be regarded as a communal responsibility even though it is, or should be, the concern of each and every stockowner.

Governments have good reason to intervene in controlling those diseases that the stockowner cannot control on his own (group b) and zoonoses and other conditions that present a risk to public health (group c) but the distinctions are not entirely clear cut. A farmer can control liver fluke infestation in his sheep flock or mange in his cattle but his efforts will come to nothing if he buys infested stock. The trade in livestock plays a crucial part in disseminating disease—a fact recognized in most animal health legislation. Similarly the distinction between potentially devastating diseases thought to be prime candidates for control and other infectious conditions not dealt with by legislation is often arbitrary. Foot-and-mouth disease can cause great economic loss in developed livestock systems but only marginal losses in extensive peasant agriculture. Despite this, public expenditure on the control of this disease is considerable in both developed and developing countries. Aujeszky's disease on the other hand is also spread by wind and by the movement of livestock but only recently has it become the subject of legislation.

The basis for a control programme

Having established this basis for governmental intervention several criteria are used to judge whether a disease is a suitable subject for control through legislation:

1. The disease must be 'important', in other words it either causes significant economic losses or it is a threat to public health.
2. The epidemiology of the disease must be thoroughly understood. Knowledge of the incubation period of the disease and its host range is essential. If there are gaps in this knowledge then the infection will find ways around the controls placed in its path. The tuberculosis control scheme was not entirely successful in South-West England because it had not been recognized that the badger (*Meles meles*) was acting as a reservoir host.
3. The disease must be clearly identifiable either clinically and/or by tests which distinguish between infected and clean animals. A control scheme for atrophic rhinitis failed partly because it was impossible to distinguish between 'normal' and 'affected' snouts.

If these criteria are met the authorities still have to make a judgement as to whether the political or social conditions are favourable to control. If a country is in the throes of civil war no amount of legislation will prevent animals being illegally traded. Rinderpest spread across sub-Saharan Africa just as the pan-African eradication programme was coming to an end simply because unrest had led to failure to control traffic across state borders. Extensive trade in livestock may make control difficult even in settled conditions—sheep scab has proved difficulty to eradicate in Great Britain because of the constant movement of sheep. Finally, if the agricultural community is poor or ill-educated it may not be in a position to support the government authorities in their efforts to eradicate disease—a farmer with only three cows is unlikely to inform the authorities if one of his cows becomes infected with foot-and-mouth disease for fear that he will lose his livelihood.

Different approaches to disease control

Once it is decided that a disease must be controlled or eradicated the next step is to devise a control programme. The structure of the programme is largely determined by the epidemiology of the disease. Three factors play an important part:

(a) The incubation period (i.e. the interval between the host animal contacting the infection and either showing clinical signs of disease or developing a measurable antibody response). This is closely linked to the interval between infection and maximum infectivity (generation time):
(b) The host range.
(c) The mode of transmission.

Incubation period

If the incubation period is lengthy, as in tuberculosis, then testing may have to be repeated several times to identify all the infected animals. If the generation time is short, as in FMD, then tests (and the elimination of reactor animals) have to be carried out quickly before the infection gets out of hand.

Host range

If the infection is host specific, as *Salmonella pullorum* is confined to poultry, for instance, then control measures and tests can be limited to the one host; breaking the chain of infection is relatively easy. If the infection has a wide host range, e.g. *Salmonella typhimurium*, then testing the livestock that are at risk and getting rid of the reactors does not prevent infection regaining entry to the herd via secondary hosts, such as rats.

Mode of transmission

If the infectious agent is airborne then a strong wind and optimum humidity may allow infection to spread over many miles as in foot-and-mouth disease and Aujeszky's disease. Control requires visiting all herds lying within the 'infective plume' (Smith 1983). If the infection is strictly contagious, i.e. it can only be transmitted by direct contact between infected and susceptible animals, as the CBPP, then control involves only the physical separation (quarantine) of infected stock. If the agent is capable of surviving for extensive periods outside the host, e.g. swine fever, then control measures must include the destruction of fomites such as bedding, keeping premises empty for a period and occasionally further visits to the repopulated farm.

All these various epidemiological factors play a part in determining the control measures that have to be put into operation. They are illustrated in Table 5.1.

Control or eradication?

Before a government embarks on a disease control scheme it must decide on the ultimate objective. Is it to eradicate the infection from the national herds and flocks? Or is it simply to control the disease in such a way that the economic loss is kept within acceptable limits?

Eradication schemes

An eradication programme is a far more attractive proposition than a control scheme because the costs are limited to the few years of the programme whilst the benefits, i.e. absence of disease, should go on *ad infinitum*. However, if the decision is taken to eradicate a disease a government must be certain that

- it has the resources, i.e. manpower and materials, to complete the task
- it has the support of the agricultural community so that illegal trade in infected animals can be firmly suppressed
- it is able to police the state borders during and after the programme so ensuring that infection is not reintroduced
- it has the scientific tools, i.e. effective vaccines and accurate tests that clearly distinguish between infected and clean stock

If an eradication programme falters for any reason the authorities may find themselves in a situation where they are controlling the disease, i.e. they have reduced its prevalence, but have little chance of eradicating it. The costs and benefits of this situation are then entirely different from those of a successful eradication programme.

Consider the situation where a government embarks on an FMD eradication programme. The disease is endemic but the direct loss due to mortality and morbidity is accepted by most of the agricultural community as a risk of the trade. However, the meat industry and some of the more advanced

Table 5.1 Epidemiological factors influencing disease control

	Incubation period		Host range			Transmission			
	Long	Short	Single	Limited	Wide	Contagious	Fomites	Vectors	Airborne
Foot-and-mouth disease (FMD)		•		•★		•	•		•
Classical swine fever (CSF)		•	•★			•	•		
(African swine fever (ASF))		•	•			•	•		
Swine vesicular disease (SVD)		•	•★			•			
Rinderpest/peste des petits ruminants (PPR)		•	•★			•			
Vesicular stomatitis		•		•★		•		•	
Lumpy skin disease	•					?		?	
Rift valley fever		•		•+★				•	
Bluetongue		•		•★		•		•	
Sheep/goat pox		•	•			•			
African horse sickness	•			•★		•		•	
Teschen			•			•	•		
Tuberculosis	•				•★	•	•		
Brucellosis	•		•★			•	•		
Contagious bovine pleuropneumonia (CBPP)	•		•			•			

★ The hosts include wildlife
† The hosts include man

stockowners realize that the presence of FMD denies them access to lucrative overseas markets.

The government decides on a ten-year eradication plan that relies on vaccination. Supplies of vaccine are limited, particularly in the early stages of the scheme, and the authorities divide the country into three zones, vaccinating each in turn. The sequence of events and the costs and benefits attached to each step of the programme are as follows.

1. *Pre-eradication* (low costs, nil benefits). The disease is endemic but the costs are borne by the industry. There are no vaccination costs. The country is denied the benefit of an export trade.
2. *Eradication Stage 1* (high costs, low benefits). Vaccination starts in zone 1. Disease continues in zones 2 and 3. The government is starting to incur substantial costs but the benefits—the reduction of the disease in zone 1—is limited.
3. *Eradication stage 2* (high costs, medium benefits). All cattle in zones 1 and 2 are vaccinated. Disease continues in zone 3. The costs of the vaccination programme are substantial but the benefits are still relatively small—the elimination of disease in zone 1 and the reduction of disease in zone 2.
4. *Eradication stage 3* (high costs, medium benefits). Vaccination ceases in zone 1 and any residual outbreaks there are dealt with by slaughter and compensation. Vaccination continues in zones 2 and 3 and there may be some extra costs due to slaughter and compensation. Although the benefits are increasing—elimination of disease in zone 1 and reduction of disease in the remainder of the country—they are still substantially less than the costs incurred.
5. *Eradication completed* (no costs, substantial benefits). Vaccination ceases and any remaining outbreaks are dealt with by slaughter and compensation. The country is recognized as being FMD free and is able to supply meat to a wide range of export markets previously closed to it.

The above sequence of events shows that a government embarking on an eradication programme faces a period (stages 2, 3 and 4) during which the costs of the programme far outweigh the benefits before it gets to the stage where the costs cease and the benefits continue indefinitely. If the eradication plan falters, perhaps because vaccination fails to combat the infection or because there is movement of infected animals into cleared zones, the authorities face the prospect of continuing massive costs unrelieved by the potential benefits. This has been the fate of a number of disease eradication programmes.

For these reasons eradication programmes should only commence when success is reasonably certain. The situation is made easier if the country is an island or otherwise geographically isolated from other livestock populations so that reinfection can be prevented. A stable social and economic structure is essential.

It is usual to assess the costs and benefits of an eradication programme on the basis that the costs are borne over the period of the scheme and the benefits accrue over a further period of 30 years. This 30-year limit on benefits is partly because it is almost impossible to forecast the benefit to the nation beyond that point as trade patterns and livestock values may change. It is also imposed because in the longer term scientific developments may provide alternative means of controlling or eradicating the disease.

Control schemes

A control scheme that does not have as its objective the eradication of the disease must be assessed on the basis that the costs and the benefits continue indefinitely and that the benefits should be substantially greater than the costs. Both benefits and costs are assessed over a 30-year period.

It is becoming increasingly difficult to justify control schemes, as distinct from eradication programmes, but they do have their place in two situations:

(a) where the livestock industry is willing to bear some of the financial burden, and
(b) where there is a risk to public health.

If the livestock industry presses for a control scheme and is willing to bear some of the costs involved it will itself help to ensure that controls are maintained, for instance by dipping animals regularly to control East Coast fever. Where there is a risk to public health, such as with salmonella infections in food animals, eradication may be technically impossible but a control programme can still provide considerable benefits in terms of human health.

Disease control and eradication campaigns in Great Britain

Bovine tuberculosis

Tuberculosis had been a major problem in human beings and animals in Great Britain for many centuries but due to lack of knowledge about the causal organism, the epidemiology of the disease and connection between human and animal cases, little was done to tackle the problem until early in the 20th century.

A Royal Commission report in 1907 for the first time drew attention to the connection between tuberculosis in children and the consumption of cows' milk contaminated with tubercle bacilli. The initial attempts to control the disease in animals were therefore aimed at combating the public health dangers, and a series of Orders, made between 1913 and 1946, were designed to remove clinically affected cattle. These Orders were intended purely as public health measures and they had no effect on the prevalence of the disease in cattle, illustrating that to control and eradicate the disease in the animal population it is necessary to identify and remove infected animals before they become infective and actively spread disease. In 1929 15 532 cattle were slaughtered under the provisions of the Tuberculosis Order and by 1936 the numbers had risen to 23 716. Clearly no progress was being made in protecting human health.

A report by the Gowland Hopkins Committee in 1934 concluded that 40% of cows in dairy herds in Great Britain were infected with tuberculosis and that at least 0.5% of cows excreted tubercle organisms in the milk. The Committee also concluded that the total eradication of bovine tuberculosis was the only complete answer.

Voluntary Attested Herds Schemes

The first Attested Herds Schemes were introduced in 1935. Under the schemes, herds which were free from tuberculosis, as judged by their having passed three consecutive tuberculin tests at minimum intervals of 60 days, or herds which had been created entirely with attested cattle, were registered as attested herds. The owner of the herd was required to give an undertaking to observe a number of rules designed to prevent, as far as possible, the reintroduction of infection into the herd. A milk bonus was paid to dairy herds—later extended to a headage payment for beef herds. The herds were tested at intervals to ensure continuing freedom from disease.

For a time progress was slow and various changes were made in the schemes to encourage farmers to clear their herds of infection. Although World War II hampered progress, by the end of 1947 1 200 000 cattle, about 14% of the total population, were in attested herds. During the same year the number of cattle slaughtered under the Tuberculosis Order fell to 6545—a clear indication of a reduction in the weight of infection in the national herd.

Compulsory Eradication and the Area Eradication Plan

By the end of September 1950, 2 042 000 cattle, comprising 22% of the cattle population, were attested and it was considered feasible to commence compulsory eradication in the areas which had made the most rapid progress.

In October 1950 an area eradication plan was introduced. The concept of the plan was to select areas in which the percentage of attested cattle was already high and which were reasonably self-sufficient in terms of stock replacements and marketing facilities. Herds in the area not already registered as attested were placed under movement restrictions and tested; reactors were slaughtered, with payment of compensation. When all such herds had been tested twice and the reactors disposed of, the area was declared an attested area.

During this phase of the campaign all movements of cattle within and into the areas were controlled by a system of official movement permits.

Periodically new areas were selected for compulsory eradication; normally these were adjacent to existing attested areas. Eventually the whole country was covered and declared attested in October 1960. During that year 28 cattle were slaughtered under the Tuberculosis Order.

Maintenance of disease freedom

Because of the chronic nature of the disease and its epidemiology—characterized by a long incubation period, resistant causal organism, subclinical infection, non-specific infection and a reservoir of infection in other animal species—it proved difficult to completely eliminate the disease from the cattle population. It was therefore necessary to continue routine testing of all herds to confirm their freedom. The interval between routine tests was periodically extended from one to three years in line with the reduction in the incidence of reactors to the tuberculin test. This was not, however, possible in areas of the country where a reservoir of infection in badgers was a source of reinfection of cattle herds, and more frequent routine testing was necessary to prevent the disease becoming re-established in the cattle population.

Undoubtedly the campaign had been highly successful and much had been learned which would be extremely useful in the planning and execution of future disease eradication campaigns.

Bovine brucellosis

During the 19th century abortion in cattle caused by *Brucella abortus* was common in most countries that had an expanding dairy industry. However, it was not until the 1940s that any positive action was taken in Great Britain to control the disease on a national scale.

Vaccination Schemes

In December 1944 the first Calfhood Vaccination Scheme was introduced in an effort to reduce the weight of infection in herds and assist in the control of the disease. The attenuated *Brucella abortus* strain 19 (S19) vaccine was authorized for use in calves with a general recommendation that animals vaccinated as calves should be revaccinated every three years when non-pregnant. In subsequent schemes the age limits were amended to take account of experimental findings which indicated that revaccination did not enhance immunity and the problems of persisting vaccinal titres in adult cattle. The final version of the Free Calfhood Vaccination Scheme, introduced in 1964, therefore restricted vaccination to calves between 121 and 240 days of age.

In 1966 925 000 doses of vaccine were used, representing 30–40% of eligible calves. The outcome was that, in herds which subsequently became infected, they did not experience the worst economic effects of a brucella abortion storm.

The vaccination schemes continued until they were systematically phased out during the course of the compulsory eradication campaign. Undoubtedly the widespread and regulated use of the vaccine had made a significant contribution to the control of the disease and paved the way for the eradication schemes which were to follow.

Surveys

Over the years a number of surveys were carried out to estimate the prevalence of brucella infection in the cattle population in the country. The most extensive and comprehensive survey was that carried out in 1960/61, *The Animal Disease Survey—Brucellosis in the British Dairy Herd* (Leech et al. 1964). The main conclusions were:

1. About 30 000 herds in Great Britain were infected, with 66 000 cows infected.
2. 7.0% of all abortions or premature calvings were due to *Brucella abortus* (0.4% of all calvings).
3. S19 vaccine reduced the frequency of infection by 50%.
4. There was no evidence that adult vaccination with S19 vaccine was beneficial.
5. Economic losses in diary cattle due to brucellosis were estimated at £1 million per annum.

A further serological survey showed that approximately 17% of cows and heifers in the country gave positive reactions to the serum agglutination test (SAT). This could be reduced to 14% by additionally using the complement fixation test (CFT).

A great deal of information was thus available on the disease situation in the country, an essential prerequisite to any eradication campaign, and this enabled plans to be formulated.

The cost of eradication and the ensuing benefits to the livestock industry made it difficult to justify a national eradication campaign purely on animal health grounds. However, the public health risk and the effect of the disease in humans was a crucial factor in the Government's decision to embark on an eradication campaign, which commenced in April 1967 with the introduction of the first Brucellosis (Accredited Herds) Scheme.

The Eradication Plan

Bovine brucellosis is a highly infectious disease with transmission of infection occurring principally at the time of abortion or, to a lesser extent, at infected normal calvings. The available laboratory diagnostic tests had to take account of residual vaccinal titres arising from the widespread use of S19 vaccine so as to avoid an unacceptable level of false positive results. The programme of testing and investigations was designed with these problems in mind. Procedures were amended as necessary during the course of the campaign in the light of continuing research and development work and epidemiological information arising out of the field operations. A full account of the eradication campaign is given in an official publication, *Brucellosis—A History of the Disease and its Eradication from Cattle in Great Britain* (MAFF 1983).

The strategy used in the eradication campaign followed the same pattern as for the eradication of bovine tuberculosis: firstly the identification through voluntary schemes of herds free of infection to serve as a 'pool' of replacement animals during the compulsory test and slaughter phase, and secondly the systematic, area by area, eradication of the disease from the country with rigid movement controls to prevent the reinfection of 'clean' herds.

Voluntary schemes

(a) The Brucellosis (Accredited Herds) Scheme:

Applications were invited from owners who wished to have their herds entered on the voluntary register of accredited herds. To qualify for acceptance the standard of management and husbandry adopted on the farm had to be such as to ensure that the herd would retain its brucella-free status after the requisite tests were passed.

In dairy herds the testing requirement was for three consecutive clear milk ring tests (MRT) (group or churn) carried out at not less than three-monthly intervals, at which stage the herd was designated as 'supervised', followed in 60 days by a serum agglutination test (SAT) on all eligible female cattle and bulls. For beef herds the MRT tests were replaced by two SATs at 60-day intervals followed by an official SAT 60 days later.

Compensation for reactors was paid once the herd became supervised and was at 100% of market value subject initially to a maximum payment of £100.

Good progress was made with the scheme and by the end of the third year 8000 herds comprising nearly 80 000 cattle were entered in the register.

(b) Brucellosis Incentives Scheme:

Introduced in July 1970, this new scheme was designed to encourage owners of herds that contained some reactors, but where there was no active infection, to undertake a programme of testing to enable their herds to be registered as attested. The scheme involved the payment of bonuses, in the case of dairy herds on the amount of milk produced, and for beef herds the number of eligible cows. Bonuses continued for 5 years after registration.

Testing procedures were changed by the replacement of the MRT with a serological screening test, the rose-bengal plate test (RBPT), which had been developed and automated by the Central Veterinary Laboratory, Weybridge. Positive samples were retested using the SAT and, if necessary, a complement fixation test (CFT). This enabled large numbers of animals to be tested rapidly and at a comparatively low cost.

Rapid progress was made and by 30 June 1971 16 134 herds were registered as accredited in the voluntary schemes with a further 22 670 undergoing testing. Total animals in scheme herds were 2 694 000, which represented about 30% of the cattle population (excluding steers).

In some counties progress had been more rapid, particularly in those with predominantly breeding herds, where up to 70%, were accredited. This then set the stage for the introduction of the compulsory phase of the eradication campaign.

Compulsory Eradication

In selecting the fist eradication areas the criteria used were:

- a low level of infection had been demonstrated
- a good response to the voluntary schemes
- general movement of breeding stock out of the area. This would assist in restocking other areas in the later stages of the campaign

• geographically suitable for extension to other eradication areas.

The first eradication areas were created on 1 November 1971. Normally a 1–2-year period was allowed between the announcement of the area and the commencement of compulsory testing and slaughter, to give owners the opportunity of joining the voluntary scheme and qualify for incentives. During this period free testing was offered. Many farmers took advantage of this concession, which in turn made a considerable reduction in the number of herds requiring compulsory testing. This is an important point in any eradication campaign where the active support of 90–95% of farmers is necessary if good progress is to be maintained.

Additional eradication areas were introduced periodically, care being taken to ensure that the available resources in terms of laboratory diagnostic facilities and field veterinary and support staff were adequate to cope with the increased workload. By late 1980 the entire country was involved in the phased eradication programme, as illustrated in Figures 5.1 and 5.2.

Attested areas

As areas reached a level of 90–95% of accredited herds consideration was given to declaring them 'Attested'. Account was taken of the number of breakdowns that were occurring which gave an indication of the level of infection remaining in the area and also the continuing threat to disease-free herds. The first areas were declared attested in August 1975 and on 1 November 1981 the whole of Great Britain was declared Attested.

In attested areas vaccination against brucellosis was prohibited, markets and shows were confined to accredited cattle, reactors could only be slaughtered at designated slaughterhouses and inter-herd movements within the area did not require movement permits.

Following eradication routine testing of all herds with eligible animals continued in order to confirm their brucellosis-free status. All abortions and premature calvings had to be notified to the Ministry and an official investigation was carried out, dairy herds were routinely monitored by MRTs and beef herds by serological testing. If any evidence of infection was diagnosed the herd was placed under movement restrictions and a programme of testing carried out to re-establish its disease freedom. The frequency of routine testing was extended as the incidence of infection was reduced in accordance with the requirements of Directive 64/432 EEC as amended by Directive 80/219 EEC.

Thus eradication, from the commencement in 1967 to the declaration of the last attested areas of 1982, had taken 14 years at an estimated cost of £203 701 575. In parallel with the gradual reduction in the incidence of infection in the cattle population there had been a similar reduction in the number of cases of brucellosis in the human population.

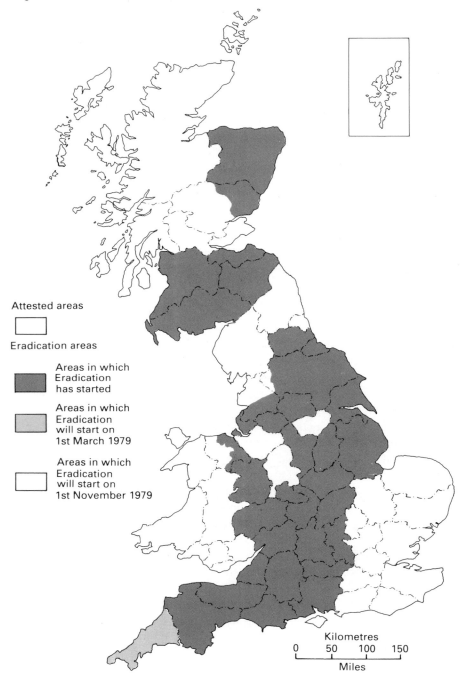

Figure 5.1 Brucellosis in Great Britain—attested and eradication areas as at 1 November 1978.

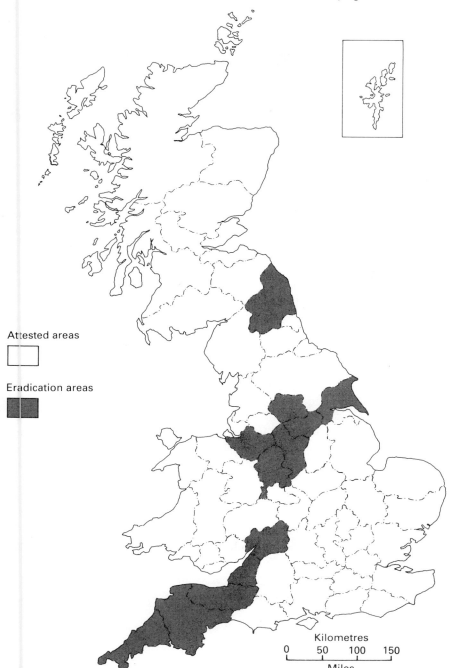

Figure 5.2 Brucellosis in Great Britain—attested and eradication areas as at 1 December 1980.

The establishment of herds or flocks free of specific diseases

The criteria that have to be considered when deciding to embark on a national eradication campaign have already been discussed. An important prerequisite for such a campaign is the identification of animals or herds which are free of the infection that is to be eradicated and which can serve as a 'pool' of healthy stock to replace infected stock slaughtered during the campaign. This can be achieved by the official registration of herds or flocks as accredited or attested.

For diseases which, although they are recognized as being of economic importance to the livestock industry, are not for the time being considered suitable for eradication, the introduction of Health Schemes may be appropriate. In this case the economic benefit may include the enhanced value of the stock in the market and/or the greater potential for exports.

Accredited/Attested Herds

The tests and testing procedures to be employed in establishing disease-free herds must take account of the epidemiology of the disease in question before they are entered on the official register of accredited or attested herds. The criteria for registration must also be based on the general principle that the system of livestock husbandry is such that the herd can be maintained as disease free after the requisite tests are passed.

Herd owners should be required to sign an undertaking to observe rules to maintain their herds free from infection derived from outside sources. These rules would include isolation from neighbouring herds at grazing and strict isolation of purchased animals until they are proven to be of equivalent health status.

To encourage livestock owners to apply for registration, incentives in the form of a bonus on the price of milk or headage payment in beef herds are often introduced as an inducement. This policy of establishing disease-free herds in advance of compulsory eradication has been used successfully in the United Kingdom. The aim should be to achieve disease freedom in 80–90% of herds by voluntary means in an area or country before the introduction of compulsory test and slaughter procedures.

Health schemes

The main purpose of health schemes is to establish a pool of herds or flocks of a recognized health status that will attract the interest of both home and overseas purchasers in addition to improving their own productivity.

Health schemes may be operated through national veterinary services where the range of expertise—field advice, laboratory diagnosis and research and development—can be channelled through a single source or through private veterinary surgeons who may have greater flexibility to cater for the individual needs of livestock owners or sectors of the industry.

Schemes may be concerned with the control of individual specific diseases or have more general aims such as the improvement of health and productivity. In practice the former have proved to be more successful and attractive to the livestock industry.

The objectives of health schemes

The objectives of health schemes can be summarized as follows:

1. To demonstrate freedom from one or more specific diseases in a herd or flock or a group of herds or flocks.
2. To reduce the national level of a specific disease as a preliminary to the possible introduction of a compulsory control and/or assuring a high level of disease control.
3. To enhance the saleability and export potential of stock by assuring a high level of disease control.
4. To raise the general standard of health and productivity in a herd or flock through general advice on the application of sound preventive medicine programmes which may include the control or elimination of one of more specific diseases.
5. To improve the expertise of those involved in raising the standards of animal health and productivity.

Factors to be considered when formulating health schemes

To ensure successful health schemes it is important that:

- a clear economic advantage can be demonstrated from participation in the scheme
- sound husbandry and management systems are practised in the participating herds and flocks
- animals are permanently marked for identification purposes
- a reliable system of record-keeping is used
- accurate diagnostic tests are available for the disease included in the scheme
- staff employed in operating the scheme are specially trained for the

purpose and are knowledgeable concerning the animal species and diseases involved

- effective communication is maintained between headquarters, field staff and participating livestock owners

An official Advisory Group should be established with representatives from farming organizations, breed societies, veterinary associations and the official veterinary services to continually monitor the operation and effectiveness of the scheme in the light of the needs of the industry and developments in disease control.

Official health schemes operating in Great Britain

Four voluntary animal health schemes covering pigs, poultry, cattle, sheep and goats were introduced in April 1987. All were based on previous health schemes but had been modified to meet the requirements of the agricultural industry and to offer members the opportunity to monitor and control a wide range of diseases. The schemes were chargeable and fees were set to recover the costs of the services provided.

An official register of scheme members is maintained centrally and available to intending purchasers of stock to check on the health status of the herds or flocks of origin if necessary.

Pig Health Scheme

The original Pig Health Scheme, which commenced in 1968, was linked to the Meat and Livestock Commission's Pig Improvement Scheme, which was set up to improve the genetic quality of British pigs and involved the performance testing of breeding animals at official stations. To protect the health status of the stations and allow the pigs under test to perform to their full genetic potential membership of the Pig Health Scheme was made obligatory.

The Scheme introduced in 1987 was based on the same principles, its aim being to maintain and improve the health and productivity of member herds. Membership is available on a two-tier basis, allowing members to opt for a higher level of monitoring to demonstrate a higher health status. In the higher category lung and snout monitoring is carried out at slaughterhouses to detect cases of atrophic rhinitis or enzootic pneumonia. All herds are subject to quarterly visits and reports by veterinary service officer and/or the owner's veterinary surgeon.

Sheep and Goat Health Scheme

The Sheep and Goat Health Scheme succeeded a Maedi-Visna Accredited

Flock Scheme. A programme of testing of the flock or herd allows it to qualify for maedi-visna (or caprine arthritis encephalitis (CAE) in the case of goats) accredited status.

In addition, members can opt for their flocks or herds to be monitored for three other economically damaging diseases, namely enzootic abortion of ewes (EAE), jaagsiekte or sheep pulmonary adenomatosis (SPA), and scrapie.

Cattle Health Scheme

The Cattle Health Scheme succeeded an Enzootic Bovine Leukosis (EBL) Attested Herds Scheme. Herds are subjected to a set programme of blood testing before being entered on a register of EBL Attested Herds. Herds can also be monitored for infectious bovine rhinotracheitis (IBR) and, if negative, classified as 'monitored—negative'.

In 1988 a further option was added to the scheme, the *Leptospira hardjo* Control Programme. In this programme herds may achieve a controlled, officially vaccinated or an elite status depending on the 'risk factors' assessed for the particular herd.

Poultry Health Scheme

The existing Poultry Health Scheme was revised in 1987. It continued to promote high standards of health and welfare in scheme flocks and ensured their freedom from *Salmonella pullorum* and *Salmonella gallinarum* infections. The scheme provides a wide range of services and benefits for members, including a diagnostic/postmortem service at special rates, testing for pullorum disease and monitoring for a range of other diseases.

Following the problems arising from the contamination of eggs with *Salmonella enteritidus* a code of practice was drawn up to control the infection at breeder and hatchery level. This provided for a standard approach to hygiene measures and uniform methods of monitoring their effectiveness.

Disease surveillance

Disease control depends on maintaining surveillance of the national herds and flocks so that new diseases are identified promptly and changes in existing disease patterns can be taken into account in control strategies.

Monitoring is the process of collecting routine data. *Surveillance* implies the collection and interpretation of data (collected during monitoring pro-

137

grammes) with a view to the detection of changes in the health status of the population.

Government departments and other public agencies are by far the most important 'customers' for surveillance returns but the co-operation of agricultural organizations, public health authorities and the veterinary profession at large is essential if the returns are to be comprehensive and reliable.

Data requirements

Veterinarians with the responsibility for advising the government require a balanced overall view of the current disease situation in the country supplemented by an appraisal of developing disease 'problems'. This 'overall view' depends not only on the output of reliable data collection systems but also on the informed opinions and experience of veterinarians working in the field.

Disease information contributing to the 'overall view' is often dismissed as being unrepresentative, i.e. it is not statistically valid, and incomplete, i.e. it does not give an account of all disease losses on farms. Nevertheless it is frequently the only kind of information that can be collected without enormous effort and expense and it plays a valuable part in decision-making at the national level.

Consideration of the surveillance evidence provided by the 'overall view' may lead to detailed analyses of specific diseases, particularly when disease policy is being reviewed. For this purpose data on specific diseases must be collected quickly, possibly through a survey and preferably using a statistically valid sample so that the results can be developed into a full appraisal including an economic analysis. Government veterinary services are particularly interested in:

(a) 'New diseases' e.g. bovine spongiform encephalopathy (BSE). Surveillance should include an 'early warning' system.
(b) The absence of disease. Countries engaged in international trade in animals and animal products have to provide their trading partners with firm evidence that certain diseases are absent from the national herds and flocks.
(c) 'Notifiable' diseases, i.e. OIE list A (see Table 5.2). These are diseases that pose an immediate and serious threat to the nation's livestock. Surveillance must include some means of immediately reporting the presence of these infections.
(d) Zoonoses. Infections that are a threat to human health, e.g. *Brucella abortus*, *Mycobacterium tuberculosis* and *Salmonella* sp., these do not always cause severe and clearly identifiable disease in livestock and may therefore be difficult to identify in surveillance programmes without laboratory tests. Surveillance is essential to protect human health.

Table 5.2 OIE List A diseases (as at 31.12.90)

Foot-and-mouth disease
Vesicular stomatitis
Rinderpest
Peste des petits ruminants
Contagious bovine pleuropneumonia
Lumpy skin disease
Rift valley fever
Bluetongue
Sheep pox and goat pox
African horse sickness
African swine fever
Hog cholera (classical swine fever)
Teschen disease
Fowl plague
Newcastle disease

Sources of information—'information costs money'

All surveillance procedures involve a cost. The cost is least where the information is already being collected for reasons unconnected with surveillance, e.g. data on laboratory examinations and tests. It is greatest where information gathering systems are being set up *de novo* with no other aim but the provision of surveillance information, i.e. collecting 'new' information.

Recording disease, as opposed to recording infections that are identifiable by serological tests, is not as easy as it may seem and numerous attempts to set up continuous surveillance systems, monitoring a sample of the national herd, have foundered. There are two main reasons for these failures.

(a) It is difficult to record clinical syndromes in such a way that they are meaningful. One nervous disease looks very much like another in the absence of pathological or serological examination.
(b) It is almost impossible to maintain enthusiasm for collecting information on a continuous basis. Busy veterinary practitioners will take part in a short-term survey but they are loath to commit themselves to the labour of record keeping if they see no direct benefit to themselves. The cost of obtaining 'new' information and the difficulty of maintaining enthusiasm for continuous surveillance are the two main factors affecting the success of surveillance projects.

Several established sources can be tapped for disease information. The main ones are considered below.

Abattoirs

Meat inspection identifies a limited range of conditions, mainly parasitic, such as liver fluke but also including some bacterial conditions such as tuberculosis and contagious bovine pleuropneumonia. Abattoirs are also a convenient point for blood sampling, e.g. for Aujeszky's disease, or for tissue sampling, e.g. for trichinosis. Tracing back infection from the abattoir to the farm of origin is difficult and expensive and is only of value in important diseases such as tuberculosis and classical swine fever.

Veterinary practices

All practices keep a day book that records visits to farms and the treatment given. Some day books provide a record of the disease encountered but this is unlikely to be anything more than a simple record of common conditions, such as hypocalcaemia, injuries, digestive complaints, etc. The exceptions to this are the detailed cattle or pig herd recording systems developed by some specialized veterinary practices.

Government veterinary services: field reports

In some countries the only veterinarians that regularly visit livestock holdings are those employed by the government; if they are trained to keep careful records of the diseases they encounter, their reports may provide a valuable source of surveillance information.

Diagnostic laboratory reports

Most developed countries are served by a network of diagnostic laboratories. Although the pathological specimens examined at the laboratories generally come from the larger farms and from those close to the laboratory, they nevertheless provide a useful source of information. They are particularly useful for identifying 'new' diseases.

Surveys

Although the sources of information described above will, between them, provide the 'overall view' that is the first requirement of a successful surveillance system they will not provide precise data indicating the prevalence and cost of particular diseases. This information can only be obtained by carrying out properly planned surveys that cover a randomly selected sample of the animal population. Surveys are beyond the scope of these pages but the reader is recommended to obtain a copy of the booklet *Livestock Disease Surveys: A Field Manual for Veterinarians* by R M Cannon and R T Roe and published by the Australian Bureau of Animal Health (Australia Government Publishing Service, Canberra, 1982).

Official animal health services

Objectives and functions

The objectives of an animal health service may be summarized as:

1. To facilitate the development of high standards of animal health and production.
2. The protection of human health.
3. The protection and welfare of animals.

The achievement of these objectives involves the effective and coordinated performance of many diverse activities which together make up the 'functions' of the service. A list of the activities of a typical service will include:

1. The development of animal health and production:
   - surveillance
   - disease investigation
   - disease prevention, control and eradication
   - quarantine
   - emergency response
   - clinical services
   - control of animal drugs and biological products
   - veterinary inspection
   - research and development
   - training
   - wildlife disease monitoring

- veterinary aspects of aquaculture
2. The protection of human health
   - control of zoonoses
   - food hygiene
   - meat inspection
   - residue testing
   - training
3. The protection and welfare of animals
   - ensuring humane treatment of animals in general
   - supervising welfare standards in markets, during transport and during slaughter
   - control of laboratory animals
   - liaison with other government departments and outside organizations

Enforcement of legislation, extension services and transfer of technology are common to all the activities and many overlap; the service must therefore be well coordinated and integrated to achieve its goals effectively.

Organization

Well-organized official animal health services are an essential prerequisite for the successful execution of animal health strategies, programmes and disease control measures. The organization should be flexible so that it can adapt to changes in animal disease situations and conditions.

Official animal health services may depend on the activities of government services, farming enterprises or private veterinarians and in many countries a combination of two or three of these agents is used. Whatever arrangement is selected it is for the provision of effective disease control measures and public health safeguards.

Experience in many countries has demonstrated that a centralized organization with a vertical command structure is the most effective way of managing national disease prevention, control and eradication programmes. The centralized organization allows for greater uniformity of action, better coordination of diagnostic procedures and control measures, and rapid mobilization of resources in emergency situations.

A decentralized organization with a horizontal operational structure offers better conditions for the identification and solution of local problems, for promoting improved productivity and for the treatment of individual or groups of animals, partly because of the enhanced opportunity for closer co-operation with livestock owners, ancillary industries and consumers.

In practice the strengths of both systems are normally combined into a mixed animal health organization which can deliver effective services at both national and local level.

Structure

The structure of animal health services usually corresponds to the general administrative, political/financial structure in the country concerned. It will, therefore, vary from country to country.

Consolidation of national veterinary resources into a single unit is desirable to prevent wasteful duplication and to enhance technical and economic efficiency. As with any organizational structure, it is essential that there is effective programming and executive liaison between government units and with non-government organizations.

In most countries the central animal health service administration under the direction of a Chief Veterinary Officer is responsible for all professional and technical activities carried out by government officers. In some countries it is also responsible for technical supervision of private and co-operative enterprises contributing to animal disease control, human health protection and animal production.

It is important that the official animal health service has, through the Chief Veterinary Officer, direct access to the administrative head of the government department or ministry and also direct access to the relevant minister when it is necessary to deal with events and emergencies which are of national importance.

At the local level, Provincial or Regional Veterinary Officers are responsible for supervising diagnostic laboratories, animal health offices and clinics and other institutions of regional importance. Similar structures could also be at a lower organizational level if such institutions exist, e.g. district or divisional level.

The most important tier of the animal health service structure is the cadre of field officers which is in direct contact with livestock producers, animals and their products. Effective action at village, farm, herd/flock and individual animal level is decisive in the success of any animal health programme.

Communications

Decentralization of administration, while it has operational advantages at local level, makes national policy application more complex and difficult. It is therefore of great importance to ensure that a communication structure and operation is in place which allows for two-way direct transmission of reporting, policy development and decision-making.

Communications must be effective both within the organization and between it and outside bodies. They include reports, policy options, public statements, advice to livestock owners, scientific papers, conferences, legislation, advice to senior administrators and ministers, and international reporting.

Legislation

Legislation on animal health and related public health matters should be drafted in a form which is clearly understood and enforceable. It should include the legal powers to enable animal health staff to carry out their duties effectively and specify the authorities responsible for enforcing the legislation.

Animal health and public health laws should give the necessary powers for the animal health service to perform its duties and also define the responsibilities of livestock owners and others in observing the law. The legislation should provide for the rapid introduction of new measures through subordinate legislation when new diseases or situations have to be controlled.

Powers of inspection

The official animal health services should have the legal powers to exercise inspection of:

- animals, including domestic and domesticated animals of all species, and wildlife for purposes of animal health control
- animal products
- products intended for animal feed
- products intended for the prevention, diagnosis or treatment of animal diseases
- anything capable of transmitting animal disease
- related premises, equipment, facilities and means of transportation, as specified in relevant laws
- the observance of regulations
- related documents as specified in relevant laws, regulations or rules

In particular, the official animal health service should have legal powers to carry out the clinical examination and testing of any animal suspected of being affected with a notifiable disease and testing or other examination of any product or thing subject to official inspection.

Notifiable diseases

The term 'notifiable disease' should only be applied to diseases which are subject to direct official measures of prevention, control or eradication. It implies that there is an obligation on the part of stockowners or keepers to notify the authorities if they suspect the presence of such a disease.

Procedures

Effective enforcement provisions should be in place to ensure that any suspected case of a notifiable disease is reported by the general public to the official animal health service without delay. In principle, every person having in his or her possession, or attendance, an animal or carcass which they suspect, or ought to suspect, of being affected with a notifiable disease should be obliged to give notice of such fact to the official enforcement authority or animal health service.

Measures should be in force to ensure that such an obligation is complied with by veterinarians, livestock owners and attendants, butchers, knackers and any other person who, by profession, trade or regular occupation, is directly concerned with animals or carcasses. Every case of serious illness or death in an animal, or alteration in a carcass, should be considered as being suspected of a notifiable disease unless the signs can be reasonably attributed to another disease which is not notifiable.

Diseases which are subject to other forms of regulatory control should not be designated as notifiable but referred to as 'reportable', 'schedule' or 'officially controlled' diseases.

Import and export controls

The movements of animals and animal products between countries that have different disease environments, of necessity, produces a potential risk of the transfer of animal disease. These risks can be minimized by the application of effective controls in the exporting and importing countries. On the other hand the acceptance of small margins of risk may result in major benefits to livestock producers through the introduction of new breeds or superior genetic material.

The conditions for importation (whether of animals or products) are determined by the importing country and to avoid ambiguity and confusion it is essential that they are clearly defined. Sanitary measures should be aimed at the important diseases that might present major animal health, human health or economic problems. The use of animal health import restrictions as a disguised barrier to trade is a matter of concern to international organizations such as the General Agreement on Tariffs and Trade (GATT). The protracted procedures employed by some countries to arrive at a decision is equally unacceptable.

Health certificates

All countries should develop an import policy based on a clear understanding of their own domestic disease situation. Even if major diseases are endemic in the importing country it may be important to prevent the entry of new strains or types of disease agents, e.g. foot-and-mouth viruses.

Whilst most diseases can be tested for pre-importation or during quarantine, for other diseases there are no reliable diagnostic tests and it may be necessary to rely on authoritative certification of history of the absence of a disease in a country, region or herd or flock. This will depend very much on a judgement of the confidence which can be placed on the knowledge and competence of the certifying veterinary authority in the exporting country.

Certification is a means of facilitating international trade and should not be used to restrict trade by requiring animal health conditions which cannot be justified. They should be kept as simple as possible and clearly set out to convey the intentions of the importing country.

The OIE International Health Code

In drawing up health certificates importing countries should make full use of the recommendations set out in the Office International des Épizooties (OIE) *International Animal Health Code* and in the same organization's *Manual of Recommended Diagnostic Techniques and Requirements for Biological Products*. The *Code* covers disease control measures, criteria for country, region/area or herd/flock disease freedom, transportation of animals, disinfection procedures, etc. The *Manual* lays down standards for diagnostic tests and the preparation and standardization of biological products, such as antigens, vaccines, etc.

Quarantine

The risk of introducing diseases through the importation of live animals can be significantly reduced by the requirement of pre- and post-import quarantine. It must be accepted that there is some possibility of disease manifesting itself at some stage between the initial clinical examination and testing on the premises of origin of the animals and their final release. The quarantine period in the importing country may therefore be the last chance to prevent its introduction.

Quarantine premises should be sited near a seaport, airport or other import point, so that there is minimum risk of contamination in transporting potentially infected animals. The points of entry to the country should be officially designated and restricted to those where proper facilities are available to inspect the animals and detain them in isolation if necessary.

Quarantine premises should not be adjacent to other livestock facilities such as farms, abattoirs and livestock markets, stock routes, etc. They should be surrounded by an animal-proof security fence so that there is no possible contact with animals from outside. The sewage system should be built so that effluent can be treated to destroy any dangerous pathogens and bedding and manure should either be retained on the premises until the end of the quarantine period or safely disposed of.

Ideally animal accommodation should be subdivided so that any potential disease problems can be isolated in small units. Animal attendants should have no contact with animals not undergoing quarantine. Veterinary surgeons carrying out tests or clinical examinations of the animals must observe strict standards of cleansing and disinfection when entering and leaving the premises. High security is the essential factor during quarantine.

Risk assessments

A recent development in the regulation of international trade in live animals and animal products is the concept of risk assessment, i.e. an objective assessment of the risks involved in importing animals and products. The factors taken into account include.

- 'Country factor'—the prevalence of the disease in the exporting country. The weight given to this factor can be modified by consideration of the quality of veterinary control in the exporting country.
- 'Commodity factor'—the likelihood of transmission of the disease agent with the commodity.
- 'Animal import units'—the number of animal units being imported.

OIE (see later) have developed a 'risk assessment' for foot-and-mouth disease and several countries that are major importers of animals and animal products are developing risk assessment systems. The intention is that these assessments shall be transparent, i.e. that the reasons for considering certain imports for certain countries as 'high risk' or 'low risk' shall be clear to all the parties involved, particularly the exporting countries.

Risk Management

Risk assessment identifies and quantifies the risk involved in importation. Risk management is the process by which the risks that have been accepted are dealt with. The main elements are health certificates to accompany consignments and quarantine conditions pre-and/or post-importation.

Role of international organizations

Improved and faster transportation systems for live animals and the animal products, introduced during the latter part of the 20th century, have resulted in a considerable increase in the volume of trade. This increased movement and the consequent increased potential for the dissemination of animal diseases has focused attention on the importance of international collaboration both to minimize the risks of spreading animal and human disease and also to provide the technical expertise to assist developing countries to improve their livestock industries. Many international organizations play a key role in achieving these objectives.

Office International des Épizooties (OIE)

Origin

The importance of the international exchange of information about the occurrence of infectious animal diseases was recognized as early as the end of the 19th century but it was not until an epidemic of rinderpest occurred in Belgium in 1920 (introduced by zebras from Pakistan in transit in the port of Antwerp) that the governments of neighbouring countries decided to take action. A diplomatic conference held in Paris unanimously decided to create the 'Office International des Épizooties'. Twenty-eight countries subscribed to the International Agreement on 25 January 1924. By 1990 the membership of OIE had grown to 115 countries.

The OIE is funded by annual contributions paid by member countries according to a contribution category selected by them upon joining the Organization.

The role of the organization

The role of the organization is defined in Article 4 of the internal statutes appended to the 1924 Agreement.

The main objectives of the Office are:

1. To promote and coordinate experimental or other research work concerning the pathology or prophylaxis of contagious diseases of livestock for which international collaboration is deemed to be desirable.
2. To collect and bring to the attention of governments and their sanitary

services all facts and documents of general interest concerning the course of epizootic diseases and the means used to control them.
3. To examine international draft agreements regarding animal sanitary measures and to provide signatory governments with the means of supervising their enforcement.

The Structure of the Organization

The International Committee

The OIE operates under an International Committee made up of Delegates of Member Countries.

The Committee meets in General Session once a year at the OIE headquarters in Paris. The Committee rules on all questions pertaining to the mission and operation of the Office. Areas of decision-making cover 'Scientific and technical orientation of the OIE, recommendations to Member Countries on procedures for the control of animal diseases, creation of Commission to assist in the operation of the Organisation; ... Signing of cooperation agreements with other International Organisations.'

The Administrative Commission

The Administrative Commission, comprising the President of the International Committee and eight Delegates elected for three-year terms, represent the Committee between General Sessions. The Commission meets twice per year to examine technical and administrative matters with the Director General, and to examine the working programme and budget to be presented for acceptance to the Committee.

Regional Commissions

Five Regional Commissions have been set up by the OIE to study specific problems and organize the coordination of Veterinary Services in each of the following five regions: Africa; the Americas; Asia, the Far East and Oceania; Europe; and the Middle East.

Each of the Commissions organizes a conference, on average every two years, when matters of particular interest to the region are discussed.

Specialist Commissions

The role of the Specialist Commissions is to study specific problems relating to the epidemiology and control of specific diseases or groups of diseases. There are currently four Specialist Commissions:

1. The Foot and Mouth Disease Commission, set up in 1946, studies the role and development of vaccines and strategies for the control and eradication of the disease. In 1988, with the reduced incidence of the disease in many parts of the world, the remit of the Commission was extended to include other epizootic diseases.
2. The Standards Commission, set up in 1949, establishes recommendations for diagnostic techniques and requirements for biological products.
3. The International Animal Health Code Commission, set up in 1960, draws up recommendations for animal health certification for the import and export of animals and animal products.
4. The Fish Diseases Commission, also set up in 1960, represents a focal point for the exchange of information in this rapidly developing area and also makes recommendations on health standards for trade in fish and fish products.

The Central Bureau

The Central Bureau, managed by the Director General, implements the decisions of the International Committee. It is assisted in this task by the Specialist Commissions and designated experts. Publications form an important part of the work of the Bureau. Most publications are available in three languages: English, French and Spanish. They include four periodicals (one monthly, one quarterly and two annual publications) and special editions devoted to conferences and symposia.

Operational arrangements

The principal function of the OIE is to inform the heads of Veterinary Services of the occurrence and development of epizootics which may endanger animal or public health.

Information is despatched with an urgency that varies according to the nature of the disease. The most contagious diseases and those which have the most serious socio-economic implications due to their possible impact on international trade in animals and animal products, are classified in List A. This includes sixteen diseases, such as foot-and-mouth disease, rinderpest, African swine fever, African horse sickness, and fowl plague. Diseases which have a lesser impact on international trade are classified in List B, which at present includes 82 diseases (Table 5.3).

The OIE has set up a warning system whereby Member Countries can take

Table 5.3 OIE List B diseases (as at 31.12.90)

Multiple species diseases
Anthrax
Aujeszky's disease
Echinococcosis/hydatidosis
Heartwater
Leptospirosis
Q fever
Rabies
Paratuberculosis
Screwworm (*Cochliomyia hominivorax*)

Sheep and goat diseases
Brucella ovis infection
Caprine and ovine brucellosis (*Brucella melitensis*)
Caprine arthritis/encephalitis
Contagious agalactia
Contagious caprine pleuropneumonia
Enzootic abortion of ewes
Pulmonary adenomatosis
Nairobi sheep disease
Salmonellosis (*Salmonella abortus ovis*)
Scrapie
Maedi-visna

Pig diseases
Atrophic rhinitis
Cysticercosis (C. Cellulosae)
Porcine brucellosis (*Brucella suis*)
Transmissible gastroenteritis of pigs
Trichinellosis

Lagomorph diseases
Myxomatosis
Tularaemia
Viral haemorrhagic disease of rabbits

Mollusc diseases
Bonamiosis
Haplosporidiosis
Perkinosis
Marteiliosis
Iridoviroses

Bee diseases
Acariasis of bees
American foul brood
European foul brood
Nosematosis of bees
Varroasis

Disease of other animal species
Leishmaniasis

Cattle diseases
Anaplasmosis
Babesiosis
Bovine brucellosis (*Brucella abortus*)
Bovine genital campylobacteriosis
Bovine tuberculosis
Cysticercosis (C. bovis)
Dermatophilosis
Enzootic bovine leukosis
Haemorrhagic septicaemia
Infectious bovine rhinotracheitis (IBR/IPV)
Theileriosis
Trichomoniasis
Trypanosomiasis
Bovine malignant catarrh
Bovine spongiform encephalopathy (BSE)

Horse diseases
Contagious equine metritis
Dourine
Epizootic lymphangitis
Equine encephalomyelitis
Equine infectious anaemia
Equine influenza (virus type A)
Equine piroplasmosis
Equine rhinopneumonitis
Glanders
Horse pox
Infectious arteritis of horses
Japanese encephalitis
Horse mange
Salmonellosis (*Salmonella abortus equi*)
Surra
Venezuelan equine encephalomyelitis

Fish diseases
Viral haemorrhagic septicaemia
Infectious haematopoietic necrosis
Salmonid herpesvirosis (Type 2)
Renibacteriosis (*R. salmoninarium*)
Ictalurid herpesvirosis (Type 1)
Enzootic haematopoietic necrosis
Edwardsiellosis (*E. ictaluri*)

Crustacean diseases
Baculovirosis (*B. monodon*)
Baculovirosis (*B. penaei*)
Baculoviral midgut gland necrosis
Infectious hypodermal and haematopoietic necrosis

The lists are amended periodically and published in the OIE *Code* and Bulletins and the FAO/WHO/OIE *Animal Health Yearbook*.

action rapidly should the need arise. Countries must notify the Central Bureau within 24 hours of the occurrence of an outbreak of a List A disease or any other contagious disease likely to have serious repercussions on public health or the economy of animal production. The OIE immediately despatches this information to Member Countries—by telex or telegram to countries directly at risk, or by letter to other countries.

In addition to this 'emergency' system, information received from Member Countries is distributed on a periodic basis in the form of a monthly 'Bulletin' which indicates outbreaks of List A diseases, month by month.

The OIE also organizes conferences and symposia on items of current interest to Veterinary Services; recent examples include, foot-and-mouth disease, rinderpest, African horse sickness, screwworm infestation, advances in biotechnology, the control and use of anabolics in animal production, and fish vaccination.

Co-operation with other International Organizations

The OIE does not intervene in the field, but through the information available to it and the spirit of co-operation of Member Countries the organization has an important decision-making role with other organizations. Accordingly, a working agreement was signed in 1953 with the Food and Agriculture Organization of the United Nations (FAO). A similar agreement was signed with the World Health Organization (WHO) in 1961 and with the Inter-American Institute for Cooperation on Agriculture in 1981. The OIE also works in close co-operation with the Pan-American Health Organization (PAHO), the World Veterinary Association (WVA), and with regional organizations responsible for operating animal health programmes.

The Food and Agriculture Organization of the United Nations (FAO)

Origin

The Food and Agriculture Organization (FAO) is an autonomous agency within the United Nations (UN) system. It was founded on 16 October 1945 and has its headquarters in Rome.

At its formation it was given four tasks:

- to carry out programmes of technical advice and assistance for agricultural communities on behalf of governments and development fund agencies
- to collect, analyse and disseminate information
- to advise governments on policy and planning

- to provide opportunities for governments to meet and discuss food and agricultural problems

Structure

FAO has a membership of 158 member countries which make up the Conference, its supreme governing body. The Conference meets every two years to review the state of agriculture and food and the Organization's work, and to approve the programme of work and budget for the following two years. The conference elects, as an interim governing body, a Council of representatives from 49 member countries who serve three-year rotating terms. The Conference also elects the Director General, who is head of the Secretariat. The Secretariat is staffed by some 3500 professional and general service personnel and a similar number are employed on field projects and at country and regional offices in the Third World.

The Council elects three main committees—the Programme Committee, the Finance Committee, and the Committee on Constitutional and Legal Matters. In addition five committees advise the Council on commodity problems, fisheries, forestry, agriculture and world food security. These latter committees are open to any member nation wishing to join them.

The funds for FAO's work come from three main sources—contributions by member nations, the trust funds of member countries and the United Nations Development Programme (UNDP).

Functions

A Development Agency

FAO gives direct practical help in the developing world through technical assistance projects in all areas of agriculture and food production. These field projects are aimed to strengthen local institutions, assist research and training, and develop and demonstrate new techniques. Projects are normally staffed by international experts and local technicians and are designed to be followed up by local or national action.

A source of information

The Organization serves as a clearing house for data which are published and made available in every medium—print, film, radio, TV, video, film strips, etc.

A mass of information, on all aspects of agriculture, is made available to farmers, scientists, technologists and government planners; this is extremely important to them if they are to make sound decisions on planning, investment, marketing, research and training. In addition, apart from providing specialist information FAO has a responsibility for increasing awareness among a wider audience of the importance of food and agriculture and the problems faced by developing countries.

Advising governments

The FAO serves as an independent source of advice to governments in developing their agricultural policies and on the administrative and legal structures needed for their implementation. Representatives, who are accredited to most developing countries, provide a ready source of information on the range of assistance and services the Organization can offer.

FAO plays a lead role in producing the annual FAO/WHO/OIE *Animal Health Yearbook* that records on a worldwide basis outbreaks of List A and List B diseases (see Tables 5.2 and 5.3).

A forum for discussion

A major forum for discussion is the FAO Conference, attended by representatives of all member nations, which meets every two years. In addition to its 'house-keeping' duties of approving FAO's work programme and budget, the Conference is able to take concerted action on issues which are of particular concern to its members and to discuss matters which have international implications; an example would be the emergency caused by the Chernobyl accident and its effect on international trade in agricultural products.

Many bodies have been set up by the FAO Conference or Council to foster co-operation in a particular subject or geographical area. Two examples of such bodies in the animal health field would be the Commission on African Animal Trypanosomiasis, established in 1979, and the European Commission for the Control of Foot and Mouth Disease, established in 1953.

Livestock disease control

FAO's greatest contributions in livestock development have been in combating animal diseases of major economic importance. Its first major field project was a campaign against rinderpest, started in China in 1947 and subsequently extended to other Asian countries. By the end of the 1950s this highly contagious disease had been eradicated from most countries of the region. In Africa the disease is still a serious problem despite much effort to control it in the past. FAO is again collaborating with other international organizations in a

Pan-African Rinderpest Campaign aimed at the eventual eradication of the disease from the continent.

Close collaboration is maintained with other international organizations, especially the other UN agencies. Special agricultural divisions have been established jointly with UN economic commissions for Africa, Europe, Latin America and Western Asia. In the field of isotopes and radiation and its potential consequence for agriculture close co-operation is maintained with the International Atomic Energy Agency based in Vienna.

The FAO European Commission for the Control of Foot and Mouth Disease

The growing international trade in animals and animal products precipitated the explosive epidemics of foot-and-mouth disease (FMD) in Europe in the early 1950s. The disruptive effect of the disease on trade was clearly apparent to governments who also realized that individual action taken by countries to combat the disease was insufficient to bring it under control. It was accepted that new initiatives were needed which would have to be coordinated on an international scale. This led to the formation of the European Commission for the Control of Foot and Mouth Disease in December 1953.

The Commission is an autonomous body, with a full-time secretariat, operating within the framework of the FAO. By 1986 27 countries were members of the Commission.

The purpose of the Commission was to encourage close collaboration between countries in the region in the fight against FMD. To achieve this objective the general functions of the Commission were:

- to assist countries in diagnostic work
- to assist countries in the organization of disease control and preventative programmes
- to maintain a register of available stocks of FMD virus
- to be aware of the evolution of the disease worldwide, particularly in the regions from which the disease could be introduced into Europe by the importation of animals, animal products, or by other means

Sessions of the Commission held in Rome, initially annually and in later years bi-annually, provided the forum whereby member countries could report on their disease position and exchange information on methods of control. In the light of these discussions countries were able to benefit from the experiences of others and amend their control programmes as necessary.

The main thrust of the Commission was to encourage regular mass vaccination of cattle in infected countries together with the application of sound zoosanitary measures. The Commission also advised on improvements in techniques of vaccine production and vaccine quality through the medium of scientific meetings and collaboration between production laboratories.

As a result of these activities there was a gradual improvement in the FMD disease position in the region. From the situation in 1951–52, when there were 860 873 outbreaks of the disease, there was a decrease in the annual incidence to 74 outbreaks in 1989 and nil in 1990. The outcome of the elimination of the disease and a cost-benefit analysis of the continuing use of prophylactic vaccination has enabled the EEC countries to decide to discontinue vaccination from the end of 1991 and thus allow for the free movement of animals between Community countries.

The successful eradication of FMD from Europe has been an outstanding example of a regional approach to the control and eradication of a highly virulent and diffusible disease of livestock which does not respect national frontiers. It sets a pattern for other regions of the world where the disease continues to be a major problem.

The World Health Organization (WHO)

The WHO, which has its headquarters in Geneva, Switzerland, plays a leading role in the animal health field by promoting international collaboration in the control and eradication of zoonotic diseases which are of public health and economic importance. The Veterinary Public Health section which deals with zoonoses and food hygiene reports to the Director of the Division of Communicable Diseases. In addition to their own technical experts the division has access to expertise in the many specialized WHO agencies. WHO collaborates closely with FAO and OIE.

In most WHO member states the public health significance of zoonoses increases in correlation with the density of the animal population, the degree of urbanization, the industrialization of husbandry, and international trade in animals and animal products. WHO pays particular attention to diseases such as rabies, enteric bacterial zoonoses, brucellosis and echinococcosis, as well as some infections of more regional and local importance such as anthrax, leptospirosis, equine encephalitis, Rift Valley fever and toxoplasmosis.

In all areas of zoonosis programmes WHO co-operates closely with animal health services. National programmes are supported through a range of technical assistance (e.g. preparation and distribution of guiding principles, promotion of research, information/technology transfer, personnel training and the mobilization of resources).

In dealing with rabies emphasis is placed on the promotion of national and international programmes for its elimination in wildlife species in certain areas. Technology for ecological studies of reservoir animals species, for carrying out mass immunization and for disease surveillance has been well developed.

The World Veterinary Association (WVA)

The WVA was founded in 1959 as a continuing Permanent Committee for the International Veterinary Congress, which is held every four years. Its aim is to unify the veterinary profession throughout the world by providing a central link for national associations, organizing congresses, improving veterinary education and establishing relations with organizations with interests similar to those of the Association. Member organizations exist in 72 countries.

The General Agreement on Tariffs and Trade (GATT)

GATT was established in 1948 as a multilateral treaty aiming to liberalize world trade and place it on a secure basis. In 1987 there were 95 contracting parties, one country had acceded provisionally and a further 29 in practice apply the rules of GATT to their commercial policy. GATT has its headquarters in Geneva with 300 permanent staff and its budget for 1986 amounted to 61.1m Swiss francs.

Organization

The Sessions of contracting parties are usually held annually in Geneva. The Session is the highest body of GATT and decisions are generally arrived at by consensus, not by vote. On the rare occasion that voting takes place most decisions are taken by simple majority.

Activities

Much of GATT's regular work consists of consultation and negotiations on specific trade problems affecting individual commodities or member countries. From time to time, major multilateral trade negotiations take place under GATT auspices. These negotiating rounds normally take 4–5 years to complete. The 'Uruguay Round', which commenced in 1986 in Punta del Este, Uruguay, was due to be completed by the end of 1990. It was largely concerned with agricultural trade and in particular disguised barriers which distorted trade. Among these 'barriers' unjustified animal health measures were cited and it was generally accepted that the recommendations in the OIE International Animal Health Code could in future serve as a basis for a dispute settlement procedure. GATT has also actively promoted risk assessment procedures as described earlier in this chapter.

Decisions

Draft agreements arrived at by the contracting parties take the form of a

Decision. The Decision enters into force within two years after acceptance and thereafter has to be respected by all contracting parties.

Regional organizations

Asia and the Pacific

Animal Production and Health Commission for Asia (APHCA)

The APHCA was founded in 1975 with its headquarters in the FAO Regional Office in Bangkok. Its overall objective is to provide a forum for developing strategies to solve important problems of livestock agriculture, based on the principles of 'collective self-reliance' and the concept of Technical Co-operation among Developing Countries (TCDC).

The APHCA collects animal disease information on a regular basis, and compiles and disseminates it to all the member countries at monthly and quarterly intervals. Reports on any unexpected outbreaks of emergency disease such as rinderpest and foot-and-mouth diseases are immediately transmitted to all countries in the region. APHCA also operates an emergency vaccine bank whereby certain member countries pledge to reserve locally produced vaccines against specific diseases, such as foot-and-mouth disease, rinderpest and duck plague, and supply these to another member country on request.

Africa

Inter-African Bureau of Animal Resources (IBAR)

The IBAR is an important African organization dealing with animal health problems. With headquarters in Nairobi, Kenya, it is a technical branch of the Organization of African Unity (OAU).

IBAR periodically issues a *Bulletin of Animal Health and Production*, which contains technical and scientific articles on disease control, research and animal production. It also issues on a monthly basis *Animal Health Statistics* giving the position on the major contagious animal diseases in Africa and information leaflets on selected topics.

In recent years IBAR has been actively involved in coordinating the Pan-African Rinderpest Campaign (PARC) with the objective of eradicating the disease from the continent of Africa.

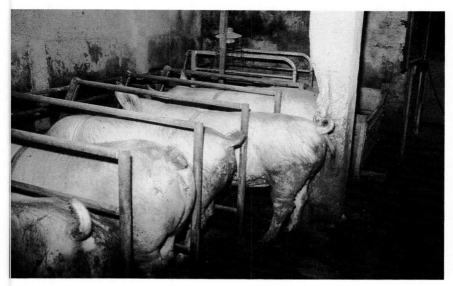

Plate 1a

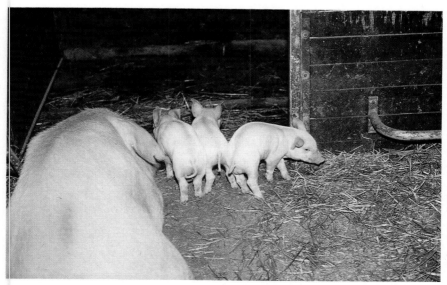

Plate 1b   Sows, dry or with litters, show a higher morbidity when kept in
confinement (a) than when loose housed (b).

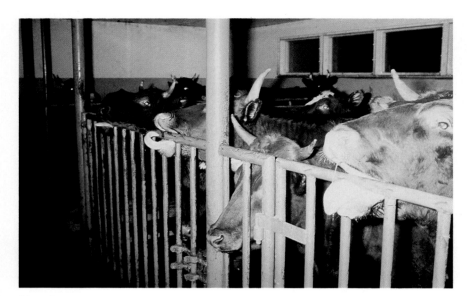

Plate 2a

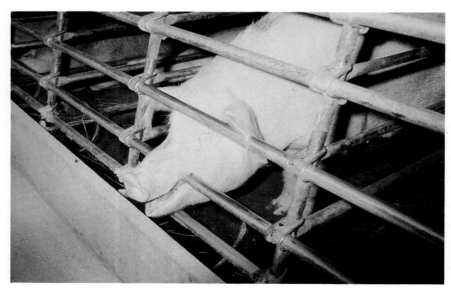

Plate 2b In barren environments cattle (a) and swine (b) show not only
aberrant behaviours but also a higher morbidity than in more
stimulus-rich environments.

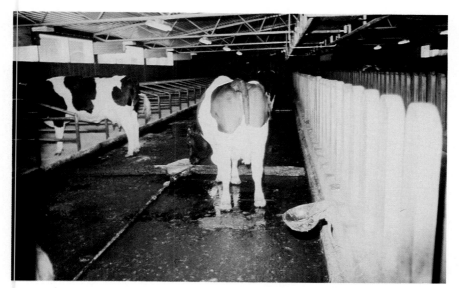

Plate 3   Feet disorders have been shown to be associated with unsuitable or dirty flooring, daily cleaning of alleys is therefore essential.

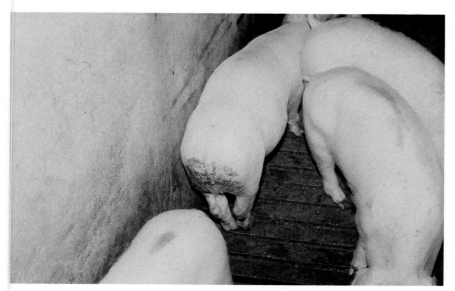

Plate 4   Tail biting in pigs is associated with barren environments.

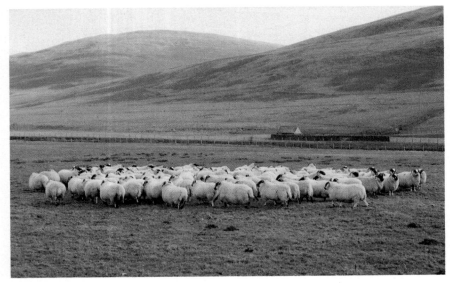

Plate 5 Blackface ewes in Scotland, an example of extensive sheep farming on a hill farm.

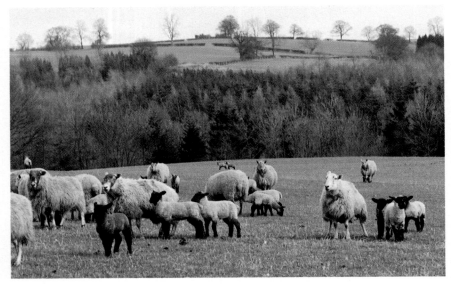

Plate 6 North of England mules with lambs by a Suffolk, an example of semi-intensive sheep farming on a lowland farm.

Latin America and the Caribbean

Pan-American Health Organization (PAHO)

PAHO, with its headquarters in Washington DC, supports the veterinary public health services in the region concerning zoonoses and sanitary inspection of livestock and fisheries products. The Pan-American Foot and Mouth Disease Centre in Rio de Janeiro organizes training courses for animal health services, the distribution of standard diagnostic reagents, identification of virus from suspect cases, vaccine quality control and publication of standardized techniques.

The Pan-American Zoonosis Centre, based in Buenos Aires, provides reference services related to zoonotic diseases for animal health services in the region.

Interamerican Institute for Cooperation in Agriculture (IICA)

IICA is the specialized agency for agriculture of the inter-American system. It is the institutional continuation of the inter-American Institute of Agriculture Sciences, which was created by the Council of the Pan American Union in 1942. Its headquarters is in San José, Costa Rica, and there are 31 member countries drawn from central and southern American countries.

In the animal health field IICA co-operates with member countries in solving the animal disease problems which have an adverse effect on the economy of their agricultural industries. They participate in multinational projects to strengthen laboratory services and epidemiological surveillance in the Central, Andean and Southern areas, including a data monitoring system for animal diseases. In addition they carry out numerous national projects dealing with specific problems of the countries concerned.

Regional Organization for Animal and Plant Health (OIRSA)

OIRSA supports the veterinary service activities of Mexico and Central American countries through specific regional activities such as epidemiological research on blue tongue virus in the region, as well as local disease control activities requested by the governments.

Interamerican Cooperation Group on Animal Health (GICSA)

Since 1984, all the international organizations which support the activities of official veterinary services in the American continent have an annual meeting under the auspices of the Interamerican Cooperation Group on Animal Health. The purpose of the meeting is to exchange information, avoid duplication and promote complementary support for specific activities.

6 WELFARE IN NATIONAL AND INTERNATIONAL LEGISLATION

R MOSS Esq., BVSc, MRCVS

Primary welfare legislation in Great Britain
Basic principles
Council of Europe
Content of primary legislation
Codes of welfare practice
Control of husbandry practices
Transport of farm livestock
Enforcement of legislation

This chapter considers the way in which legislative provisions can improve the welfare of livestock. It cannot hope to include all the regulations which have been enacted but can illustrate the principles involved by reference to some of them.

In Great Britain, the philosophy behind much of 19th century legislation, or lack of it, was that of individualism. The judiciary and parliament agreed that the only legislative function of government both within and outside this country was the maintenance of law and order.

The reasons for this emphasis on the freedom of the individual were many. Most importantly it was in line with the interests of the new emerging middle-class of industrialists. In addition it accorded with John Locke's views on the sanctity of private rights and property. The emphasis of the common law was on freedom of property, freedom of contract and freedom of the person. Interference with these rights was not acceptable.

However, the very success of this *laissez-faire* philosophy led to the need for government to intervene in the interests of both public safety and health. Such an interference, although inconsistent with unlimited freedom of property and of the person, was inevitable, particularly in regard to the way society dealt with domestic animals.

The control of disease in domestic farm livestock was not only important for the maintenance of the satisfactory health and productivity of the national livestock population; it was also important for public health. These controls have been successful over the intervening years in eradicating many of the very serious livestock epidemics (e.g. tuberculosis) and zoonoses (e.g. rabies) which plagued the 19th and first half of the 20th centuries. The introduction and implementation of disease controls are dealt with in detail in Chapter 5.

Primary welfare legislation in Great Britain

Protection of Animals Act 1911

Welfare, apart from its disease aspects, is another matter. In Great Britain the second schedule to the Protection of Animals Act 1911 lists the enactments repealed when it became law:

• The Knackers Act 1786	Sect. 4
• The Knackers Act 1844	Sect. 3
• The Cruelty to Animals Act 1849	The whole Act
• The Cruelty to Animals Act 1854	,,
• The Poisoned Grain Prohibition Act 1863	,,
• The Poisoned Flesh Prohibition Act 1864	,,
• The Drugging of Animals Act 1876	,,
• The Wild Animals in Captivity Protection Act 1900	,,
• The Injured Animals Act 1907	,,

The list indicates that some attention to cruelty to animals had been present in Great Britain's society from as early as the late 18th century. However, it was not until the middle of the 19th century that an Act of Parliament specifically related to cruelty (note welfare has yet to be mentioned) was placed on the statute book.

In Great Britain the Protection of Animals Act 1911 as amended is still an important if not a central piece of legislation relating to the treatment of livestock. It must be remembered that when it was first enacted the horse was an animal in everyday use—a work animal and a means of transport both commercially and for defence. Thus, although not specifically stated much of the Protection of Animals Act 1911 when it first became law dealt with the prevention of cruelty to horses and its terminology reflects that bias. Thus Article 1(1)(a) states:

If any person—

shall cruelly beat; kick; ill-treat, over-ride, over-drive, over-load, torture, infuriate, or terrify an animal, or shall cause or procure, or, being the owner, permit any animal to be so used, or shall, by wantonly or unreasonably *doing or omitting to do* any act, or causing or procuring the

> *commission or omission*, or, being the owner, permit any unnecessary suffering to be so caused to any animal; . . .

Such a person shall be guilty of an offence of cruelty within the meaning of this Act. One further very important point should be noted with regard to Article 1(1)(a). Underlined are two phrases which not only set out the principle of something being done which leads to an offence of cruelty, i.e. commission, but also something not being done, i.e. omission.

This principle has been debated for many years. In essence the debate centres round the question of whether welfare legislation should be positive or negative in its content. Should it require things to be done or should it simply require that certain things should not happen. So on one side there is the argument that systems of husbandry shall be approved, down to the smallest detail—in effect saying 'this shall be done'. On the other side is the argument that it is sufficient to state 'thou shalt not inflict unnecessary suffering or be cruel to any animal in thy care'. It is claimed this latter argument is deficient in many respects not least of which is that it leads to so many interpretations of what is 'unnecessary'.

The Protection of Animals Act 1911 also enshrined one other important principle, i.e. that an animal is property, and that in Great Britain without due process of the law no one can be deprived of any animal in their ownership without proven cause.

Agriculture (Miscellaneous Provisions) Act 1968

In Great Britain farm animals are afforded further protection in Part 1 Para 1(1) of the Agriculture (Miscellaneous Provisions) Act 1968. Part 1 has the heading 'Welfare of Livestock'; note the use of the word 'welfare'. Part 1 Para 1(1) states:

> Any person who causes unnecessary pain or unnecessary distress to any livestock for the time being situated on agricultural land and under his control or permits any such livestock to suffer any such pain or distress of which he knows or may reasonably be expected to know shall be guilty of an offence under this section.

Very similar 'animal protection' legislation is present in almost every developed country in the world. Such legislation, which has been built up in rather piecemeal fashion, covers all the main areas of man's use and exploitation (not necessarily used in the pejorative sense) of animals in both the domestic situation and in the wild. In this book we are primarily concerned with animals used for farming purposes and it is on legislation relating to farm livestock that this chapter will concentrate.

Basic principles

Essentially, the legislation can be divided into the various practical situations in which man finds himself dealing with farm livestock. These are:

- on the farm
- in the market place
- during movement from one location to another by all means of transport
- at the slaughterhouse

Each situation has a body of regulations covering the daily handling of livestock and many of the specific activities such as routine husbandry practices which can, even if correctly carried out, inflict pain and/or suffering on the animals involved.

However, before examining this body of legislation in more detail it must not be forgotten that the one principle which virtually all countries enact in primary legislation is that of the prevention of cruelty, and although some countries do not in the first instance specifically define cruelty many do have similar statements as embodied in Art. (1)(a) of Great Britain's Protection of Animals Act 1911 (as amended).

Thus in Northern Ireland, Part 1 Para. 1(1) The Welfare of Animals Act 1972 states:

> ... any person who causes unnecessary pain or unnecessary distress to any livestock for the time being situated on agricultural land and under his control or permits any such livestock to suffer any such pain or distress of which he knows or may reasonably be expected to know shall be guilty of an offence.

Part III of the same Act, which has the title 'Protection of Animals' sets out in a very similar manner to the Protection of Animals Act 1911 in Great Britain the categories of action which by implication are considered to cause unnecessary pain or unnecessary distress and thus constitute an offence:

- (a) cruelly beats, kicks, ill treats, over-rides, over drives, over loads, tortures, infuriates or terrifies any animal; or
- (b) conveys or carries any animal in such a manner as to cause that animal any unnecessary suffering; or
- (c) wilfully, without reasonable cause or excuse, administers to or causes to be taken by an animal any poisonous or noxious substance; or
- (d) uses rubberbands or any other form of constriction for the purpose of dehorning any animal; or

(e) without reasonable cause or excuse, abandons, whether permanently or not, any animal of which he is the owner or has charge or control, in circumstances likely to cause the animal any unnecessary suffering; or

(f) exposes for sale any animal bearing unhealed wounds from castration or other operation; or

(g) causes, procures or, being the owner, permits any of the acts of cruelty specified in paras (a) to (f) or causes or procures or, being the owner, permits the causing of any unnecessary suffering to any animal;

The Swedish Animal Protection Act promulgated on 2 June 1988 makes a very simple direct statement of intent in Section 2: 'Animals shall be treated well and be protected from unnecessary suffering and disease'. There is no explanation of the scope for interpretation of the word 'unnecessary'. The Swiss Federal Animal Protection Act dated 9 March 1978 sets out in Art. 2 the Principles which the Act seeks to satisfy. Thus:

1. Animals shall be treated in the manner which best accords with their needs.
2. Anyone who is concerned with animals shall, insofar as circumstances permit, safeguard their welfare.
3. No one shall unjustifiably expose animals to pain, suffering, physical injury or fear.

Notice there is no use of the word cruelty although the word exists in both the French and German language. In addition use is made of such modifying (and unexplained and often difficult to interpret as to intention) phrases as 'the manner which best accords with their needs', 'in so far as circumstances permit' and 'no one shall unjustifiably'.

The Finnish Animal Protection Act issued in Helsinki on 27 January 1971 is written in similar vein to both the Swiss and Swedish legislation. Section 1 states: 'Animals shall be treated well, so that they are not caused unnecessary suffering.' Section 2 confirms 'It is forbidden to cause an animal unnecessary pain or suffering.'

The French within their legislation protecting nature deal in Chapter II with the protection of animals. Art. 9 sets out the principles to be followed: 'All animals being sentient beings must be kept by their owner in conditions compatible with the biological needs of their species.' Art. 13 amends part of article 453 of the French penal code and uses the word cruelty in the statement: 'whoever, without need, publicly or not, ... commits an act of cruelty against a domestic animal ... will be punished'.

Luxemburg, in a law of 15 March 1983, states its objective as the protection of life and well-being of animals and sets out in Chapter 1 Art. 1 the principles to be observed:

> The present law has for its objective to assure the protection of the life and well being of animals. It is forbidden to anyone, without necessity to kill or to cause to be killed an animal, or himself cause or permit to be caused pain, suffering, damage or wounds (to an animal).
>
> All suffering animals, wounded or in danger must be succoured with all possible means.

So the principle that animals shall not be treated cruelly nor caused unnecessary pain or distress or suffering and their well-being sought by providing them with their biological needs is generally agreed. The fact that the use of such words as 'unnecessary', 'needs', 'distress' and 'suffering' is open to interpretation (see Chapter 1) does make not only for some confusion but engenders a great deal of argument even among veterinary surgeons.

Council of Europe

It should be no surprise that these principles are found in most, if not all, legislation. Countries which have ratified the European Convention for the Protection of Animals kept for Farming Purposes are expected to adopt the principles of that Convention within their own country by administrative or legislative means. The General Principles of the Convention are set out in Chapter I Articles 1 to 7:

Art. 1. This Convention shall apply to the keeping, care and housing of animals, and in particular to animals in modern intensive stock-farming systems. For the purpose of this Convention "animals" shall mean animals bred or kept for the production of food, wool, skin or fur or for other farming purposes, and "modern intensive stock-farming systems" shall mean systems which predominantly employ technical installations operated principally by means of automatic processes.

Art. 2. Each contracting party shall give effect to the principles of animal welfare laid down in Arts. 3 to 7 of this Convention.

Art. 3. Animals shall be housed and provided with food, water and care in a manner which—having regard to their species and to their degree of development, adaptation and domestication—is appropriate to their physiological and ethological needs in accordance with established experience and scientific knowledge.

Art. 4. 1. The freedom of movement appropriate to an animal, having regard to its species and in accordance with established experience and scientific knowledge, shall not be restricted in such a manner as to cause it unnecessary suffering or injury.

2. Where an animal is continuously or regularly tethered or confined, it shall be given the space appropriate to its physiological and ethological needs in accordance with established experience and scientific knowledge.

Art. 5. The lighting, temperature, humidity, air circulation, ventilation, and other environmental conditions such as gas concentration or noise intensity in the place in which the animal is housed shall, having regard to its species and to its degree of development, adaptation and domestication, conform to its physiological and ethological needs in accordance with established experience and scientific knowledge.

Art. 6. No animal shall be provided with food or liquid in a manner which may cause unnecessary suffering or injury.

Art. 7. 1. The condition and state of health of animals shall be thoroughly inspected at intervals sufficient to avoid unnecessary suffering and in the case of animals kept in modern intensive stock farming systems at least once a day.

2. The technical equipment used in modern intensive stock-farming systems shall be thoroughly inspected at least once a day, and any defect discovered shall be remedied with the least possible delay. When a defect cannot be remedied forthwith, all temporary measures necessary to safeguard the welfare of the animals shall be taken immediately.

Two phrases which occur in the above articles are of considerable importance both to the drafter of primary and secondary legislation and to veterinary surgeons and livestock producers. The phrases are open to a considerable breadth of interpretation and without due regard being given to all the circumstances surrounding particular cases can be open to gross misrepresentation. The phrases in question are 'having regard to their species and to their degree of development, adaptation and domestication' and 'is appropriate to their physiological needs in accordance with established experience and scientific knowledge'.

It is accepted that these phrases do allow for modification and amendment to recommendations relating to specific species which are promulgated by the

Standing Committee of the Convention. Thus new practices, new scientific knowledge and perhaps even at a later stage genetic changes can be taken into account in formulating specific legal requirements for the treatment of domestic farm livestock.

Most, if not all countries in their primary legislation do attempt to expand on the principles set out in their first chapters. They also as signatories of the Council of Europe Convention embody either in their primary legislation or in rules and regulations (or codes of practice) made under that legislation the principles set out in Arts. 3 to 7 of the Convention.

So, the Swedish Animal Protection Act 1988 requires in Section 3(1) that 'Animals shall be provided with sufficient food and water and adequate care. Stables and other premises shall provide animals with adequate space and shelter, and they shall be kept clean.' Section 7(1) requires that 'Animals which are bred and kept for the production of food, wool, skin or furs shall be kept and handled in a good environment for animals and in such a way as to promote their health and allow natural behaviour.' Section 5 states: 'Animals must not be over strained ... Nor may they be beaten or driven with implements which may easily wound or otherwise injure them.' Section 6(1) requires that 'Animals must not be kept tied in a painful way or in a way that does not allow them necessary freedom of movement or sufficient shelter against wind and weather.' Sections 3, 4 and 6 above also contain a paragraph which states: 'The Government or, upon authorisation by the Government, the National Board of Agriculture may issue further directions concerning the treatment of such animals.' Swiss legislation contains similar articles.

As has been stated the law relating to animal welfare and farm livestock in all countries covers the protection of such livestock from birth to slaughter. In this chapter we deal almost exclusively with the legislation covering such animals when on the farm, during transport and in markets. The legislation relating to these particular aspects of the life of a farm animal—on farm, in the market, during transport, in the slaughterhouse, etc.—may or may not derive from one principal Act. In Sweden, Switzerland, Finland and a number of other countries it does so. In Great Britain, as has been seen, there are a number of primary sources.

Content of primary legislation

We can now consider some of the separate sectors in greater detail. All primary legislation and the regulations derived from that legislation cover a number of aspects of the welfare of the animals concerned. This principle is well illustrated by reference to Chapter 1 of the Norwegian Welfare of Animals Act of 20 December 1974. Thus Section 2 covers the general treatment of animals to which the legislation applies. Section 3 denotes the persons and organisations who have the power to inspect animals and premises in which they are kept. Section 4 sets out the principles which must be followed in providing 'suitable quarters with sufficient space. Suitable warmth, enough light and access to fresh air, etc. as appropriate to the needs of the kind of animal in question'. Section 5 deals with the provision of the care and attention of the animal. Section 6 requires any animal 'sick, injured or helpless' to be assisted. Section 7 prohibits persons other than veterinarians to carry out surgical procedures or initiate medical treatment of animals 'when there is reason to believe that the procedure or treatment may cause the animal to suffer'. This section also requires the veterinarian to employ total or local anaesthesia, unless there are contraindications, if there is reason to believe that the procedure or treatment will cause the animal 'considerable pain'. Notice how much subjective judgement is required in this section. Section 8 sets out 'Prohibited ways of treating animals' and Section 13 lists prohibited operations. Thus under Section 13 it is forbidden to castrate dogs, cats and poultry unless there are special circumstances, and to insert a ring in the snout of pigs and dehorn animals.

Codes of welfare practice

Mention has already been made of the two main pieces of legislation in Great Britain which relate to the welfare and protection of farm livestock whilst on the farm: the Protection of Animals Act 1911 and the Agriculture (Miscellaneous Provisions) Act 1968. Under Section 3(1) of the latter Act:

> The Ministers may from time to time, after consultation with such persons appearing to them to represent any interests concerned as the Ministers consider appropriate:

> a. Prepare codes containing such recommendations with respect to the welfare of livestock for the time being situated on agricultural land as they consider proper for the guidance of persons concerned with the livestock;

> and

> b. revise any such code by revoking, varying, amending or adding to the provisions of the code in such manner as the Ministers think fit.

The codes issued under this legislation have all been initially drafted by a government advisory body, The Farm Animal Welfare Council. Members of this Council are appointed by the Government and bring to the deliberation of the Council varying expertise.

Status of Codes of Practice in Great Britain

The Codes themselves have a unique status in law. A note at the beginning of each Code explains:

Art. 3(4) of the Agriculture (Miscellaneous Provisions) Act 1968 states:

A failure on the part of any person to observe a provision of a code for the time being issued under this section shall not of itself render that person liable to any proceedings of any kind; but such a failure on the part of any person may, in proceeding against him for an offence under Section 1 of this Act, be relied upon by the prosecution as tending to establish the guilt of the accused unless it is shown that he cannot reasonably be expected to have observed the provision in question within the period which has elapsed since that provision was first included in a code issued under this section.

All of these codes are divided into four basic sections:

1. Housing, which includes the control of the ventilation and temperature of both climatic and totally controlled environment housing, lighting equipment and services.
2. Space allowance for individual animals depending upon their species, age, sex and systems of husbandry.
3. The provision of food and water, in both intensive and extensive systems.
4. Management, which includes: the provision of isolation facilities, the loose housing of cattle and the housing of calves, sow farrowing quarters, the tethering of sows, and the outside shelter of sows kept in extensive systems; the cleansing and disinfection of buildings, the facilities for handling deer and for cattle during routine tuberculin testing, vaccination, etc. and the provision of facilities to cover the risk of fire.

All the codes also refer to the need for the rapid diagnosis and treatment of injury and disease which in turn depend on a high level of stockmanship, the type of management system in use and the frequency of inspection.

The publication and purpose of these Codes of Practice in Great Britain are mirrored in Switzerland by regulations, which the Federal Council having consulted specialists 'shall issue on keeping of animals, covering such matters as the minimum dimensions, lay-out, lighting and ventilation of accommodation provided for them, stocking density for housing in groups and tethering arrangements.' (Art. 33 Federal Act on Animal Welfare, 9 March 1978).

Sweden: subordinate legislation

Similarly in Sweden in Section 3 of the Animal Protection Act, 2 June 1988, it is stated:

1. Animals shall be provided with sufficient food and water and adequate care. Stables and other premises shall provide animals with adequate space and shelter, and they shall be kept clean.
2. The Government or, upon authorisation by the Government, the National Board of Agriculture may issue further directions concerning:

    1. Stables and other premises for animals,
    2. obligations to have such premises inspected prior to use, and
    3. obligation to have new technology relating to animal husbandry pre-tested.

Here is a novel concept—the prior inspection and approval by competent authorities of existing and new housing and equipment (see Chapter 2).

A similar provision is applied in Switzerland which in Art. 5 of the Federal Act on Animal Welfare of 9 March 1978 requires:

1. Mass produced housing systems and installation for the keeping of animals for purposes of profit may not be advertised and sold without prior authorisation from a service designated by the Federal Council. Authorisation shall only be granted if such systems and installations provide proper living conditions for animals. The costs of the authorisation procedure shall be paid by the applicant.
2. The Federal Council shall fix a transitional period during which housing-systems and installations already on the market may continue to be sold.

The implications of this form of legislation as contrasted with the greater flexibility of the code of practice approach and the consequences for the ways in which the implementation of animal protection and animal welfare legislation is carried out will be discussed later in this chapter.

Control of husbandry practices

Most, if not all countries, either in their principal legislation, or in subsidiary regulations, prohibit or control certain husbandry practices. Thus in Great Britain the following legislation has been made under the Agriculture (Miscellaneous Provision) Act 1968.

1. The Welfare of Livestock (Intensive Units) Regulations 1978.
   These Regulations require livestock on agricultural land in an intensive unit and the automatic equipment of such units to be thoroughly inspected not less than once daily by a stock-keeper (or other competent person in the case of equipment), and for appropriate measures to be taken to safeguard livestock from suffering unnecessary pain or unnecessary distress if any problems are found.
2. The Welfare of Livestock (Prohibited Operations) Regulations 1982 and (Amendment) Regulations 1987
   These regulations prohibit a number of operations in relation to livestock on agricultural land. The prohibitions do not, however, apply to the provision, in an emergency, of first aid for the purpose of saving life or relieving pain, nor to the carrying out by a veterinary surgeon of an operation which is, in the veterinarian's opinion, necessary for reasons of injury or disease.

   The regulations prohibit the following:

   (i) penis amputation and other penile operations;
   (ii) freeze dagging of sheep;
   (iii) short-tail docking of sheep, unless sufficient tail is retained to cover the vulva in the case of female sheep and the anus in the case of male sheep;
   (iv) tongue amputation in calves;
   (v) hot branding of cattle;
   (vi) tail docking of cattle;
   (vii) devoicing of cockerels;
   (viii) castration of a male bird by a method involving surgery;
   (ix) any operation on a bird with the object or effect of impeding its flight, other than feather clipping;
   (x) fitting any appliance which has the object or effect of limiting vision to a bird by a method involving the penetration or other mutilation of the nasal septum;
   (xi) tail docking of a pig unless the operation is performed by the quick and complete severance of the part of the tail to be removed and either:

a. the pig is less than 8 days old, or

b. the operation is performed by a veterinary surgeon who is of the opinion that the operation is necessary for reasons of health or to prevent injury from the vice of tail-biting;

(xii) removal of any part of the antlers of a deer before the velvet of the antlers is frayed and the greater part of it has been shed;

(xiii) the tooth grinding of sheep.

Further protection is provided for the docking of pigs more than 7 days of age and the removal of antlers which are in velvet, if that becomes necessary, which can only be carried out with the use of an anaesthetic; this is enshrined in the Docking of Pigs (Use of Anaesthetics) Order 1974 and the Removal of Antlers in Velvet (Anaesthetics) Order 1980.

Similar legislation is to be found in other countries. The German Law on Animal Protection 1986 Section IV article 5 states:

1. Painful operations may not be carried out on vertebrates without anaesthetic. In the case of warm blooded vertebrates, the anaesthetic must be administered by a veterinarian. Whenever evidence can be produced that there is good reason to do so, the competent authorities may grant exemptions from the previous sentence if the anaesthetic is administered in cartridge form.

2. No anaesthetic shall be required if:

a. no anaesthetic is usually administered for comparable operations on human beings; [An interesting criterion! Also to be found in Belgian legislation!]

b. in the judgement of the veterinarian, it does not seem possible to administer anaesthetic in the specific case in point.

3. In addition, no anaesthetic shall be required for:

a. castration of cattle, pigs, goats, sheep and rabbits under two months old provided their anatomy shows no sign of deviation from normal;

b. the removal of horns or prevention of horn growth in cattle under six weeks old;

c. the docking of tails of piglets under four days old or lambs under eight days old;

d. the docking of tails of lambs under eight days old using elastic rings;

e. the docking of tails of puppies under eights days old;

f. the docking of the horny parts of the beak of poultry;

g. the removal, during the first days of the chick's lives of the claws of bail chickens intended for breeding.

In Sweden Section 25 of the Animal Protection Ordinance, 2 June 1988, reads:

1. It shall be permitted to castrate domestic animals, dehorn cattle and goats and tail lambs without veterinary justification.
2. The above measures may be taken without recourse to a veterinarian provided that:

   a. castration is performed on male animals, in the case of cattle and sheep before the animal has reached the age of two months and in the case of pigs before the animal has reached the age of six weeks.
   b. cattle are dehorned before the animals have reached the age of one month and goats before they have reached the age of two weeks; and
   c. lambs shall be tailed before they have reached the age of one week.
3. Male reindeer may be castrated without recourse to a veterinarian.

Note there is no reference here or elsewhere to the use of anaesthetics.

So much for protection of livestock whilst on farm. Such animals are also moved from farm to farm, from farm to market and from farm to slaughter. This movement is effected by the use of many forms of transport—road, rail, sea and air. Each form is covered by legislation and recommendations both nationally and internationally.

Transport of farm livestock

In principle all the legislation concerning the transportation of animals is essentially protective. It prohibits the carriage of animals that are sick and/or injured except under very special conditions and in some cases only with the specific approval of a veterinary surgeon. The legislation may also describe in minute detail the construction requirements of the mode of transport to be used together with the space required for each type of animal and the need for access to that animal during transport. Thus, Section 8(1) of the Swedish Animal Protection Act 1988 states:

> The means of transport used for the transportation of animals shall be suitable for the purpose and provide shelter against heat and cold and protect the animals from shocks and abrasions and the like. To the extent necessary, the animals shall be kept separate from each other.

Section 8(2) of the same Act allows the Government or the National Board of

Agriculture to issue further directions concerning the transportation of animals.

European Community Directive

Most countries follow similar provisions, although some set out requirements in very great detail while others merely set out principles. These latter are well illustrated in the Annex to the Council Directive of the European Communities (77/489/EEC) dated 18 July 1977, which covers the protection of animals during international transport. This in turn derives from an earlier Convention of the Council of Europe, the European Convention for the Protection of Animals during International Transport, dated 13 December 1968.

The Annex is divided into five chapters. Chapter 1 covers domestic solipeds and domestic animals of the bovine, ovine, caprine and porcine species e.g. Horses, Asses, Mules etc. It has five sections, one covering general provisions and the remaining four dealing respectively with special provisions for transport by rail, road, water and air. Chapter II relates to domestic birds and rabbits, Chapter III to domestic dogs and cats, Chapter IV to other mammals and birds, and Chapter V to cold-blooded animals.

Section A of Chapter I, dealing with General Provisions is of prime importance; apart from requiring all livestock to be inspected by an official veterinarian before export from their country of origin, it totally prohibits 'the carriage of animals likely to give birth during carriage or having given birth during the preceding 48 hours.'

Sections 4 to 12 of Section A then set out what are in effect basic principles for the transport of all species with the occasional reference to specific cases. Thus:

4. a. Animals shall be provided with adequate space and, unless special conditions require to the contrary, room to lie down.
   b. The means of transport and containers shall be constructed so as to protect animals against inclement weather conditions and marked differences in climatic conditions. Ventilation and air space shall be adapted to the conditions of transport and be appropriate for the species of animals carried.
   c. Containers in which animals are transported shall be marked with a symbol indicating the presence of live animals and a sign indicating the upright position. Containers shall be easy to clean, escape proof and shall be so constructed as to ensure the safety of the animals. Containers shall also allow for inspection and care of the animals and shall be stowed in a way which does not interfere with ventilation. During transport and handling, containers shall

always be kept upright and shall not be exposed to severe jolts or shaking.

d. During transport animals shall be offered water and appropriate food at suitable intervals. Animals shall not be left more than 24 hours without being fed and watered. This period may, however, be extended if the journey to the destination where the animals are unloaded can be completed within a reasonable period.

e. Solipeds shall wear halters during transport. This provision need not apply to unbroken animals.

f. When animals are tied the ropes or other attachments used shall be strong enough not to break during the transport under normal conditions, and long enough to allow the animals, if necessary, to lie down and to eat and drink. Bovines shall not be tied by the horns.

g. Solipeds, unless in individual stalls, shall have their hind feet unshod.

h. Bulls over 8 months should preferably be tied. They shall be fitted with a nose-ring for handling purposes only.

5. a. When animals of various species travel in the same truck, vehicle, vessel or aircraft, they shall be segregated according to species. Furthermore special measures shall be taken to avoid adverse reactions which might result from the transport in the same consignment of species naturally hostile to each other. When animals of different ages are carried in the same truck, vehicle, vessel or aircraft, adult and young animals shall be kept separate; this restriction shall not, however, apply to females travelling with their young which they suckle. With regard to bovine, soliped and porcine animals, mature uncastrated males shall be separated from females. Adults boars shall also be separated from each other. This shall also apply to stallions.

b. In compartments in which animals are transported, goods shall not be loaded which could prejudice the welfare of the animals.

6. Suitable equipment for loading and unloading of animals such as bridges, ramps, or gangways shall be used. The flooring of this equipment shall be constructed so as to prevent slipping, and the equipment shall be provided with lateral protection if necessary. Animals shall not be lifted by the head, horns or legs during loading or unloading.

7. The floor of trucks, vehicles, vessels, aircraft, or containers shall be sufficiently strong to bear the weight of the animals being transported, close boarded and so constructed as to prevent slip-

ping. The floor shall be covered with an adequate amount of litter to absorb excrement unless this can be dealt with a different way presenting at least the same advantages.

8. In order to ensure the necessary care of the animals during transport, consignments of livestock shall be accompanied by an attendant, except in the following cases:
   i. where livestock is consigned in containers which are secured;
   ii. where the transporter undertakes to assume the functions of the attendant;
   iii. where the sender has appointed an agent to care for the animals at appropriate staging points.

9. a. the attendant or sender's agent shall look after the animals, feed and water them, and if necessary milk them.
   b. Cows in milk shall be milked at intervals of not more than 12 hours.
   c. To enable the attendant to provide this care, he shall, if necessary, have available a suitable means of lighting.

10. Animals which become ill or injured during transport shall receive veterinary attention as soon as possible, and if necessary be slaughtered in a way which avoids unnecessary suffering.

11. Animals shall only be loaded into trucks, vehicles, vessels, aircraft, or containers which have been thoroughly cleaned. Dead animals, litter and excrement shall be removed as soon as possible.

12. Animals shall be transported to their destination as soon as possible, and delays, particularly in transshipment and marshalling yard, shall be reduced to a minimum.

These provisions as part of a European Community Directive have been incorporated into the legislation of all Community Member States. Although they only apply to animals that are moving from one country to another within and into and out of the European Community the principles set out will be found in one form or another in the domestic regulations of most countries whether within the European Community or not.

Other transit legislation

Swiss transit legislation

The Swiss, in Part 6, Articles 52 to 56 of the Federal Act on Animal Welfare of 9 March 1978, set out:

(i) Responsibilities of the sender (Art. 52).
(ii) The way in which animals shall be prepared for and cared for during the journey (Art. 53).
(iii) The requirements which the mode of transport shall satisfy (Art. 54).
(iv) The design and mode of construction of the transport containers themselves (Art. 55).
(v) Exception for 'postal and air transport' providing the animals are caused neither suffering nor injury (Art. 56).

Norwegian transit legislation

Norway, in Section 3.1 of its Transport of Live Animals Regulations issued by the Ministry of Agriculture on 10 May 1984, prohibits the transport of certain classes of animals:

a. large, pregnant animals during the last two weeks before birth is expected to take place;
b. other pregnant animals likely to give birth during transport;
c. animals which have given birth during the 48 hours prior to transport;
d. ill or injured animals;

However, these prohibitions:

> ... do not apply if veterinary or animal welfare considerations dictate that the animal should be transported, or if there are no veterinary or animal welfare doubts connected with such transport. This exemption also applies in the case of seasonal transfer to other areas of reindeer by boat.

So principles and then details are set out, prohibitions are made but exceptions are granted to enable traditional husbandry providing the overriding need to safeguard the welfare of the animals involved is not breached.

IATA regulations

With regard to the transport of all animal species by air, it is interesting to note that the International Air Transport Association (IATA), through their Live Animals Board, issue 'regulations' covering air transport which are binding on all member airlines. These regulations have been adopted by the Office Internationale des Épizooties (OIE), in Paris, and have become 'recommendations' to all member countries of the OIE within the Zoo Sanitary Code issued by that organization.

Markets

Farm animals are in a very few countries exposed for sale in markets as known in the UK. The welfare of animals in these situations is covered by the same principles of legislation which related to the on-farm situation and during transport. Thus in Great Britain the Markets (Protection of Animals) Order 1964 (as amended) protects cattle, sheep, goats and swine while being exposed for sale or awaiting removal. The orders also allow a Veterinary Inspector to treat or cause to be treated, or cause to be removed from the market to a suitable place for treatment, any such animal which is being caused or likely to be caused, unnecessary suffering. Furthermore, the orders provide for feeding and watering during the marketing process and require animals to be penned so as to avoid injury and overcrowding. They also allow for the separation of some categories of animal and for certain categories of animal to be kept under cover and protected from the weather.

Enforcement of legislation

With all this legislation there is a need for effective implementation or the legislation is liable not only to be disregarded but to be held in contempt.

In all countries central government has the overall responsibility for enacting the principal legislation relating to animal welfare. Central government is also responsible for ensuring that such legislation and any subordinate legislation is publicized and enforced. Usually enforcement is delegated to a specific authority. In Great Britain enforcement is the responsibility of the State Veterinary Service of the Ministry of Agriculture, Fisheries and Food, and at local level of the County Councils.

In Sweden central government delegates authority to the National Board of Agriculture, which according to Section 24(1) of the Animal Protection Act 1988:

> shall exercise central supervision in compliance with this Act and, unless otherwise stated, the directions which have been issued under the provisions of this Act. The National Board of Agriculture shall co-ordinate the activities of other supervisory authorities and, if necessary, give advice and assistance in these activities.

Section 24(2) of the same Act states: 'The local Environment and Health Protection Committees shall exercise supervision in municipalities unless the Government has prescribed that supervision shall be exercised by other means.' Section 24(3) adds: 'other supervisory activities shall be exercised by the authority or authorities so empowered by the Government' and Section 24(4) completes the enforcement provisions by stating: 'The Police Authorities shall if so requested give such assistance as is necessary in the exercise of supervision.'

In Norway the police have a primary responsibility in the enforcement of the Welfare of Animals Act 1974. However, they are by virtue of Section 23 of that Act assisted by animal welfare boards appointed by each local authority (borough, urban or rural district). Each board has three to five members. The District Veterinary Officer or another veterinarian appointed by the Ministry of Agriculture may join the Board. Members, and an equal number of substitutes, are elected by the local authority council for a period of four years. Primarily it is persons with practical knowledge of animal husbandry and animal care that are elected to the board.

A similar mixture of enforcing authorities is found in most countries. Voluntary welfare organizations also play a part in animal protection generally, although mainly in the field of companion animals.

Yet it is true to say that even with this large body of legislation and considerable activity on the part of enforcing authorities instances of cruelty, neglect and poor animal welfare still occur. In the brochure on animal protection published by the German Federal Minister of Food, Agriculture and Forestry, issued in 1986, under the heading 'everyone is responsible' one reads:

> Legislation alone cannot create animal-lovers. All it can do is to delimit the reasonable and permissible and lay down basic standards for protecting animals.
>
> No doubt even in the future, public opinion will remain divided on such fundamental issues as livestock farming or experiments on animals. However, compromises must be reached to impose at least minimum standards to protect the interests of animals; they will not please everyone.
>
> Government measures such as laws and regulations alone cannot protect animals. Responsible, considerate behaviour by every citizen is far more important.
>
> Every law and regulation is only as good as the measures taken to enforce and observe it. This is the job not only of the authorities but also of every individual citizen.

Approval of housing and equipment

It is interesting to note that two countries, Sweden and Switzerland, go further than most others in their efforts to improve animal welfare. These two countries require prior approval of livestock housing and systems.

Legislation in Switzerland is very specific. Articles 27, 28 and 29 of the Swiss Federal Regulations on animal protection cover the authorization of, and the procedure for, the approval of 'mass produced housing systems and in-house installations for cattle, sheep, goats, rabbits and domestic poultry.'

Article 28 requires a local manufacturer or the importer to apply to the Federal Veterinary Office, submitting such documents as are necessary for the assessment of the item or items. Where a test of the actual item proves necessary then this is carried out at one of the Swiss Federal Research Stations; in the case of cows, pigs, sheep and goats this is at the Research Station for Farm Management and Agricultural Engineering at Tanikon, while for poultry and rabbits it is at the Research Station at Zollikofen. The applicant has to pay a certain amount towards the examination of the housing system or installation concerned but the main cost is borne by the Federal Government. The procedure to be followed when an application for approval is received is set out in Figure 6.1.

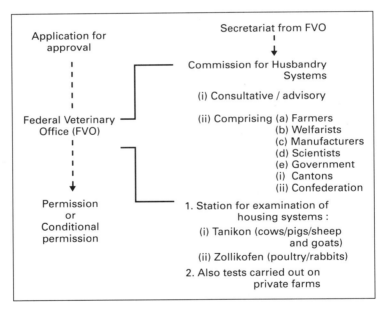

Figure 6.1 Procedure for approval of livestock housing and equipment in Switzerland.

If permission is refused, or only conditional permission given, and this is challenged by the applicant then an attempt is made by the Federal Veterinary Service to resolve the objections. If that is unsuccessful a formal appeal can be made to the Ministry of Public Economics which has a special section to deal with such matters. It may or may not require the Federal Veterinary Service along with the Advisory Commission to reconsider the matter. Ultimately the whole question can be referred to the Federal Courts.

Enforcement or education?

Recently in Great Britain the Farm Animal Welfare Council (FAWC), a government appointed advisory body, has published a report on the enforcement of farm animal welfare legislation and their related codes of welfare practice (Farm Animal Welfare Council 1990). The report recommended some change in legislation to enable better enforcement. It recommended new enforcement initiatives by all the statutory bodies concerned with the welfare of animals on the farm, in-transit, at markets and at slaughter. In effect the report found there was a need for more attention to be paid to animal welfare legislation by all those involved from the State Veterinary Service of the Ministry of Agriculture, Fisheries and Food to the local authority inspectors, which the report recommended (Para. 9.29) 'are fully trained and competent in animal welfare'.

The same report emphasized that the FAWC did not regard the number of prosecutions to be the sole indicator of enforcement activity. The report authors stated: 'we believe that education, advice and good stockmanship are the key to improved welfare' (Para. 8.2). Indeed, these are surely crucial to any improvements in animal welfare that are to be achieved in the coming years.

International initiatives

Progress will almost inevitably be spurred by existing and future initiatives, from the Council of Europe's Standing Committee for the Welfare of Animals Kept for Farming Purposes and from the Commission and Council of the European Community. The former has already published the Convention for the Welfare of Animals Kept for Farming Purposes (see Chapter 1) and under it has issued a number of recommendations dealing with laying hens, pigs and calves. The Council of Europe has also promulgated a Convention dealing with the transport and slaughter of livestock.

These latter two Conventions have already been taken up by the European Community and have been agreed as Community Directives, which have now been incorporated into law in each of the Community Member States.

This will almost certainly become the trend with the realization of a Single European Market. The Commission has already published draft Directives dealing with the keeping of calves and pigs. These drafts bear a close resemblance to the Recommendations concerning the same species agreed and published by the Council of Europe.

Yet in the end questions still remain. Is legislation the correct way to improve the welfare of animals? If it is how do we ensure that not only is the content of such legislation appropriate for the purpose but that such legislation is flexible enough to enable changes to be made in the light of scientific findings?

Perhaps there are no easy answers to either question. It will remain the responsibility of everyone involved in livestock production to ensure they are well informed and capable of making valid judgements on situations they find themselves faced with in their working life. To that end it could be argued that education is probably the key to animal welfare improvements with legislation kept for the, hopefully, few recalcitrants.

PRIVATE HEALTH SCHEMES
R G EDDY Esq., BVetMed, FRCVS

History
Objectives of herd health schemes
Factors affecting the uptake of herd health schemes
Requirements of a herd health scheme
Components of a herd health scheme
Marketing herd health schemes
Other agency health schemes
Herd health packages
Pigs
Sheep
Appendices

Humans need to eat. The production of food of both animal and plant origin, at affordable prices, is an essential requirement of human society. A balanced diet is also essential for optimum human health, and this diet will include meat, milk and milk products. It is therefore not surprising that much effort has been directed in this century to improve the output and efficiency of production from livestock that are intended to produce food, whether in the form of meat or milk. At the same time, much effort has been directed at improving the health characteristics of food in terms of both its composition, e.g. increased lean/fat ratios, and reducing the risk of transmission of zoonotic infectious disease.

The veterinarian, at all levels, has made a major contribution to this improved productivity, whether working in research, industry, public laboratory, state veterinary service or in practice.

During the first half of this century the main veterinary input into food-producing animals was in the control of the major epizootic infectious diseases, such as rinderpest, tuberculosis, brucellosis, foot-and-mouth disease and swine fever. Although the main stimulus for controlling these diseases was their negative effect on animal productivity, there was also an incentive from the human health aspect, especially with tuberculosis and brucellosis.

History

The evolution of health schemes operated by the practising veterinary surgeon (PVS) began in the 1940s. Previous to 1940, the PVS was primarily concerned with the equine species, and when called to farm livestock it was to assist at parturition or treat the individual sick or injured animals, what more recently has been called a 'fire brigade service'. During the 1940s in the UK, when there was an urgent need to rapidly improve the productivity from British farms, the first structured health scheme was introduced, known as the four disease scheme. This scheme was a valuable attempt to involve the PVS on the farm to help reduce the economic losses that were then attributable to mastitis, abortion, sterility and tuberculosis. The practitioner was supported with technical expertise from specialists within the State Veterinary Service. This was a valiant attempt to develop an advisory partnership between the farmer, PVS and the State Veterinary Service to the ultimate benefit of the farmer, the PVS and the nation.

During the period 1945–1960, there was an unprecedented growth in farm animal practice, at a time when society was enjoying increasing affluence and meat and milk consumption was rising rapidly. Because farm animals were in demand and their value rose, it became economical to treat sick animals and, together with introduction of chemotherapy and antibiotics, the PVS was in great demand. However, this demand kept the PVS extremely busy with 'fire brigade' work, helping with tuberculosis eradication and state-controlled vaccination schemes, for example swine fever and brucellosis. There was no incentive for the PVS to promote the concept of preventive medicine and herd health advice, although the advent of vaccines, such as clostridia and oral parasitic bronchitis, did allow some preventive medicine to take place.

During the early 1960s, fertility control programmes began to evolve in the USA (Morrow 1966) as it was already well recognized that poor fertility was a major constraint on the productivity of most dairy farms. Similar control programmes were introduced into the UK in 1963–64 by forward-looking practitioners, such as J Nicol and Wood (personal communication). These early workers recognized the importance of cow identification, data recording and a record system where cows requiring attention could be easily identified and analysis of herd performance could be regularly performed.

During the 1960s farmers were learning to treat their own sick animals and to carry out more procedures, including dystocia correction, castration, calf debudding and routine vaccination. At the same time, there were attempts to control specific diseases, such as mastitis, parasitism and infertility. The definition of the word disease was beginning to take on a broader meaning and to include inefficiencies of management and stockmanship.

A major landmark in the history of herd health and veterinary involvement in preventive medicine was reached in 1968 when the Mid-West pilot exercise in preventive medicine was completed. This pilot exercise was a collaborative exercise between the University of Bristol, the practitioners of the Mid-West Veterinary Association and 14 Somerset farmers (Grunsell et al. 1969). This was an attempt to take a whole farm approach to the economic use of veterinary expertise. The starting point was a study of the profit and loss account to identify aspects of the farm that were underperforming. Economists, agricultural advisers and nutrition chemists would be part of the advisory team and brought in as and when required. The timing of the involvement of these experts would be decided by the practitioner in consultation with the farmers. Land use, alternative livestock strategies, fertilizer use and nutrition policies as well as herd health status, would all be discussed at quarterly advisory meetings where the effects of previous advice would be monitored. The success of this exercise led to the establishment in 1970 of a national pilot scheme called the Joint Exercise in Health and Productivity (Jointex), which was a collaborative scheme organized jointly between the British Veterinary Association (BVA) and the Agriculture Development and Advisory Service (ADAS). This involved a minimum of four joint advisory visits to the farm per year for three years. The joint visits were conducted by the practising veterinary surgeon (PVS) and the Agriculture Advisory Officer of ADAS and expert advisers consulted as and when necessary. To be eligible farmers had to be members of the ADAS farm financial analysis services which were used to monitor progress of the scheme.

A small fee of £60 per year was payable to the PVS on completion of the necessary health reports. The joint exercise did have a number of individual successes, some of which were dramatic, but unfortunately there were too many farms where there was insufficient data to accurately assess the impact of the joint advice on subsequent profitability. The scheme suffered from not recognizing the need for a health recording scheme which could analyse data and monitor performance. Some recording of disease incidents was performed by the farmer each month but no analysis was carried out.

Although on pig and poultry farms the whole-farm approach to preventive medicine continued to evolve, the development of herd health in the ruminant sector of livestock production took a new direction after the joint exercise. In dairy cattle practice fertility control became the main area in which the PVS was involved in preventive medicine and regular visits to the farm to carry out reproductive examinations and advise on improving reproductive performance of the herd became more common.

The introduction of fertility control programmes in the early 1960s also marked the debut of individual cow cards for recording health and fertility data. With a colour tag system these cards could be used to identify, at a glance, cows at various stages of the annual production cycle. Unfortunately, it was not possible to analyse the data on a herd basis so information on the health and fertility performance of the herd was not readily available. This deficiency had been recognized by Wood, a practitioner in Gloucester (personal communication), who set up a card index database at the practice which would supply action lists to be used at veterinary fertility visits, and would analyse herd fertility performance quarterly and annually. Thus records and record systems became valued by stockpersons and veterinarians alike and objective analysis of health and production became possible, particularly with the advent of computerized recording schemes.

One of the earliest workers in the field of computerized recording was R S Morris, at the Melbourne Veterinary School, who, with his co-workers, developed a fertility and health recording scheme using a mainframe computer, two-digit numerical codes, and post-in/post-out delivery system for the reports which were produced monthly and annually (Blood et al. 1978). This software was further developed at the University of Reading by Esslemont, his co-workers and a small number of practitioners, and in the UK became known as Melbread (Eddy and Esslemont 1973).

It became clear during the development of Melbread that a mainframe-based, post-in/post-out service for fertility and health had a number of constraints which prevented its widespread adoption. These included:

1. Slow turnround time, which made the reports out of date by the time they arrived back at the farm.
2. The voluminous nature of the reports. Large quantities of paper, tables and statistics were a major disincentive for the widespread adoption of this system.
3. Duplication of recording. A new system requiring the farmer to record many events in yet another place increased the time spent in on-farm recording.
4. There was a need to integrate health, fertility and production into one recording scheme, not only to reduce duplication of recording but also to be able to demonstrate the effects of health and fertility on production.
5. There was a need to validate data at the input stage, to avoid errors in the reports (Eddy 1982b). Errors in computer printouts were a major disincentive to the adoption of such schemes by herdsmen in the early days of computerized recording.
6. The two-digit coding system also became a serious constraint to those farmers who wanted to record detailed health events.

With the constraints recognized with rapid advances in computer technology, development of Melbread, the mainframe system, led to the production of DAISY, the dairy information system, which could operate on a mini-computer (Stephens et al. 1982). DAISY was purchased by two veterinary practices in 1979 and in the UK was the beginning of veterinary practice becoming involved in herd health and production recording. Similar developments were taking place throughout the world, and the 1980s saw the advent of numerous computer-based health and productivity recording schemes around the world.

Many notable advances in the knowledge of animal health control were made during the 1970s which enabled the PVS to increase his or her ability to successfully improve herd productivity by improving the health and fertility status of livestock production. Some of these were:

1. The report of the third mastitis field experiment (MFE3) in 1972, which showed the way forward to successful control of mastitis in dairy cows due to staphylococcal or streptococcal infections.
2. The quantification by Esslemont (1973) of the importance of oestrus detection in dairy herd fertility. At that time Esslemont calculated that for every day a herd calving index exceeded 365 days, the potential loss in production in the subsequent lactation would be 30 pence × the number of cows in the herd. In 1990 this loss is estimated to be £3.00. per cow per day the calving index exceeds 365 days.
3. The understanding of the epidemiology of parasitic gastroenteritis in sheep and calves was also a major advance in animal health knowledge which could be of considerable value to the PVS when advising on parasite control.
4. The introduction in 1976 of the synthetic prostaglandins was a major advance in fertility control, enabling planned breeding with fixed time AI in cattle.
5. The availability from 1985 of simple kits for assessing progesterone levels in milk, which has been shown to be a valuable aid in improving oestrus detection efficiency and accuracy (Eddy and Clark 1987).
6. Considerable advances in the immunology have led to the production of some effective vaccines in all farm livestock, for example *Leptospira hardjo*, rotavirus, intra-nasal respiratory virus vaccines for cattle, porcine parvovirus in pigs and Marek's disease in poultry. The availability of these vaccines has increased the role of the PVS, as their successful application invariably means changes in husbandry techniques are often required to obtain the greatest protection from the vaccines.

Thus, at the end of the 1980s, practitioners are equipped better than they have ever been to offer effective planned health and productivity schemes to their clients. The availability of sophisticated data processing and analysis systems, the increased knowledge of animal nutrition and animal husbandry and its effect on health, the availability of effective pharmaceutical products and vaccines leave the modern PVS in a position of great influence with livestock keepers. This chapter will analyse how effective this influence has been and possibly how it can be increased in the future.

Objectives of herd health schemes

Optimum production is rarely achieved in livestock units and a major constraint to this is the presence of disease, suboptimal fertility or management practices that either encourage diseases to become manifest or directly restrict the level of production achieved. This premise is the cornerstone on which veterinary activity is based, to the benefit of the PVS, the farmer and the animal. The ever present goal is to control and manage animal health and production at a high level of efficiency and, at the same time, to seek and introduce new techniques that will continue to improve efficiency (Blaxter 1979). Many farmers are continually striving to introduce new techniques to their units; some improve health and productivity and are widely adopted, whereas others apparently at first improve productivity but later health and welfare problems emerge and any initial gains in productivity achieved are not always maintained. It is the veterinarian's role to oversee the introduction of new techniques, monitor their effect and identify any deleterious effects on health and welfare. The role of the PVS is exemplified by Muirhead (1980) and shown in Figure 7.1. Although this example refers to pig production the principles remain the same for all species. Besides the maintenance of optimum production, through the control of health and fertility, there are other roles for the PVS on all livestock units. These include ensuring that high standards of animal welfare are maintained at all times, identifying zoonotic diseases that may occur and preventing these entering the human food chain, and ensuring that pollution of the environment from animal wastes is minimized.

Factors affecting the uptake of herd health schemes

It is essential that the veterinary input is financially beneficial to the livestock owner. Without an economic benefit, the farmer will not continue to employ and pay for veterinary services and advice. The use of the veterinary surgeon will then be limited to emergency treatment of sick and injured animals.

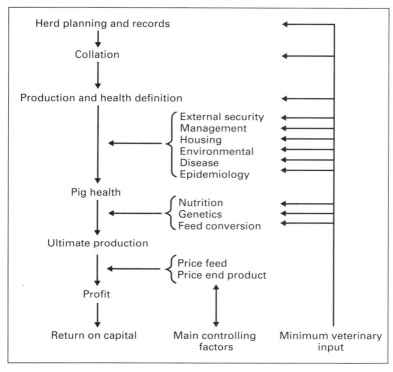

Figure 7.1 The role of the veterinary surgeon in intensive pig production (from Muirhead 1980).

However, the farmer, like any other businessman, will pay for a service which improves his productivity. The most frequent obstacle to this development is the lack of information of the effects of disease on herd productivity, and to overcome this it is necessary for the PVS to demonstrate to the farmer the benefits that have accrued following veterinary intervention. Hence the requirement of a sophisticated recording and analysis system. Many failures by practitioners to continue to operate herd health programmes are not due to lack of improved productivity but more often to lack of measurement of the productivity before and after intervention.

Costs and benefits

Farmers perceive veterinarians primarily as providers of clinical services only (Goodger and Ruppanner 1982). This view has subsequently been confirmed in the UK by the Lancaster University survey on the future of farm animal practice (Hopwood and Christie 1986). The reason, of course, is historical. Veterinarians in practice have traditionally provided a valued clinical service to the livestock industry and with the rapid development of an armoury of therapeutic agents since 1945 they have continued to keep one step ahead of most disease situations as far as therapy is concerned. The subsequent use by farmers of veterinary services will largely depend on the experience of the outcome of previous encounters with employing veterinary services. There is always a relatively small cadre of farmers who are reluctant to seek veterinary help for sick or injured animals and frequently delay calling for veterinary intervention until an effective cure is impossible or extremely difficult. These farmers may be judging the value of veterinary help on the basis of previous experience where the outcome was less successful than expected or where the veterinarian gave an incorrect diagnosis, prognosis or treatment. In marketing terms this is called the repeat order phenomenon. For any business to succeed, repeat orders are essential and repeat orders only come following successful experiences. The PVS is also providing a service which requires payment of a fee. It has been the assumption of many veterinarians that farmers will only pay for procedures carried out or for products, i.e. medicines supplied, and that farmers are unwilling to pay for advice alone. This attitude among veterinarians is more perceived than actual and has been shown to be an incorrect perception. Advice should be considered by the PVS in the same way as other service professions provide advice and successfully charge a fee. Livestock owners will pay for successful advice and will return for more help if the previous advice was successful. The repeat order phenomenon applies as much to advice as it does to skills and products.

One particular problem with herd health advice is that there often exists a considerable time lapse between paying for the advice and the benefits appearing in the form of improved productivity. For example, a lame cow can be attended, her foot abscess diagnosed and treated, and the cow will be walking normally within 3–5 days. The farmer is pleased and willingly pays for the service. However, if the farmer seeks veterinary advice to prevent a laminitis and solar ulcer problem, which is present in the herd, the advice may well involve considerable expenditure in alterations to the buildings, the bedding used or the method of effluent disposal, and even if the advice is effective the benefits in terms of the reduction of lameness incidence and subsequent improved milk production may take several months. In dairy herd fertility control any improvements that may be achieved by reducing the calving-to-conception interval and culling rate will not be rewarded financially until after the beginning of the subsequent calving season, i.e. 10–12 months following veterinary intervention. An added complication in fertility control is that milk output of the herd actually declines 9–10 months after the start of successful intervention as cows are dried off earlier in preparation for the subsequent calving season. The result is often that the dairy farmer is faced with a bill from his PVS for a fertility control programme but will not have seen the benefits and will not see any for several months to come.

There are also a large number of other advisory services to which the livestock farmer has access, such as feed company nutrition advisers, milking machine manufacturers, artificial inseminators, and staff of the milk purchasing co-operatives. Much of this advice is apparently without direct cost, although the cost must inevitably be incorporated in the cost of the service or product being supplied. Nevertheless, much advice relating to health and productivity is dispensed by such people in spite of the fact that the advice is rarely impartial. Accountants, bank managers and other financial consultants are also involved in advising farmers on profitability. The main problem with these people is they see veterinary and medicine costs on the profit and loss account as an unnecessary expense and one which should be reduced. Their advice for improving financial performance is too often to simply reduce expenditure rather than to look at benefit/cost ratios of the various cost items in the accounts. Perhaps the veterinary profession should spend more time educating financial advisers on the benefits that can be obtained from veterinary inputs.

Requirements and attitudes of individual farmers

Livestock enterprises vary enormously in size within any country and more so between countries. Smallholder farming is present to some degree in all developed countries and is still a predominant force in some Southern European countries. These farmers are generally employed full time in nearby towns and attend to the small number of animals before and after their day's work. In Germany, for example, the average dairy herd size is only 19 cows. Even in the more developed agricultural economies, such as the UK, there still remains a large number of relatively small farms in the less favoured areas such as Wales, Scotland and some parts of the West Country and where survival still depends on government support in the form of subsidies to assist production. Veterinary intervention would undoubtedly benefit many of these small enterprises but as the benefit/cost ratios will necessarily be less than with large livestock holdings, the task of convincing such farmers of the benefits of veterinary advice is more difficult.

It is also to be remembered that many farmers see their farming as just a 'way of life'. They value their independence, their freedom and just being able to live and work in the countryside. For many, their requirements from life are few and relatively inexpensive and as a large number are owner-occupiers with no outstanding mortgages and run farms which have been in the family for generations, they have no real incentive to increase their disposable income. These farmers perceive their veterinary surgeon as a friend of the family, who is always at hand when needed, but is only needed when there is trouble. Although they will usually require help to prevent the recurrence of disease, they find it difficult to understand the importance of subclinical infections and reduced performance due to management or nutritional inadequacies.

The profitability of some sectors of livestock farming is also maintained at an artificially high level, due to central government policies to support agriculture. In the EC some national governments, notably France, Germany and Italy, are intent on maintaining a profitable existence for their main small-holders and peasant farmers. This allows a living to be made from a small number of animals. This situation results in medium to large farms being very profitable in spite of many inefficiencies existing within the unit. This also explains the different attitudes towards herd health schemes as regards the different species. Poultry farming, for example, has become almost entirely conducted in large intensive units, which, because of consistently falling profit margins, have continually strived to look for ways of improving productivity. This has included the seeking of veterinary advice to reduce or minimize the effects of subclinical or clinical disease on production. In the UK pig farming is following the model set by poultry. Small, inefficient pig producers are now rare in the UK and here the cyclic fluctuations in the profitability of the industry have resulted in increased demand for veterinary advice. This demand has not always been met by the profession (see below). It is interesting to note that neither the poultry nor pig industry receives any significant government support in the UK.

At the other end of the scale, the beef and sheep farmers receive the most government support, generally because of the desire of governments to maintain the social fabric of rural areas, but neither of these sectors has historically been involved to any great extent in seeking veterinary herd health advice.

The dairy industry has always been the sector that employs the largest proportion of veterinary time. This is because of the diseases which result from the intensification of dairy cow production, such as mastitis, foot lameness, metabolic diseases and failure of reproductive performance. This sector also provides the greatest scope for veterinary involvement in the field of herd health control because of the constraints the various problems mentioned above have on milk production. However, in the last 20 years or more, dairy farming in Europe has always been profitable, even for the least efficient producers. Until the introduction of EC milk quotas in 1984, dairy farmers throughout Europe were paid a guaranteed price for all the milk they produced. This of course, led to overproduction, stockpiles of surplus butter and skimmed milk and the introduction of quotas in 1984. The introduction of quotas led to a fall in the number of dairy cows throughout Europe and the emphasis among dairy farmers in the UK switched to finding ways of increasing the efficiency of the production of their quota of milk, whereas before 1984 the emphasis was always to increase total production. This change in attitude has not resulted in a reduction of demand for veterinary services, except in areas where dairy cow numbers have fallen. The use of veterinary help to improve the efficiency of production is still a viable option to dairy farmers in the UK. However, within the dairy farming sector there remains a significant number of farmers, with units of varying sizes, who see no need for veterinary advice because of the relatively good level of profitability they currently achieve.

The inefficient producer can still achieve a reasonable income and a standard of living to suit his family's requirements.

However, there still remains a large number of livestock holdings which are motivated to improve their performance. This motivation may be economically based or simply a natural desire to improve performance and to improve the standard of living for the family. Many who are motivated for economic reasons need to achieve high levels of productivity and financial performance because of varying levels of debt, incurred to finance land purchase or building development. Many of these farmers, and their staff, have received further or higher education in agriculture where the benefits of veterinary advice are often taught. Also, in the larger dairy units most employed herdsmen have received further education and also are motivated to achieve a high level of performance. This motivation often stimulates the herd owner to seek herd health advice.

For the varying reasons postulated above, one can speculate on the proportion of each livestock sector which is likely to require or accept veterinary intervention in the form of herd health advice. In the poultry industry flock health advice is adopted in virtually 100% of the industry in the UK. In the pig sector the total market for herd health advice is probably in excess of 80% Muirhead (1980), which suggested that up to 15% of pig farmers are not receptive to advice. In dairy farming, the total market is probably no more than 50%. Although the market in the beef and sheep sectors is probably growing because of more economically motivated farmers entering the sectors in recent years, the market for herd or flock health schemes is probably no more than 20% at the moment.

Farm size

The trend of the last 50 years towards increased size of all livestock holdings has been apparent in all developed countries. Economies of scale can undoubtedly be achieved in larger units, particularly in the use of machinery and the employment of labour. This is most apparent in the poultry industry, followed by pigs and then dairy cattle. However, larger units invariably result in increased problems from disease and management inadequacies; for example, increased stocking densities are likely to increase the risk of infectious disease.

It is also apparent that disease patterns change with increased unit size. Intensive indoor beef or pig production, for example, may not be troubled with internal parasitism but the risk of respiratory disease is increased, and the increasing incidence of coccidiosis and parasitic gastroenteritis in grazing lambs in recent years is a direct result of increased stocking densities.

Inadequacies of management are also a feature of increasing unit size and the the reduction in the number of persons employed. In the 1960s it was normally accepted in dairy farming that 50 cows was the maximum that could be successfully managed by one herdsman, whereas in the 1990s, with the improvements made in milking machines, feeding equipment and effluent disposal, it is a common experience in the UK to find one person in charge of 150 cows.

While one individual can certainly milk 150 cows and carry out the daily routine procedures required in a dairy herd, he or she will find it difficult to find the time necessary to observe and inspect the cows frequently enough to detect abnormalities in behaviour that may be the signs of impending disease or even to detect the signs of oestrus. One-and-a-half hours a day are required for oestrus detection alone (Esslemont 1973). A busy herdsman in charge of 150 cows may not find the time required for good oestrus detection, resulting in depressed reproductive performance.

Building design

The trend of amalgamation of farms and development of larger livestock units in the last 30 years was stimulated in the UK by government and EC grants, particularly for livestock buildings. It is unfortunate that many buildings were erected without any scientific knowledge of the animals' requirements, particularly in the areas of temperature control, ventilation and comfortable lying areas. Respiratory and enteric diseases have become severe problems in intensive pig and cattle herds because of poor building design and high stocking densities. The high stocking densities have also been required because of the high capital cost of many of the buildings erected. Low-cost buildings, e.g. for calf rearing, are available where low stocking densities are acceptable, but unfortunately when buildings were grant aided, such structures frequently did not qualify for grant. The adoption of slurry systems for effluent disposal has resulted in inadequate bedding being used in pig, beef and dairy cow buildings. Adequate bedding is incompatible with slurry disposal systems; furthermore, the straw is considered by many farmers to be too expensive for use as bedding. Thus, changes in behaviour are frequently encountered, which lead to increased disease problems. For instance, cubicles or free stall systems were installed in the late 1960s to conserve bedding. Not only were many of these cubicles too small but the lack of a comfortable bed resulted in dairy cows spending longer periods of the day standing than normal, resulting in an increased incidence of solar laminitis and ulceration (Colam-Ainsworth et al. 1989). Currently the annual incidence of lameness in UK dairy cows is of the order of 25% (Kelly 1990). The main problem with inadequate building design is that once erected and in use, alterations can be very expensive and farmers are usually reluctant to make the necessary changes unless they can be convinced of the economic benefits that may accrue.

Veterinary competence and attitudes

The education and training of veterinary surgeons has always been heavily biased towards the production of clinicians to attend individual sick or injured animals. The artificial division within veterinary schools of departments of pathology, animal husbandry, medicine and surgery maintains this emphasis on treatment of individual animals. The division of the clinical teaching departments into medicine and surgery has evolved from a similar approach in medical education, and in veterinary education is ideally suited to the teaching of companion animal medicine and surgery. However, for farm animal teaching, the profession would be best served if clinical farm animal medicine were taught from one department which encompassed animal husbandry, medicine and surgery. Thus, the importance of animal husbandry in the whole field of herd medicine would be enhanced and greater emphasis on preventive medicine in the curriculum would be the result. It is also to be understood that the rate of advancing knowledge is such as to produce severe constraints on the teaching timetable. Perhaps undergraduate specialization should be considered. There is no doubt that the modern veterinary graduate is extremely well versed in the basic sciences and has a good grounding in clinical techniques but knowledge and skills in herd medicine are limited. This, of course, is not a new phenomenon. It has always been this way and those practitioners that have successfully employed herd health schemes are largely self-taught with the help of some continuing education courses, provided by the species veterinary associations.

The PVS has also suffered from a lack of objective analysis of the costs and benefits of herd health schemes which could be used in marketing his or her services. There have been relatively few publications in this field. The Mid-West Pilot Exercise in the UK (Grunsell et al. 1969) was a start in this direction but because the approach on the farm was all embracing, accurate cost/benefit evaluations were not possible. The approach by Blood et al. (1978) at Melbourne was the first to provide cost/benefit evaluations of various aspects of dairy herd health schemes and was a major step forward in understanding the requirements of herd health control. Nothing similar has been produced in the UK.

To succeed in the application of herd health schemes, the PVS needs to have a thorough understanding of the economics of agriculture, farm management and its effect on production, and of nutrition and its effect on livestock performance. Also a thorough understanding of epidemiology and the use of recorded data to help monitor herd performance and to measure the effect of disease and suboptimal management on production are required.

The problem is compounded by the attitude among many teachers in some veterinary schools that the future of veterinary practice lies with companion animals and that farm animal practice is in decline (Kyle 1990). This attitude is likely to increase the emphasis in the clinical teaching departments on companion animal teaching and reduce the teaching time for farm animal medicine. Herewith is another reason for separating farm and companion animal clinical teaching into different departments and the universities should ensure that the farm animal departments are properly staffed.

The structure of veterinary practice in Europe is not wholly conducive to the development of a high level of herd health expertise. In the average mixed practice all species, farm and companion animals, are usually attended. To develop the necessary expertise required to provide a high-quality herd health service, species specialization is necessary. It is not possible with the current state of scientific knowledge to develop skills in companion animal medicine and surgery and acquire the necessary knowledge and experience required in the field of dairy herd health, let alone all other farm species. In the UK veterinarians specializing wholly in poultry, pig or cattle medicine have evolved and these have successfully promoted herd health schemes which are now established within British agriculture. It is difficult to develop species specialisms within a 2–3-person mixed practice because there will be insufficient farms to provide the necessary experience to develop herd health expertise. Larger practices in the UK, in areas where livestock density is greatest, have been able to allocate species specialization to various members of the practice and these have successfully promoted herd health schemes to their clients.

Attitudes of practitioners will also be affected by the availability of work. During the period of tuberculosis and brucellosis eradication in the UK, practice income was generally buoyant with income from clinical work and the disease eradication schemes. Many practitioners did not perceive a need to further educate themselves within the fields of herd medicine. This has been compounded in the UK over recent years by the relative shortage of veterinary graduates and the declining income from eradication schemes has been compensated by the rapidly developing companion animal practice. Many practitioners who operated almost full-time farm animal practice in the 1960s and 1970s are now spending in excess of 80% of their time with companion animals. The increasing income derived from dispensing medicines in recent years has also been a disincentive to develop further expertise among some practitioners. If both the farmer and veterinary surgeon are content with their income, there is no incentive to develop. In a recent survey of UK veterinary practices involved with cattle work, Wassell and Esslemont (1991) found that only 3.12% of dairy herds received a full herd health scheme from their practitioner. This included regular visits to the farm and a recording service. A further 12% of herds did receive routine visits but without any recording service.

Requirements of a herd health scheme

Blood et al. (1978) identified the following as essential requirements of any successful herd health scheme:

1. A farmer willing and able to receive advice.
2. A competent veterinary surgeon willing and able to supply herd health advice.
3. Animal identification.
4. An efficient and effective recording scheme.
5. The necessary facilities for restraining animals.

The farmer

The willing farmer will be one who is always seeking to improve the performance of his farm. By definition this excludes that group described above who have no inclination to change or adopt new methods. In any defined community there is always a group who can be called the innovators (or 'group 1'). They are always seeking and exploring new techniques, only a proportion of which are likely to succeed. However, with these people the excitement of success will outweigh the disappointments of the inevitable failures. A second group comprises those who adopt new techniques only when they have been tried elsewhere. These 'group 2' farmers tend to be knowledgeable people who keep up to date by reading widely and attending meetings, courses and conferences. The majority of the community ('group 3') will only adopt techniques which have been tried and tested by both groups 1 and 2. The farming community is much the same as any other in the way it adopts new techniques, although there are probably more late or non-adopters ('group 4') than in many other communities. This is because, as described above, national and EC subsidies have allowed this category to maintain a living without the need to greatly improve efficiency, or the price of agricultural land has risen to such a level that they can sell their assets to neighbouring farmers and enjoy a comfortable retirement.

The willing farmer will also be one who is prepared to pay for advice. There will be no problem in convincing the innovator, or lead farmer, of the need to pay for advice or to adopt a herd health scheme. However, such people will also be critical of the exercise, will evaluate its performance and, if it does not succeed, will terminate the arrangement or not seek further advice from the same source, i.e. repeat orders will not be forthcoming. The second group in the farming community, the early adopters, are less easy to convince to adopt herd health schemes or to pay for advice but will do so if they can see success elsewhere. It is therefore important to succeed with the Group 1 farmers as failure here will make it extremely difficult to convince group 2 of the benefits of joining herd health schemes.

It is important with all groups that a relationship of confidence develops between the farmer and the veterinarian. This confidence will arise from the farmer's previous experiences of the veterinarian, and within a practice this may only apply to one particular veterinarian. When the farmer is confident of the veterinarian's expertise and advice he will be more willing to pay for advice and adopt new techniques such as herd health schemes.

If success has been achieved with the group 1 and group 2 farmers, the growth in the development of herd health schemes will gain momentum as the group 3 farmers (being the majority) learn of the successes. Attitudes of the farmers and previous experiences with their veterinary services will also be important.

The concept of paying for advice will, however, be a new experience for both farmers and veterinarians. However, the veterinarian must not under-value his services, even at the outset of a new exercise. Once fee levels have been set between him and farmers in group 1 and 2, these will be known by the group 3 farmers. It is always possible to reduce fees but to increase them, even once success has been proven, is extremely difficult.

Another factor which affects the willingness of farmers to adopt new techniques is age. Frequently the ageing farmer, who has made a success of his farming, is unwilling to make any more changes to his system. However, many such farmers will allow their sons to innovate and adopt new methods. With the increasing tendency for farmers' children to receive further or higher education, on return to the farm they are more receptive to the adoption of new techniques and to listen to external advice.

The adoption of a herd health scheme is only the beginning. To be success-ful for the PVS the maintenance of the scheme is essential, not only for the success of the practice but to convince the later adopters within the farming community. It may be necessary to restrict the scheme to one area of herd performance to convince the farmer of the value of the herd health advice. It would be wise to assess which area needs the greatest attention and select the one where success is most likely. For example, in a dairy herd it may be wise to concentrate on reproduction, obtain data on the previous year's performance, calculate the fertility indices and if there is scope for improvement institute a control programme and leave other problems until the farmer is convinced of the value of veterinary intervention. Once a confident relationship has been established between veterinarian and farmer and, assuming the reproduction control programme was successful, embarkation on other disease control schemes can be considered, such as mastitis, lameness, calf scour and calf pneumonia. Once success has been established in these areas the herd health scheme should develop into areas related to nutrition, housing, milk production (both yields and milk quality) and farm management. By this time the farmer–veterinarian relationship will have developed to the point where the farmer will consult the veterinarian whenever he plans any development, expansion or change in management. To the farmer the veterinarian has become indispensible to the success of his operation.

Competent veterinarians

The PVS is ideally suited to provide advice to farmers on a wide variety of topics, being geographically near to the farm and usually a frequent visitor to the farm. Apart from the artificial insemination technician he is probably the most regular visitor the farmer receives. In some countries, for instance in Austria, the PVS also carries out insemination so is an even more frequent visitor. On emergency or 'fire brigade' calls to the farm, the observant PVS will be looking at the stock for signs of illness of suboptimal production. Body condition, coat colour, coughing and diarrhoea are readily observed even in groups of stock which were not the prime reason for the veterinary visit.

A detailed knowledge of the value of stock, current market prices and a good understanding of the economics of production for the particular livestock sector can be obtained from agricultural magazines. The PVS should be able to discuss and comment on management accounts, gross margins, margin over feed costs and other such parameters used to measure production performance, and develop a working knowledge of the parameters used to measure physical performance in the sector, such as litres of milk per hectare, total butterfat per cow, growth rates in grams per day or feed conversion ratios for different age groups within the particular sector. Some of this may be taught at a basic level at veterinary school but mostly it will be learnt after graduation. Competence at clinical diagnosis, prognosis and providing effective therapy is of course essential and this does need at least 2–3 years postgraduate experience to develop. The PVS is not likely to enter the field of herd health until at least 2–3 years after qualifying. However, this is not to say that if the occasion arises he or she should not attempt to advise on prophylaxis for disease occurrences encountered in the course of clinical work. He or she would be expected to do this as an essential part of the training period.

Competence at certain technical skills is also essential; for instance, in dairy cattle practice good rectal technique is essential. Accurate diagnosis of pregnancy at 35 days post-service, detection of uterine abnormalities, and palpation and detection of normal and abnormal ovarian structures are all essential prerequisites of a fertility control programme. Competence at semen collection and evaluation from bulls, rams and boars will also be a useful attribute.

In other species, e.g. poultry and pigs, a competent postmortem technique needs to be developed and preferably, but not essentially, access to a practice laboratory. Whatever laboratory is used it must offer speedy turn round of results. These and other skills will take some time post-graduation to develop to the level required for successful participation in a herd health scheme. The use of milk progesterone assay to assess the accuracy of ovarian palpation is a useful technique and should be encouraged.

In the post-graduation period the PVS will also be developing a specialized interest in one or possibly two farm species with membership of the species veterinary association and regular attendance at Continuing Professional Development (CPD) courses for at least 5 days per year. This does mean that, for mixed practice, at least three veterinarians need to be employed in the practice; alternatively, single species practices will develop, as has happened in poultry and pig practice in the UK.

A detailed knowledge and understanding of epidemiology is also essential. Collection of data, data processing and interpretation of reports are also essential features of PVS-operated herd health schemes, and the schemes are only likely to succeed if the practice has access to data processing facilities.

Above all, the competent PVS will be able to communicate well with farmers and their employees. He or she must explain the findings, the advice and reasons for the advice in a manner which can be readily understood by all the farm personnel. Advice must always be followed by a written report, which will be readily understandable and not written using scientific jargon.

Punctuality is also important; arrival for farm visits should always be prompt and the same veterinarian should, wherever possible, make the visits to the farm whether for herd health work or for emergencies.

Technical input into the farm advisory programmes will be at different levels. Some PVSs will restrict their activities to prevention of disease and aspects of management which impinge directly on disease or reproductive performance; when specialist advice is required on certain aspects of the farm's development the PVS will seek specialist advice from other agencies or advise the farmer to do so. For example, in a mastitis control programme, the PVS may request assistance from a specialist agency to carry out the required tests on the milking machine or specialist advisers in building design may be consulted if alterations are required to existing buildings or a nutrition specialist consulted for ration formulation. If outside agencies are consulted for specialist advice this should be arranged by the PVS, who will consult the specialist for an exchange of information before making a joint visit to the farm. Reports from specialist advisers should be submitted to the PVS who will then discuss and interpret the advice with the farmer. In the UK specialist advice on infectious diseases is always available from the Veterinary Investigation Service, which will need to be consulted from time to time. Consultation with colleagues in other practices is not common but as specialized expertise develops among practitioners this should be encouraged.

Other practices, usually the larger group practices, will, for example, develop expertise in areas of management advice, building design, nutrition and milking machine testing, and will need to consult outside agencies much less frequently. If a high level of competence is achieved in these areas, there is no reason why this should not be of benefit to practice income. The larger group practices could well afford to allow at least one member of the practice to develop expertise in one or more of these areas and he or she would be consulted within the practice.

Animal identification

It is surprising that there still exists a number of farms where animals are not readily identifiable. Breeding animals such as dairy cows, beef cows and sows should be identified individually so that a lifetime history of breeding, production and disease occurrences can be recorded and readily available for analysis. The identification should also be easily read at all times without the need to restrain the animal. Freeze branding is now a proven technique with black- or dark-red-skinned cattle, but large plastic ear tags, with the animal number clearly written, are suitable for cattle and sows. Small metal ear tags used for unique identification for tuberculosis or brucellosis schemes are unsuitable for normal farm management requirements.

Members of commercial sheep flocks are rarely identified individually. However, rams must be identified and the breeding ewes should at least be identified by breeding group. Weaned animals for meat production can be identified by pen number or age group.

If animal identification is not practised on the farm, a herd health scheme should not be offered as it will not be possible to measure performance, and this will severely restrict the ability of the PVS to offer any sound advice.

Recording scheme

Analysis of data, to measure herd performance and to continually monitor performance, is the cornerstone of any herd health scheme. Before embarking on a herd health scheme, historical performance analysis needs to be performed to identify the areas of suboptimal productivity where action is required to improve the performance.

Many farms will have recording schemes in place, and efforts should be made to utilize these whenever possible. However, many recording schemes are designed for a specific purpose and may be of limited use in a herd health scheme. In the UK the most widely used dairy cow recording scheme is National Milk Records (NMR) operated by the Milk Marketing Board of England and Wales (MMB). This scheme provides excellent analysis of milk yield and quality performance for individual cows. However, disease recording is non-existent and the analysis that is available for reproductive efficiency, known as Herdwatch, is severely limited in its scope. It does provide analysis of heat detection efficiency, pregnancy rates and calving index but there is no detailed analysis to help the PVS diagnose reasons for inadequate performance in these three parameters. Approximately 35% of dairy farmers subscribe to the NMR.

Recording schemes operated by the Meat and Livestock Commission (MLC) for pig breeding and fattening herds, recorded beef herds and sheep flocks do provide valuable information on production and should always be consulted by the PVS and used to monitor continuing performance.

Duplication of record-keeping is a real problem on many livestock units, particularly dairy farms, as several systems may be in place, each designed for a specific purpose. In the UK all cattle farmers are required by statute to keep records of purchases and sales of all cattle in a Movement Register and in 1990 a regulation requiring farmers to record the identification of all calves born and their dam's identification was introduced. Other on-farm records frequently kept include: a farm diary where all events are recorded daily; individual lifetime cow cards; a book where calving dates are recorded; a card or book to record artificial insemination or service dates; and a variety of rotary wall boards on which, using pins or magnets, the stage of the breeding cycle of each cow can be readily identified. Therefore, events may be recorded in up to five places. Apart from NMR, no herd analysis is performed from these other systems; they act solely as a reference source for each event. The rotary wall boards are a valuable aid to management as they will predict impending events, e.g. dates due to calve, due for service, due for pregnancy diagnosis and due for drying off. However, such records are not permanent—when one event supersedes another, the previous record is lost.

The need for an integrated recording scheme to encompass production, lifetime history, reproduction events and disease recording and to produce comprehensive analysis of health, fertility and production, was identified in the late 1970s with the advent of mini- and micro-computers. In the UK a number of recording systems were developed for cattle and pigs, of which the most comprehensive were DAISY (Stephens et al. 1982) and PIGTALES

(Oldham, personal communication). Similar systems have been introduced in most developed countries, for example Dairy CHAMP (Udomprasert and Williamson 1990).

These integrated systems, designed for use on microcomputers, can be sited on the farm, or are often run as a bureau service to local farmers by agricultural advisers or veterinary practices (Eddy 1982b). The operation of the recording scheme by the veterinary practice is to be recommended. This allows the PVS to control the records, to advise on which events to record, to control which reports are required and to produce relevant analyses of performance whenever required. Furthermore, software developments are absorbed by the bureau when available, and errors are dealt with by the bureau operator, who can also be available for the interpretation of the reports. The added advantage is that the farmer becomes dependent on the practice and this encourages further involvement in herd health schemes. Practices who operate and control the recording schemes are more likely to succeed in the operation of herd health schemes.

Components of a recording scheme

The requirements for a recording scheme will vary between classes of live-stock. It is important that the system is simple to use and the amount of recording on-farm raw data is minimized. It is possible to record each event in one place only, in chronological order as events occur. Individual cow cards are still used for small herds of 50 or so cows, but the time required to analyse the data manually generally deters comprehensive analysis. As computer systems are now widely available, discussion within this chapter will concentrate on these.

Before adopting a computerized or manual recording scheme, it is important to use standardized terminology, without which it will not be possible to produce analysis which can be meaningfully compared with standard targets or the performance of other farms or livestock units. In the UK standard termino-logy has been produced for dairy cattle reproduction and pig production. These were published by the Ministry of Agriculture, Fisheries and Food (MAFF) and were produced after extensive consultation with MAFF person-nel and veterinarians active in the respective sectors. They are reproduced here as Appendices 7.1 and 7.2 and are available in booklet form from Her Majesty's Stationery Office (HMSO).

If the computer is sited on the farm, data can be entered daily by the farm secretary or farmer's wife. It is important that a discipline is established for data entry and that data is not entered by the herdsman. Experience in the UK has shown that if the herdsman operates the computer this reduces the time spent observing and working with the animals. If the computer is based at the veterinary practice office the discipline is established and weekly data entry is quite satisfactory.

Speed of turnround of reports is paramount to prevent the information being out of date. National schemes, like the NMR, suffer from a turnround time of up to 14 days. If the computer is practice located, data transfer can be by telephone, collected by the visiting PVS or actually taken to the bureau by messenger. It is now possible to process the data and produce the necessary reports within 30 minutes so the messenger can wait for the reports to be produced, consequently they may be back at the farm within 1 to 1½ hours. Even by telephoning in the data and posting out the reports turnround need not exceed 24 hours.

The recording system should be able to:

1. Store the lifetime history of production, reproduction and disease and pedigree information where required.
2. Store the current (lactation for dairy cows and farrowing parity for breeding sows) detailed and summary of individual animal production, reproductive and disease events.
3. Record medicines used, offspring identification and details of livestock sales and purchases.
4. Provide lists for action whereby the next event for individual animals is predicted in list form, e.g. for cows, dates due to dry off, to calve, due for service, or for sows, due to farrow, due to wean, due to serve, etc. In particular the action lists should identify animals that are past their target date for any event so that corrective action may be taken. This may involve presenting the animal at the next veterinary visit.
5. Provide analysis of production performance (both current and lifetime), reproduction efficiency and disease. The analysis should be available as and when required but generally summary analysis can be available for each veterinary health visit and detailed analysis prepared once or twice a year. The analysis should also be able to establish the effects that disease or fertility efficiency is having on production.

The design of the output reports is important. Minimum quantities of paper should be used and, where possible, graphs and histograms used for the analysis reports. The action lists should be printed on A5 size paper, so they can be used as pocket reports, always being carried by the herdsman. Voluminous computer printouts, with copious tables and statistics, are a disincentive to the adoption of computerized recording on farms.

Errors in the reports are also a disincentive to the use of computer-based systems. However, it has been shown that if all data are validated thoroughly at the entry stage the majority of errors originate in on-farm recording of the raw data (Eddy 1982b). Once the source of the error has been thus identified and a correction sought, the accuracy of the on-farm recording rapidly improves. Farmers instinctively attempt to find faults in computer printouts and then apportion blame to the computer. However, if it can be demonstrated the error is with their own record-keeping, they will make a determined effort to improve their own recording accuracy.

Once such an integrated system is in use on the farm and confidence is established by running it in tandem with existing systems for two or three months, the farmers should be persuaded to stop using the other recording books, wall charts, etc. so that the time spent in on-farm recording is reduced and more time is used to study the computer reports and take the necessary action with the animals. On some farms this has been shown to be difficult to achieve. For reasons of tradition or perhaps mistrust, many herdsmen are reluctant to abandon their traditional recording systems. An education exercise is therefore required by the PVS to explain and interpret the reports, identify their benefits and how best to use them and tactfully show that relying on the new system and abandoning all other recording will be to the herdsman's or farmer's benefit.

Flexibility of report production is also essential, if only to reduce the quantity of paper. The stock-person will require the action lists on a regular basis but the farmer or herd owner may only require some summary analyses. Once again the PVS will be required to spend time to determine what is required by the different farm personnel and which reports will benefit them the most.

Facilities for animal restraint

The facilities for restraining animals will vary considerably with the species being handled. For breeding beef and dairy cattle herds suitable crushes or stalls are required for rectal examinations. Pens for separating groups of animals for examination and treatments are also required for all mammalian species as is the provision of isolation and quarantine pens.

Components of a herd health scheme

The components of any herd health scheme are as follows:
1. Historical analysis of herd performance. This will include reproductive efficiency and disease incidence to identify areas of low productivity or where disease is affecting the herd's performance. Prepare a written report for the farmer and file a copy for future reference.

2. Identify areas which need immediate attention and for which reasonably simple solutions are available.

3. Identify other economically important problem areas which need improvement and set up an order of priority for the problem areas. Do not attempt to control all problems from the outset.

4. Set target performance figures for the identified problem areas.

5. Ensure that the recording scheme will provide the necessary information to regularly monitor the scheme.

6. Agree with the farmer the frequency of farm visits to be made by the PVS. The frequency will vary with species and according to which elements of the scheme are adopted. For dairy cattle where fertility control programmes form the core of most herd health schemes, visits should be made weekly or fortnightly. Dairy herds of 200 cows or more require weekly visits, at least during the breeding season. For herds of less than 200 cows, fortnightly visits should suffice. For pigs, frequency of visits are discussed on page 241. For sheep and beef suckler herds visits will need to be planned in relation to the production cycle. For sheep pre-tupping, pre-lambing and pre-weaning would be considered suitable by most operators of sheep health schemes.

7. The structure of each herd health visits (HHV) will also vary with the species but should contain at least the following:

   a. Review performance since the last visit, and review any production analysis reports available to the farmer.

   b. Check the list of animals being presented to ensure all required animals are presented, in particular animals requested for re-examination at the previous visit.

   c. Examine the animals.

   d. Record the findings and treatments following the animal examinations.

   e. Undertake any routine work such as vaccinations, foot trimming, debudding, etc.

   f. Inspect all stock on the unit and discuss current performance, body condition and nutrition.

   g. Carry out any necessary postmortem examinations and collect samples for laboratory examination where required, e.g. milk, faeces or blood samples.

   h. Discuss disease incidents since the last visit and examine records to ensure medicine use is recorded.

   i. Summarize the findings of the HHV.

   j. Collect data for the recording scheme and advise where necessary on recording accuracy.

   k. Produce a written report summarizing the visit and advice provided.

8. Emergency or 'fire brigade' visits to attend sick or injured animals

between herd health visits, or to investigate disease occurrences or disease outbreaks in groups of animals.

9. Consultations by telephone also become an important element of a herd health scheme. Farmers will wish to consult either their PVS increasingly by telephone and this should not be discouraged, even if the calls are made out of normal working hours. However, if advice is given, notes should be made and followed up by a written letter or report. This is particularly important if the advice involves medication.

10. The close relationship that develops between farmer and PVS should enable the PVS to persuade the farmer to obtain all his medicine supplies from the PVS. This will allow the PVS to control medicine use, to ensure they are used effectively and to supervise medicine recording.

11. For dairy herds, purely advisory visits once or twice a year, depending on herd size and calving pattern, should also be made where an up-to-date analysis of performance will be available. The discussion will review performance, identify whether targets are being met and where necessary adjust or set new targets. The costs of the health scheme will usually be questioned by the farmer at these visits and the PVS should be prepared to quantify the improvements made and make an economic assessment of the benefits of the scheme to date.

Even after the initial advice has been offered, it will be necessary to continually monitor performance, fine tune the advice and set new targets as shown in Figure 7.2.

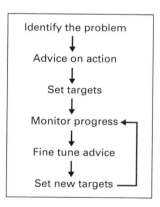

Figure 7.2 A schematic illustration of herd health control in practice.

These visits will present an opportunity to check the priority list and where problems have been overcome, to identify new areas for action. Also detailed discussion on economics of production, nutrition and other management inputs may be included so that the scope of the health scheme may be broadened and the veterinary involvement in the whole farm enterprise increased. Although these visits will primarily be discussions with the farmer, for at least part of the visit it is wise to involve the herdsman and all other staff who work with the animals. Again these visits must be followed by a written report with copies filed for future reference.

12. The account for services rendered. Although some workers suggest that a written signed contract should be drawn up at the outset of any herd health scheme, most veterinarians do not. The success of any herd health scheme depends on trust and confidence between farmer and PVS and a written contract should not be necessary. If a farmer is not satisfied with the progress being made, he will cease to employ the PVS, whether a contract exists or not. The method of payment should, however, be clearly stated at the outset, so that no misunderstandings arise. Most PVSs operate on a time-chargeable basis, plus medicines at retail prices and a small turnout or visit fee. Others set a capitation fee or charge per animal per year. Although, for historical reasons, the author practises the time-chargeable system he is of the opinion that a capitation charge per animal per year might be more acceptable to many farmers. A herd fertility programme for dairy cows takes 7–15 minutes per cow per year, with a mean of 9.9 minutes (Eddy 1981), therefore using the practice hourly rate a capitation fee per cow could be readily calculated. This would exclude visits for emergency work and medicines supplied.

Marketing herd health schemes

The British Veterinary Association (BVA) in 1983 was of the opinion that the failure of private herd health schemes to develop at a faster rate was due to lack of marketing by the profession of the services it has to offer the farming community. The BVA commissioned the University of Lancaster to conduct a survey of farmers and veterinary practices to evaluate the attitude of veterinarians to marketing their services and to seek the view of farmers on the operation of herd health schemes. A report was published and a series of actions undertaken to help the PVS understand the basic requirements of marketing farm animal practice and herd health schemes. One initiative was a joint one with the National Farmers Union (NFU) to set up an Animal Health Management Scheme (AHMS), which consisted of a series of one-day seminars for veterinarians and their clients at which papers were presented on the benefits of herd health schemes. Seminars were presented for cattle, sheep and pigs. In the first year the subject was reproduction and in the second year the young animal. Booklets were also produced to assist the PVS in the technical aspects of fertility and health control (AHMS 1 1984; AHMS 2 1985).

Marketing has been defined as the:

RIGHT PRODUCT

in the

RIGHT PLACE

at the

RIGHT TIME

at the

RIGHT PRICE

That veterinarians do not promote the services they can offer has been identified (Goodger and Ruppanner 1982; The Lancaster Survey, Hopwood and Christie 1986). There are a variety of reasons, among which is a lack of confidence by veterinarians in their own technical ability. However, other reasons discussed previously, such as a ready income from other sources, act as a disincentive for promotional activities.

Another marketing slogan is 'Buyers Buy Benefits not Features'. To promote herd health schemes, the benefits must be quantified and cost/benefit projections made.

(1) Newsletter	– stimulates interest
(2) Identify target market	
(3) Practice client meetings	– features discussed
(4) Small group meetings	– benefits discussed in detail
(5) One to one discussions	– discuss adaption to individual circumstances
(6) Produce league tables	– for discussion meetings

Figure 7.3 Stages in the marketing of herd health schemes.

Practice newsletters (Figure 7.3) are a starting point for informing farmers of services available. At least these can act to stimulate interest. However, practice newsletters must be regular, well presented and in a uniformly identifiable format (Hopwood and Christie 1986). Practice client meetings are best used once or twice a year to promote in detail a single aspect of herd health. These meetings have more impact if at least one member of the practice makes a presentation and they are not obviously financed by pharmaceutical companies (Hopwood and Christie 1986). Again these will further stimulate interest. However, if a specific herd health scheme is to be promoted this is best done with small groups (five to six farmers only) followed up by discussions on a one-to-one level (Eddy, 1982a).

Financial incentives may be necessary to encourage some farmers to join specific schemes. However, if these involve offering veterinary time and expertise for no, or reduced, fees, they should always be avoided. However, if for example a computerized recording scheme is being promoted to farming clients, incentives such as recording for 2–3 months either free or at reduced cost or a percentage discount for the first six months may be helpful in convincing farmers to join the service. Any farmers who fail to continue with the service can be seen as a failure on the part of the PVS to demonstrate adequately the benefits that exist.

In the right time and place also means identifying the target market for the scheme. As discussed previously, some members of the community, the innovators, will usually adopt new schemes more readily than others. However, it must be established that the scheme will be of benefit to the potential customer. There is little point therefore in attempting to set up a fertility control scheme for a dairy herd which already consistently achieves a calving to conception interval of 85 days and a culling rate of less than 18% or to attempt to market a computerized recording scheme to a farmer who owns an on-farm computer or who is completely happy with his national recording scheme. Although the principle of marketing first to the innovators or lead farmers is sound, exceptions do exist as were identified by Eddy (1982a) when promoting computerized recording to dairy farmers. He found that the majority of the early adopters of his DAISY recording scheme were those farmers that had no structured recording scheme for milk production or reproduction in place. Such farmers would not normally be considered lead farmers or innovators.

To maintain interest in a scheme and to promote the scheme to waiverers, a scheme club should be formed at which members regularly meet and to which interested non-members but potential clients can be invited. League tables of performance will be identified only by code but this does present the opportunity for farmers and stock-persons to compare their own herd's performance with their peers, and in discussion they may identify methods by which they can improve their herd's performance in one or more of the parameters in the league table. Such discussion needs tactful chairmanship by the PVS to avoid unnecessary embarrassment to those present whose performance is well below average. These meetings will also further stimulate non-members present to consider seriously whether to adopt a similar scheme.

Other agency health schemes

A number of individual schemes are operated in the UK by agencies other than the private practitioner, although involvement of the PVS is encouraged or in some cases is obligatory. These schemes will be briefly identified here but are discussed in detail later:

1. The mastitis control service operated by the MMB involves visits by trained technicians to dairy farms to discuss mastitis control. A bacteriology service is also offered and copies of reports may be submitted to the farmer's veterinary surgeon.
2. Foot trimming is also offered as a service by the MMB with the objective of reducing lameness by regular foot trimming for dairy cows. There is no involvement of the PVS in this scheme.
3. A dairy herd health and productivity service is offered by the Royal (Dick) School of Veterinary studies in conjunction with a national feed compounding company, Dalgety Agriculture Ltd. Involvement of the PVS is obligatory.
4. ADAS offers a dairy cow fertility analysis service known as Datamate, which is used in conjunction with advisory visits to discuss fertility efficiency by livestock husbandry advisers. There is no PVS involvement although the PVS may call in the service of a specialist adviser if he wishes.
5. The Pig Health Control Association (PHCA) exists to list herds which have been tested for the absence of specific infections, e.g. enzootic pneumonia, swine dysentery, Aujeszky's disease, atrophic rhinitis, mange and streptococcal meningitis.
6. Sheep health schemes have been developed at the University of Liverpool Veterinary School by Clarkson for teaching purposes and the education of private practitioners.

Herd health packages

This section will discuss individual herd health packages. As already stated, any veterinarian embarking on a herd health scheme would be advised to identify areas for improvement and offer herd health advice in the form of packages, concentrating on separate problems or disciplines.

Dairy cows: reproductive efficiency

Reproductive efficiency is the area where veterinarians are most frequently involved in dairy herds in developed countries. Many PVSs offer what are apparently herd health schemes. These should be considered as operating at varying levels:

1. Regular visits to the farm to conduct rectal examinations on cows presented by the farmer or stockperson. If a recording scheme exists, it is operated by the farmer or some external agency and any monitoring of performance or analysis is carried out by the farmer, the veterinarian having little or no input into policy decisions or diagnosing reasons for inadequate performance. These are frequently called 'routine visits'.
2. At a second level, the PVS will have access to the on-farm recording system for analysis or report production. This will enable the PVS to receive the information on the herd's performance from which he or she can monitor progress. The quality of the information will depend on the system adopted by the farm so the PVS is often still constrained by inadequate information.
3. At the third level the PVS will control the recording system, will identify cows that require attention at the herd health visit (HHV) and will decide when analysis of herd performance is required. Usually at this level the recording system will be installed at the veterinary practice.

Wassell and Esslemont (1992) from their survey of veterinary practices estimated that 12% of dairy farms in the UK received veterinary herd health visits at level 1 or 2 and only 3% at level 3.

Level 1 will not be considered further, as this cannot be called a herd health scheme and will frequently fail because no system is in place to ensure that the progress is monitored or the farmer is informed of any benefits that may accrue, and no information is available to the PVS on which he or she can offer sound advice. Such advice can only be based on reliable information and this is only likely to be available if the PVS has considerable input into the operation of the recording scheme.

Economics

It is important to realize the relationship between herd productivity and reproductive efficiency. Esslemont (1973), using a computer model, calculated that for every day the herd calving-to-conception interval exceeded 85 days, the average milk yield loss was 16 litres per cow. Thus, on milk yield alone and using a margin over concentrates of 13p per litre, a 1 day improvement in calving-to-conception will yield an increased margin of £2.08 per cow in the herd if the culling rate remains unchanged. However, there are other indirect economic effects on production, as described by Williamson (1987). As the calving-to-conception interval is reduced, the number of calves born increases, thus the number of replacement heifers available increases as does the number of bull calves available for sale. Improved reproductive efficiency is normally associated with reduced culling for reproductive reasons. This results in an increase in the average herd age or an increase in the number of cows culled for low yield. In either case, the effect will be an increase in average herd yield as the production level of cows increases with age up to the 6th or 7th lactation (Williamson 1987).

Williamson (1987) compared the performance of 21 dairy herds that used the Dairy CHAMP programme, with the average performance achieved by dairy herds participating in the Dairy Husbandry Improvement Association (DHIA) recording scheme. The results are summarized in Table 7.1.

Table 7.1 A comparison of performance-related indices and livestock inventory of Minnesota average DHIA and average Dairy CHAMP recorded herds (from Williamson 1987)

Herd size	Average DHIA herds	Average CHAMP herds
Herd size	56	56
Calving to conception (days)	126	107
No. of cows culled	19	15.5
Calves born per year	50	53
Males born per year	25	26.5
Females born per year	25	26.5
Calves died	4	4
Bull calves for sale	23	24
Females raised	24	25
Heifer replacements required	19	15.5
Heifers to sell	1	6

It is important to note that both calving-to-conception interval and culling percentage are critical indices when measuring reproductive efficiency. They should always be looked at together as frequently calving-to-conception interval can be seen to improve at the expense of increasing culling rate. In fact the two indices are inversely related. A reduced culling rate will yield an increased calving-to-conception interval if reproductive efficiency is not improved.

Using partial budgeting, Williamson (1987) measured the financial implications of the improved reproductive efficiency in the Dairy CHAMP herds and this is shown in Table 7.2. It is important to note the relatively high

Table 7.2 Budgeted returns from improved reproduction in Minnesota dairy herds
(from Williamson 1987)

Additional returns		Value $
Increased milk production due to improvement in calving–		
conception interval	17252 lb	
Increased milk production due to increase in average cow age	19430 lb	4219
In-calf heifers sold	4	4037
Bull calves sold	1	101
Total extra returns		8357
Additional costs		
Increase in veterinary costs		840
Feed for extra production		1067
Costs of raising extra heifers		1590
Total added costs		3497
Less returns no longer obtained		
Decreased cull cow sales	3.5 cows	1575
Net return from improvement		3285
Net return per cow		$58.66

By kind permission of N. B. Williamson

contribution to production income from the increase in herd age and the availability of heifers for sale following the reduced number of cows culled. If the herd policy was to purchase herd replacements then similar financial benefits would be achieved by a reduction in the number of cows needed to be purchased and the increase in number of calves available for sale.

Also in this example, the benefit/cost ratio of veterinary intervention can be seen to be 3285:804 or approximately 4:1. This kind of return should convince any dairy farmer of the benefits of herd fertility control.

Measuring herd fertility

The components of herd fertility and parameters used for analysing reproductive performance have been described in detail elsewhere (Eddy 1980) and are summarized in Figure 7.4. 'Farm policy' encompasses two factors. Firstly, the decision when to serve following calving. Some farmers wait until 70 days or more before considering 1st service and others may serve at the first oestrus after calving. The former will result in unnecessary delays in conception and the latter will result in reduced pregnancy rates. Service at the first oestrus after 50 days calved is a compromise that will result in a mean interval to first service of 65 days if oestrus detection is over 80%. Secondly, in seasonal or block calving herds, there is an involuntary delay in the interval to first service

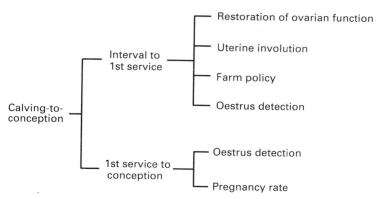

Figure 7.4 Components of the calving-to-conception interval.

in the cows which calve in the first 4 weeks of the calving season. In such herds an overall mean interval to first service of less than 70 days is difficult to achieve.

The fertility indices which need to be calculated are shown in Table 7.3. The interference levels are also included and are arbitrary levels at which action should be taken. If the indices calculated are better than the interference levels but still short of the desired targets, it is probably uneconomic to attempt to make improvements as there is unlikely to be a beneficial benefit/cost relationship. However, these are arbitrary and a final decision will need to be taken when the individual circumstances of each farm have been assessed.

While overall culling rate must be calculated, culling specifically for reproductive problems, as recommended by some workers, is difficult to calculate in practice. Cows are generally culled for more than one reason—e.g. a moderate yielding cow will be served once or twice but if she returns again she will be culled if there are sufficient replacements. The same may be said for cows with poor conformation or advancing age, or a cow returning for the third time that has recently become lame may be culled for a combination of failure to conceive and lameness. To overcome this difficulty, and to be able to make comparisons between herds, it is more useful to analyse the percentage of cows calved which are served at least once and the percentage of cows served which eventually conceive. It can be reasonably assumed that if cows receive a first service it is the intention they should calve again and if they fail to conceive this is an indication of reproductive inefficiency.

Measuring oestrus detection efficiency directly is difficult. It is wise to first make an assessment of oestrus detection accuracy by measuring the percentage of interservice intervals that are less than 18 days. In normal herds with accurate oestrus detection, less than 10% of interservice intervals will be less than 18 days. In such an event oestrus detection rates (ODR) can be calculated:

Table 7.3 Fertility indices that need to be recorded in dairy herd reproduction analysis with target and interference levels

	Target	Interference
Calving-to-conception interval (days)	85	95
Calving to 1st service (days)	65	70
Mean interval 1st service to conception (days)	20	25
Pregnancy rate to 1st service (%)	60	50
Pregnancy rate to all services (%)	60	50
Overall culling rate (%)	<18	>23
Per cent served of cows calved	95	<90
Per cent conceived of cows calved	85	<80
Per cent conceived of cows served	95	<90
Per cent of interservice intervals 18–24 days	60	45
Per cent of interservice intervals <18 days	8	12
Submission rate (%)	90	<75

$$ODR = \frac{No. \ of \ interservice \ intervals}{No. \ of \ interservice \ intervals + No. \ of \ missed \ heats} \times 100$$

To calculate the number of missed heats interservice intervals of:

$$30–50 \ days = 1 \ missed \ heat$$
$$50–70 \ days = 2 \ missed \ heats$$
$$70–90 \ days = 3 \ missed \ heats$$

Wood (1976) suggested the following formula:

$$ODR = \frac{21}{Av. \ inter\text{-}oestral \ interval} \times 100$$

This formula will be influenced by oestrus detection accuracy and a high percentage of short intervals. A commonly used parameter is the ratio of 3-week (18–24 day) to 6-week (36–48 day) inter-oestral or interservice intervals, with a target figure of 7:1. Also when calculating oestrus detection rates, interservice intervals (i.e. intervals after 1st service) should be used as on many farms recording of oestrus dates before first service is sporadic and it is normal to find many intervals between 1st and 2nd oestrus post-calving to be less than 18 days. The various methods of assessing oestrus detection efficiency and oestrus detection rates are summarized in Table 7.4.

Oestrus detection accuracy must also be assessed because of its detrimental effect on the herd pregnancy rates, and it always needs to be considered when assessing the reasons for poor pregnancy rates. The percentage of total heats recorded which are inaccurate is approximately:

$$\frac{per \ cent \ of \ intervals < 18 \ days}{2}$$

Table 7.4 Six methods for assessing oestrus detection efficiency

---

1. $\text{ODR} = \dfrac{\text{No. of interservice intervals}}{\text{No. of interservice intervals} + \text{No. missed oestruses}} \times 100.$

2. $\text{ODR} = \dfrac{21}{\text{Average inter-oestral interval}} \times 100.$

3. Per cent of all interservice intervals that are between 18 and 24 days.
   Target $> 60\%$

4. Ratio of 18–24-day intervals to 36–48-day intervals.
   Target $= 7{:}1$

5. Per cent of cows demonstrating oestrus by 60 days post-calving.
   Target $> 85\%$

6. Per cent of cows served by ESD + 21 days.
   Target: 90%

The initial historical fertility analysis should be conducted for the previous two calving seasons whenever the data are available. The calving season should be identified and for autumn-calving herds the indices for all cows calving 1 July to 30 June calculated for each of the two previous years. For spring-calving herds, the indices are calculated for cows calving 1 January to 31 December.

For genuine all-year-found calving herds, the indices for cows calving in the period 30 months to 6 months before the date of investigation should be calculated. Thus, at least 6 months will have elapsed to allow the last cows in the analysis to conceive although the culling rate for cows currently in lactation will still not be complete.

Having completed the analysis, priority areas for setting the targets should be discussed with the farmer. Experience has shown that the one parameter which is most easily influenced is calving-to-1st service interval and a target of 65 days should be set, with the exception of block calving herds where the target would be 70 days.

Investigation of low pregnancy rates should first involve an assessment of oestrus detection accuracy and secondly a look at whether some cows are being served too early after calving. The third action for investigating pregnancy rates is to construct Cu sums, in service date order (Eddy 1980). This will indicate whether the poor pregnancy rate is consistently low throughout the year and thus if the reason may be difficult to establish or whether there are fluctuations within a season which can be attributed to changes in management or feeding practices. Here reference to the farm diary will be necessary to identify dates of management changes which may affect pregnancy rates. Pregnancy rates appear to be very sensitive to changes in feed practices or feed quality with abrupt pregnancy rate changes occurring within one or two days of changes in feed management, e.g. from grass to silage in the autumn, or changes in silage clamps of different quality or a sudden reduction in concentrate input, e.g. to reduce milk yield to quota levels. Such management effects on pregnancy rate may then persuade the farmer to alter his feeding practice for the following season.

The fertility Herd Health Visit (HHV)

The action lists will identify the following groups of cows for examination at the HHV together with their relevant reproductive history.

1. Cows for pregnancy diagnosis (served > 42 days).
2. Cows not served by the earliest service date + 21 days (no visible oestrus) (NVO).
3. Cows with a history of abnormalities at calving, such as:

   a. dystocia
   b. abortion
   c. retained afterbirth
   d. observed abnormal discharges

   These should be presented at the first HHV following 21 days calved for a postnatal check (PNC), which should include both vaginal and rectal examination.
4. Cows with inter-oestral intervals less than 18 days—palpation will determine whether this is due to inaccurate detection of cystic ovarian disease, which requires treatment.
5. Cows that have returned to service four or more times.
6. Cows identified at a previous HHV that require further examination.
7. Cows previously diagnosed not pregnant and not yet re-served.

Postnatal checks or pre-breeding examinations on all cows are not considered to be economically beneficial as so few of these cows are found to be abnormal and if they are abnormal they will be detected at the NVO examination. Whether the recording is computerized or manual an action list of cows should be prepared prior to the visit (see Appendix 7.3).

Interval to 1st Service

Uterine involution: Prompt and effective treatment for cows in category 3 above, which show signs of endometritis, is essential, as these cows normally produce extended calving-to-conception intervals due to delay to 1st service and reduced pregnancy rates. Uterine irrigation is not considered to be effective. However, recent work indicates that a single injection of prostaglandin $F_{2\chi}$ (Lutalyse, Upjohn) will result in reduced calving-to-conception intervals for cows treated 14–28 days after calving (Young and Anderson 1986).

Oestrus detection and restoration of ovarian function: The number of cows presented in category 2 above will indicate whether ovarian inactivity or oestrus detection is a problem. No more than 2% of cows in the herd should be acyclic at this time. Two rectal examinations at least 10 days apart will be required to establish true acyclicity. Cows with a functional corpus luteum (CL) present may be injected with prostaglandin and a Kamar heat mount detector applied at the same time. Cows with no palpable CL should have a Kamar applied and be re-presented at the next HHV if not served in the interim. If more than 20% of the herd are being presented at this examination an education exercise should be set up to train the herdsmen on methods of oestrus detection. The Agricultural Training Board (ATB) oestrus detection courses are ideal for such purposes.

Interval from 1st service to conception

The main influence on this interval by the PVS is the pregnancy diagnosis (PD) examination, i.e. cows in category 1 above. Opinions vary on the optimum time or stage of pregnancy for manual pregnancy diagnosis. This should be performed as easily as possible, which is conducive to a high level of accuracy and no foetal attrition. Some clinicians can manually detect pregnancy at 35 days, with a high degree of accuracy, while others at this stage appear to cause a considerable number of foetuses to die (Abbitt et al. 1978).

A target figure of 97% of cows diagnosed pregnant producing a calf is reasonable. The advantage of 35-day pregnancy diagnoses is that all negatives can be identified before the 6-week return interval and with the help of Kamar heat mount detectors, 80% or more should be re-served at this time. If PDs are performed after 42 days' gestation then the actual time is not critical as long as they are performed before 60 days, to ensure that non-pregnant cows can be served at the 9-week interval. A suggested regime is:

For weekly visits PD at 49–56 days served
For fortnightly visits PD at 45–59 days served

The number of cows failing PD will depend on both pregnancy rate and oestrus detection rate. The relationship between PD failure rate, pregnancy rate (PR) and oestrus detection rate (ODR) can be seen in Figure 7.5. PD failure rate is frequently the first indicator that pregnancy rate may have changed some 6 weeks earlier, although if PD failure is a consistent problem, poor oestrus detection is probably the cause. An approximate ODR calculation can be made once the PR is known by referring to Figure 7.5.

Cows in category 5 above, frequently known as repeat breeders, do cause

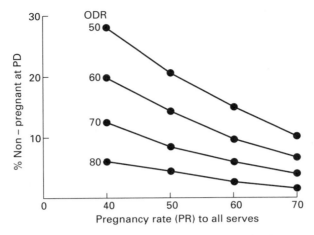

Figure 7.5 The relationship between oestrus detection rate (ODR), pregnancy rate (PR) and percentage of cows failing pregnancy diagnosis (PD−).

problems for many farmers and veterinarians. The first action is to examine the service history of such cows, as surveys have shown that 45% of repeat breeder cows have a history of at least one mistimed insemination, i.e. they have suffered from inaccurate oestrus detection and been inseminated when not in oestrus. Calculation of the interservice intervals will indicate whether this may be the case. The cows should then receive both a vaginal and a rectal examination. Both uterine horns and both ovaries, including ovarian bursae, need to be palpated.

The ovarian structures palpated should be consistent with the last observed oestrus date and, if not, inaccurate oestrus detection should be suspected. If no abnormalities are detected on rectal and vaginal examination, no treatment is necessary.

Body condition score

While conducting the examinations the PVS should make a note of body condition score (see p. 225) of the cows examined. Lower than expected condition scores may be indicative of inadequate nutrition, which could explain certain failures in reproductive efficiency, e.g. high PD failure rates, more than 20% of the herd being presented for NVO examination or more than 2% of the herd exhibiting acyclicity at the NVO examination.

Hormonal treatment of such cows should not be considered until the nutritional status has been shown to be adequate.

Recording HHV findings

When all other routine work has been completed, and other groups of animals inspected (see p. 205) time should be allocated to write in the raw data recording book the findings of the day's HHV, together with all treatments administered and notes made of cows required for examination at future HHVs. At this time, the results of the visit can be discussed. Is oestrus detection being maintained? Has there been a change in pregnancy rate? Is cow condition adequate? Is nutrition adequate? What is the current level of milk production? What disease occurrences have there been since the last HHV? What is the latest situation regarding mastitis and somatic cell count (SCC).

If any further investigations are required, e.g. metabolic profiles, mastitis bacteriology or calf disease investigation, these can be arranged at this time.

The data in the recording book should be coded and a copy taken for entry into the computer, pending production of the next set of action reports. If the PVS oversees the on-farm recording and the transfer of data to the computer the number of errors is generally low.

HHV report

A summary report may be produced by the computer, following an HHV. If there are any observations that need the attention of the farm owner, they should form the basis of a short report or letter to be sent immediately following the visit.

Examples of analyses which can be performed and included in HHV reports throughout the breeding season in a block calving herd, with a breeding season of 13 weeks are:

Week 4   *Submission rate* for first 24 days of the breeding season, using all cows that were eligible for service on day 1, i.e. past their earliest service date.   Target 90%

Week 7 and thereafter following each HHV.   *Pregnancy rate* for the first and subsequent weeks of the breeding season.   Target 65%

Interval to 1st service for cows calved in the 1st 8 weeks.   Target <70 days

No. of cows calved and not served by the earliest service date + 24 days.   Target <20%

Week 20   A full fertility analysis for the whole breeding season.

Advisory Visit

At least once a year, and in larger herds twice, yearly advisory visits should be made. A full fertility analysis should be available with the parameters calculated for the year and by month of calving (see Appendix 7.4) and to include histograms of oestrus detection efficiency and Cu sum (Eddy, 1980) graphs of pregnancy rate. The agenda for this meeting will be the report on the previous advisory visit, on which targets were set; the discussion will start on whether the targets were met, whether further action is required and then on setting new targets. Management ability of the herdsman, the quality of the forage and the milk production (both yield and quality) will all enter the discussion and their effects on the seasons reproductive performance assessed. A full written report should follow this visit.

Other aids to fertility control

Planned breeding programmes

Cows calving in the first 4 weeks in a seasonally calved herd will, on average, be 70 days calved on day 1 of the breeding season. Even if oestrus detection is 100% during the first 3 weeks, by the time these cows are all served, the mean interval to 1st service will be 80 days. with 70% oestrus detection, the mean interval to 1st service will be 88 days.

Planned breeding programmes, using prostaglandins, will enable all cows to be served in the first week of the breeding season.

It has been demonstrated that double injection, followed by fixed time double AI (2 + 2) reduces pregnancy rates by around 10% in most dairy herds because, for varying reasons, approximately 15% of cows do not synchronize (Eddy, 1978). However, other regimes have been successfully applied, including the 10-day regime:

Days 1–6   Serve cows normally on observed oestrus.
Day 6   Inject unserved cows with 1 dose of prostaglandin
Days 7–11   Serve all cows on observed oestrus

Experience has shown that up to 92% of eligible cows will be served in the 11 days with a peak number served on days 9 and 10. The herdsmen need to be involved in the planning and be prepared to make extra time available for oestrus detection. The mean calving-to-conception intervals will be reduced by 10–12 days in treated cows (Esslemont et al. 1977).

Progesterone-releasing intravaginal devices (PRIDs)

Experience has shown that cows which calve in the last 6 weeks of the season suffer culling rates of up to 50% on some farms, particularly in autumn-calving herds when calving takes place at the end of the grazing season or when being housed. The use of PRIDs (Sanofi Animal Health) applied 21–28 days after calving, will ensure an early return to cyclicity. Such cows can then be served by fixed time insemination 2 and 3 days following PRID removal. Although pregnancy rates of around 35% will be achieved at this service, good pregnancy rates can be expected at the repeat service and overall calving-to-conception intervals of 55–60 days can be expected with over 75% of the group conceiving (Drew 1980)

Induction of parturition

As an aid to maintain a short calving season in seasonally calved herds, and to reduce the culling rate, induction of parturition is widely practised in some countries, e.g. New Zealand and Australia, where calf value is minimal. The object is to allow the breeding season to extend by 4–6 weeks longer than normal, thus allowing time for more cows to conceive. These cows are then induced to calve at approximately 7–8 months of gestation, using long-acting corticosteroids, such as dexamethasone trimethyl acetate (Opticortenol, Ciba Geigy) (Welch et al. 1979). In the UK induction of parturition is limited to dystocia prevention when cows are pregnant to bulls known to produce elongated gestations or relatively oversized calves. The object is to use long-acting corticosteroids to induce cows to calve at 275–280 days of gestation by administering the injections at 260–270 days of gestation. Various regimes and combinations of pharmaceutical agents have been used and are summarized by Welch et al. (1979)

Milk progesterone assay

The introduction of ELISA test kits for milk progesterone assay has been a major step forward in the control of reproductive performance, although to date the uptake by the farming community is disappointingly low. That economic benefits can be achieved with their use has been clearly demonstrated (Eddy and Clark 1987). Their application can be summarized as follows:

> Day 24: To detect cows not pregnant which can be treated with prostaglandin at the subsequent HHV. If more than 10% of cows consistently fail PD by rectal palpation, at 45–59 days after service, 24-hour milk progesterone should be considered.
> Days 19, 21 and 23: For predicting returns to oestrus for cows not pregnant. If the day 24 test reveals more than 15% of cows to be negative, progesterone assay on days 19, 21 and 23 should be considered.
> Day of oestrus: If accuracy of oestrus detection is a problem, proges-

terone assay on the day of suspected oestrus will help in determining whether or not a cow is truly in oestrus.

Bull semen evaluation

If natural service is practised, all bulls should undergo semen evaluation on a sample of semen collected in an artificial vagina before the bull is used. A clinical examination of the bull should be made at the same time.

Dairy cows: dry cow management

Very few dairy farmers manage their dry cows. They are frequently turned out on pastures some distance from the farmstead and, apart from being counted daily, no further attention is given. An example of a dry cow programme would be:

1. At drying off, all quarters should be infused with dry cow antibiotic and the body condition score recorded (see Figure 7.6).
2. Cows with condition scores of 3 or more will need restricted feed during the dry period and those with scores 2.5 or less will need a higher quality feed. Condition scoring should be repeated at 3-week intervals and feed availability adjusted as necessary. The feed available needs to be largely composed of long fibre. Old mature grass is ideal. If this is not available, the grass should be supplemented with hay or straw. This ensures rumen size is maintained to allow intakes of large quantities of forage after calving.
3. Fly control measures will need to be applied as necessary and during the summer, if summer mastitis is a problem, cows should be reinfused with antibiotic 4 weeks before calving.
4. At monthly intervals, particularly during late summer or autumn, a metabolic profile of six cows within 3 weeks of calving should be conducted, measuring beta-hydroxybutyrate, glucose, calcium, magnesium and copper (where appropriate). This will provide information to help prevent milk fever and to assess whether nutrition is adequate. Dairy farmers need to be made aware that lactation performance and subsequent fertility can be affected by dry cow management.

Mastitis Control

Considerable success has been achieved in some aspects of mastitis control over the past 30 years or so (Booth 1988). Quoting other workers, Booth suggests the prevalance of clinical mastitis in the UK has fallen from 120–150 cases per

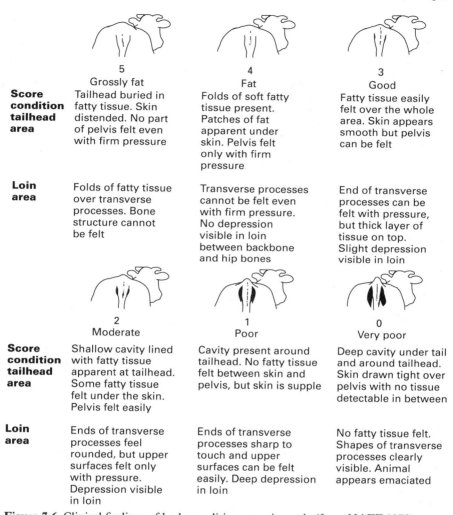

Score condition tailhead area

	5 Grossly fat	**4** Fat	**3** Good
	Tailhead buried in fatty tissue. Skin distended. No part of pelvis felt even with firm pressure	Folds of soft fatty tissue present. Patches of fat apparent under skin. Pelvis felt only with firm pressure	Fatty tissue easily felt over the whole area. Skin appears smooth but pelvis can be felt

Loin area

	Folds of fatty tissue over transverse processes. Bone structure cannot be felt	Transverse processes cannot be felt even with firm pressure. No depression visible in loin between backbone and hip bones	End of transverse processes can be felt with pressure, but thick layer of tissue on top. Slight depression visible in loin

Score condition tailhead area

	2 Moderate	**1** Poor	**0** Very poor
	Shallow cavity lined with fatty tissue apparent at tailhead. Some fatty tissue felt under the skin. Pelvis felt easily	Cavity present around tailhead. No fatty tissue felt between skin and pelvis, but skin is supple	Deep cavity under tail and around tailhead. Skin drawn tight over pelvis with no tissue detectable in between

Loin area

	Ends of transverse processes feel rounded, but upper surfaces felt only with pressure. Depression visible in loin	Ends of transverse processes sharp to touch and upper surfaces can be felt easily. Deep depression in loin	No fatty tissue felt. Shapes of transverse processes clearly visible. Animal appears emaciated

Figure 7.6 Clinical findings of body condition score in cattle (from MAFF 1978).

100 cows in the late 1950s and early 1960s to less than 50 cases per 100 cows by the mid 1980s. The national mean somatic cell count (SCC) has been reduced from 573 000 in 1971 to 320 000 in 1991. A survey by Marshall (cited by Booth 1988) also revealed the percentage of dairy herds practising mastitis control measures in 1983:

Teat disinfection	68%
Dry cow therapy on all cows	74%
Dry cow therapy on some cows	16%
Milking machine testing	66%

In any evaluation this must be considered a major success story and much of this has been the result of a concentrated national campaign, involving MMB and ADAS in particular, but also involving other interested agencies, including the veterinary practitioner.

It is impossible to quantify the effect the PVS has had in the achievements so far. However, there remains much to be achieved in the control of mastitis. The current average incidence is 30–50 cases per 100 cows per year, which still represents considerable wastage.

Moreover, the infectious patterns causing mastitis have changed over the years. Whereas streptococci and staphylococci accounted for over 90% of clinical cases prior to 1970, they now account for less than 50% of cases. Environmental or opportunist infections, e.g. *E. coli*, *Pseudomonas* and *Streptococcus uberis* now account for over 50% of cases of clinical mastitis in the UK.

One can speculate as to the reasons for this change but the reduction in the SCC has certainly reduced the natural resistance of the mammary gland to new infections and the opportunity for environmental infections to gain entry to the teat is also widespread. The standard of hygiene in many dairy farms is very poor, with inadequate bedding, infrequent cleaning of yards and passageways, and unhygienic calving accommodation—all result in a high challenge from environmental organisms.

The selection over the years for such traits as milk yield and quality, udder conformation and ease of milking has ignored mastitis incidence. In fact, selection for such traits as ease of milking may be inadvertently selecting for an increased susceptibility to mastitis.

Practitioner involvement

The level of practitioner involvement in mastitis control advice has varied enormously. Apart from treating acute clinical cases and advising on suitable therapy for subacute cases and dry cow treatment, many practitioners have not been involved. When requested to investigate a mastitis problem they will seek the services of a specialist, for example from the Veterinary Investigation Service, to visit the farm and advise on the implementation of control measures. At the other extreme a few practices in the UK offer a mastitis advisory service, which includes monitoring clinical cases and intramammary therapy tube usage, regular advisory visits, bacteriology and, in some practices, a milking machine testing service.

Recording

In the UK the milk of every dairy herd has been sampled and tested for SCC monthly since 1977. For a small fee and with the permission of the herd owner, the MMB will supply a veterinary practice with dairy farmers' SCC figures each month. This is known as the Veterinary Cell Count Information Service (VCCIS). Currently 123 practices subscribe to this service, representing approximately 4000 of the 34 000 dairy herds in England and Wales.

Traditionally, recording of clinical cases has been recommended as a method of monitoring mastitis incidence. This is important not only to monitor incidence but also to identify cows which repeatedly exhibit clinical mastitis and need to be culled. It is the author's experience that many herdsmen lose interest in mastitis recording and, on most farms, recording is incomplete. The simplest way to stop an outbreak of mastitis is to stop recording cases!

However, since 1988 in the UK, it has been obligatory for farmers to record the use of all medicines used in food-producing animals. This regulation, although not widely adopted to date, should be used to encourage the recording of clinical cases.

Recording by the practice of intramammary tube usage for each herd should be possible in most practices. This can be a valuable aid in identifying herds where the incidence of clinical mastitis suddenly increases. It can also be used to assess whether the herdsman is actually recording clinical cases.

If a herd is recorded with DAISY, the drying off action list will identify the number of clinical occurrences that have occurred during the lactation and this information can be used to make a decision as to whether to cull or not.

Analysis of mastitis occurrence by time of year, number of cases in the lactation, month of calving, stage of lactation, age of cow (lactation number) and feeding group, is available from DAISY. This or similar formats for analysis are valuable in demonstrating to the farmer the epidemiological pattern for mastitis occurrence (see Appendix 7.5).

The mastitis investigation

A mastitis investigation should start by identifying the organisms responsible for the clinical cases observed. This will involve bacterial culture from milk samples of clinical cases. Farmers usually require instruction on how to take uncontaminated samples. Separate samples from at least six cows should be cultured to establish the range of organisms responsible. At the same time, a sample of milk from the bulk tank should be cultured for total bacterial count, coliform count, culture identification and a lab pasteurized count to indicate the efficiency of the milking plant sterilization routine. Overall the bulk sample investigation will indicate the standard of hygiene practised, the efficiency of plant sterilization and the range of pathogenic organisms present on the farm. It is important to establish whether clinical cases are being caused by infectious (e.g. streptococci or staphylococci) or environmental organisms. Correct application of the accepted control measures, including dry cow therapy, teat disinfection, culling cows with recurrent cases, prompt treatment of clinical cases and regular milk machine maintenance, should reduce clinical mastitis and SCC to acceptable levels.

If *Streptococcus agalactia* is identified, 'Blitz therapy' of the whole herd may be considered and has been shown to be cost effective (Edmondson 1989). The presence of *S. agalactia* would also indicate that the accepted control measures of teat disinfection and dry cow therapy are not being applied or their application is intermittent or incomplete.

If it is established that the main causal organisms are environmental the investigation will need to examine pre-milking hygiene, cleanliness of the cows, cleanliness of the lying accommodation and yard management. The milking machine may also need to be examined if there is evidence of damage to the teats during milking which could result in entry of organisms during or after milking.

The visit

Having identified the causal organisms, a visit to the farm should be made at milking time, arriving at the farm approximately 30 minutes before the start of milking. The visit should be structured and follow a predetermined format to avoid omissions. A checklist, as shown in Appendix 7.6, may well prove valuable but the visit will follow the following pattern:

1. Examination of the records.
2. Milking routine.
3. Examination of the cows and teats.
4. Visual assessment of the machine function.
5. Measurement of machine function (only a small number of practices have the necessary equipment to conduct vacuum testing).

   If the equipment is available, tests can be performed during milking to assess the vacuum at various points in the parlour when in use, i.e. dynamic testing. If the PVS does not have access to the necessary equipment he or she will call on the services of specialized agencies to carry out this part of the investigation.
6. Inspection of housing accommodation. This element will be essential if environmental organisms have been identified by the bacteriological test previously performed. Particular attention should be paid to the cleanliness of the yards and lying areas and the quantity and quality of bedding used. The cleanliness of the cows when inspected in the parlour will already have indicated whether attention to housing hygiene is required.
7. The report. Following the visit a typed report of the investigations to date, the deficiencies found at the advisory visit and recommendations

should be sent to the farmer and the herdsmen. An example of a mastitis report is shown in Appendix 7.7.

Monitoring progress

It is important, as with all health schemes, to monitor the progress that is made and this will involve follow-up visits on a regular basis. Machine testing should be performed twice yearly and advisory visits at milking time should follow two or three times a year. These visits will follow the same format as the initial visit and should always be followed by a report.

Monitoring of mastitis, using the monthly SCC reports, intramammary tube usage and monthly clinical case reports, should continue. Farmers should also be encouraged to sample clinical cases on a regular basis to identify changes in the prevalence of the various causal organisms. If a practice-based health recording scheme is in operation all four parameters should be included in the regular reports produced by the system.

Non-PVS mastitis control services

In most countries, the milk purchasing agencies offer a variety of mastitis advisory and control services. In England and Wales, the MMB offers a service to all milk producers which encompasses the following features:

1. Mastitis bacteriological service. This tests milk samples for bacterial presence and antibiotic sensitivity. Reports are copied to the farmer's veterinary surgeon.
2. Individual cow cell count service.
3. Bulk milk mastitis bacteriology
4. Milking machine testing using both static and dynamic tests.
5. Regular visits by a trained mastitis technician, who advises on most aspects of mastitis control. Four visits are undertaken in the first year followed by visits three times a year thereafter.

These services are all chargeable to the farmer; if the farmer wishes and the PVS is receptive, liaison with the farmer's veterinary surgeon is generally encouraged. Some practices have encouraged farmers to use this service in preference to providing their own mastitis advisory service.

Calf scour package

Diarrhoea in calves is still very common, particularly in the winter housing period and does account for considerable economic loss on some farms. There are a number of infectious agents involved in the aetiology of calf scours as well as numerous defects in management, particularly related to the hygiene of calving accommodation. The following would form the main points of a calf scour prevention package.

The calving accommodation should be clean and dry and every effort should be made to ensure that calves suckle and drink 3 litres of colostrum within 6 hours of birth. If the dam's colostrum appears to be of poor quality frozen colostrum should be available and administered by stomach tube. It is common in high yielding Friesian cows for colostrum leakage to occur before calving. All navels should be dipped in a strong iodine-based solution. At the first evidence of scouring, faeces samples should be tested for viruses and bacteria, and blood samples from calves 1–7 days old assayed for immunoglobulins to assess colostrum status. If rotavirus is present, vaccination of the dry cows should be implemented. This vaccine has proven extremely effective in both beef and dairy herds in the UK.

If cryptosporidia or coronavirus are identified, calves must be weaned at 2 days old and reared on bucket or machine-supplied milk. If cryptosporidia are identified in beef calves born out doors, a new, clean paddock should be provided for cows calving subsequently. Glycine electrolytes should be made available for early treatment of all calves that scour. Calf scouring is an example of problems that can be identified at any farm visit by an observant PVS. Many farmers accept scouring calves as inevitable because previous attempts to seek veterinary advice have failed to prevent the problem and they are reluctant to seek help again. The PVS needs to make the farmer aware that he can offer preventive advice.

Youngstock

To calve replacement heifers at 2 years old, targets have to be set for weight for age. The ratios of weight and height for age for Friesian Holstein heifers can be seen in Figure 7.7. To ensure optimum growth rates, advice will be required on pneumonia prevention, parasite control and service management.

Dairy replacement heifers are frequently served in the autumn, a time of declining grass quality. Advice on nutrition prior to service will be required to prevent weight loss at this very important time. Planned breeding programmes using prostaglandin and fixed time insemination will work well with heifers if they are being fed adequately, and 60% pregnancy rates can be expected. This will give the opportunity to inseminate with Friesian semen using bulls known to produce short gestations and ease of calving. Heifers are genetically the most

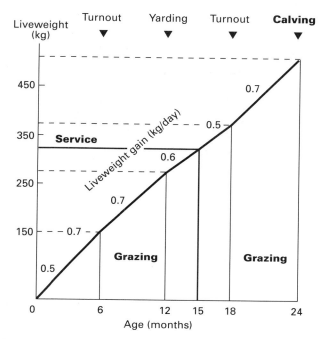

Figure 7.7 Weight for age for Friesian heifer replacements calving at 2 years old (from MAFF 1982).

superior age group in the herd, and inseminating them with proven semen will increase the rate of genetic improvement in the herd as well as providing a crop of calves early in the calving season, which themselves can be easily managed to calve at 2 years old. Body condition should be regularly assessed as calving approaches, and heifers close to calving should be blood tested for magnesium levels. There is considerable wastage in the rearing of youngstock and a recording scheme could prove to be useful in helping reduce this wastage, as has recently been shown by Williamson (1988) using a recording program developed at Minnesota. The University of Reading has also developed a youngstock program that has the advantage of being compatible with DAISY. This should prove valuable in helping the PVS to become more involved with the health control in youngstock rearing.

Foot care

The increasing incidence of lameness in dairy herds is cause for great concern, if only from a welfare point of view. Frequently advocated preventive measures of foot trimming and foot bathing have not proven to be effective in reducing lameness. Cubicle comfort has recently been shown to be related to cubicle use, particularly by heifers, and lack of cubicle use can result in laminitis and solar ulceration (Colam-Ainsworth et al. 1989).

The recent observations by Blowey and Sharp (1989) of the presence of digital dermatitis in the UK and studies of the effect of lameness on fertility (Collick et al. 1989) have increased the understanding of the epidemiology of lameness in dairy cows. It is likely that considerable changes in cubicle design, bedding use and effluent disposal will be required before the incidence of lameness can be substantially reduced.

Behaviour of cows in cubicles has been studied by Cermak (1987), who observed that the type of bedding used in the cubicles influenced the time spent lying; the results are shown in Table 7.5. It can be seen that attention to

Table 7.5 The effect of cubicle beds on time spent lying down by Friesian dairy cows (from Cermak 1987)

Cubicle floor surface	Occupation time (hrs)
Concrete	7.0
Insulated screed	8.3
Rubber mat	9.8
Enkamat-K	14.3
Chopped straw (50 mm) on concrete	15.3

bedding will have a considerable effect on the time spent lying down and therefore resting the feet. Colam-Ainsworth et al. (1989) postulated that if straw were to be used for bedding approximately 1/10th of a bale per cow per day would be required.

Cermak (1987) has also made recommendations on the size of cubicles and design of cubicle partitions. He suggests that cubicle partitions should be set 1200 mm clear, that there should be a 75 mm fall from front to back and the cubicle length can be determined by reference to the average body weight of the heaviest 50% of the herd, as shown in Table 7.6.

In the meantime, the PVS is only able to treat cases as early as possible in the disease process and therefore limit the effect lameness has on production and welfare.

Leptospira control

The importance of *Leptospira hardjo* infection and its effect on reducing milk yields, particularly in 1st lactation heifers, cannot be over-emphasized. This is as well as losses from abortion, which are preventable. The risk factors for any herd have been identified by Pritchard (1989):

Table 7.6 Calculation of required cubicle length with respect to the body weight, chest girth and diagonal body length of cows

Cow body weight (kg)	Chest girth (m)	Body length (m)	Cubicle length (m)
375	1.68	1.36	2.00
425	1.75	1.41	2.04
475	1.81	1.46	2.08
525	1.87	1.50	2.12
575	1.93	1.54	2.16
625	1.98	1.58	2.20
675	2.04	1.62	2.24
725	2.09	1.65	2.28
775	2.14	1.68	2.30
825	2.18	1.72	2.33

1. The presence of rivers or streams on the farms.
2. Purchasing replacement animals.
3. The use of natural service.
4. The simultaneous grazing of pastures with sheep.

If one or more of these risk factors apply to a herd, appropriate action should be taken. This would start with a representative sample of the herd (from 20 cows rising to 28 cows for herds over 100 cows) being blood tested for *Leptospira hardjo*. If there is a high proportion of the herd with positive titres, the herd should be treated with streptomycin at 25mg/kg and vaccinated annually for 3 years. If the test confirms the presence of leptospires but in only a small number of cows, vaccination of the herd annually for 3 years should be implemented; if the test shows no infection, then security measures should be applied to prevent the introduction of infection and perhaps consideration given to joining the MAFF Cattle Health (Leptospira) scheme.

Production and nutrition

Monitoring milk yields weekly or fortnightly and adjusting feed intake as necessary is now a feasible proposition with the use of computerized recording schemes. If the veterinary practice operates a bureau recording service to its clients, using software such as DAISY, milk recording and concentrate feed monitoring can be offered with the result that the PVS becomes involved in advising on the nutrition of the herd. Milk output is very sensitive to nutritional input and if yield production graphs are produced following each milk recording, any group of cows whose milk yield falls by more than 2.5% per week can be quickly identified and corrective advice offered regarding quality or quantity of the feed input.

Metabolic profiles

Since Payne et al. (1970) described the use of metabolic profiles as an aid to nutrition management in dairy herds, much has been published on their use and value. Their use now is much less widespread than in the early 1970s. The reasons for the decline are difficult to determine, other than to say that in practice their value as an assessment of nutritional status in relation to production has not proved as useful as first thought. However, there is one scheme in the UK which is a structured use of the technique; it is offered by the University of Edinburgh Veterinary school as a Dairy Herd Health and Productivity Service (DHHPS) (Kelly et al. 1988). Only dairy farmers who are customers of Dalgety Agriculture are eligible to take part in the scheme. The main component of the scheme is for the nutrition adviser of Dalgety Agriculture, the PVS and farmer to agree when blood sampling is required, usually 2 weeks following a major dietary change. Blood samples taken from up to 17 cows (seven cows calved 2–6 weeks, five cows in late lactation and five dry cows) are submitted to the University of Edinburgh for assay. The results and written report are supplied within 3 to 4 days to the farmer, nutrition adviser and PVS. At the time of blood sampling, individual cow body condition score and body weight (using a weighband) are assessed, together with a record of milk yield and estimated feed intake. Herd milk quality and analytical results of the forage are also recorded, as are disease incidents. Following receipt of the reports (see Appendices 7.8 and 7.9) an advisory meeting is arranged between the farmer, nutrition adviser and PVS to discuss the results and make recommendations for any modifications required to the feed input for the various groups of cows within the herd. In 1988, 127 veterinary practices were involved with this scheme. Farmers who are given positive advice in relation to herd health and productivity remain members of the scheme for longer (Kelly et al. 1988) demonstrating that positive veterinary and nutrition advice stimulates farmer interest and results in continuing use of a service.

Pigs

In contrast to the application of herd health schemes in dairy herds, the whole-farm approach to herd health control, as envisaged by Grunsell et al. (1969) is more readily applicable to pig production. The principal output is pigs for meat production, so reproductive performance is the most important aspect of pig production. Management, housing, nutrition, disease and welfare are so inextricably linked in all stages of the production cycle that to operate the 'package' approach as in dairy cattle is inappropriate. Also the value of individual pigs is much less than individual cattle at all ages and veterinary visits to attend sick pigs are relatively uncommon. However, losses from disease in groups of pigs can be quite considerable and reduction in performance due to disease is recognizable and extremely costly.

A suitable approach would be to subdivide pig production into the five main production areas:

1. Farrowing and suckling
2. Weaning and growing (up to 30 kg body weight)
3. Fattening (30 kg body weight to slaughter)
4. Service and reproduction
5. Dry sow

However, the same broad approach, as described on page 205 under 'Components of a herd health scheme', still apply to pig production.

Standards of production

Muirhead (1976) lists the standards of production which are achievable in a well-managed sow unit of 100–250 sows (Table 7.7). The interference levels are levels at which investigation should be instigated to identify the cause of poor production. No single figure should be read in isolation since, for instance, high numbers born could also raise the number of stillbirths and piglets of low viability, while the numbers reared could well remain satisfactory. When monitored over a period of time and examined collectively, the figures give a measure of the management and disease standard, which can be graded as high, satisfactory, low or fluctuating (Muirhead 1976).

Muirhead (1976) also lists the range of production and disease data extracted from 4017 farrowings in ten herds, under a variety of intensively managed situations, which clearly show scope for improvement (Table 7.8).

Targets and standards are determined by evaluating the performance of a large number of herds. The recording scheme for pig producers operated by the Meat and Livestock Commission (MLC) is a valuable aid to management advice at individual farm level but it also produces information from all recorded herds which can be used to set targets for production on individual farms. Results for one UK breeding herd, are shown in Appendix 7.10. Other agencies in the UK offer similar recording schemes for pig producers, such as the Universities of Exeter and Cambridge.

Table 7.7 Standards of reproductive efficiency and piglet mortality per 100 sows with 28-day weaning (reproduced by kind permission of M R Muirhead)

	Suggested targets	Action or interference level
No. of gilts available for service	6	4
Age at first service	220 ± 10 days	240 days
No. of sows—productive	100	95
Weaning to effective service (days)	7 days	9 days
Regular return (18–22 days)	6	10*
Irregular return (23 days+)	3	5*
Empty days per sow	12	14
Abortion (%)	<1	>1.5*
Sows not in pig (%)	1	>2*
Culled pregnant (%)	<1	>2
Deaths pregnant (%)	1	>2
Farrowing rate (%)	89	85
Vaginal discharge—>7 days post-service %	1	>1.5*
Sows culled per year	38	42
Sow parity at culling	6–7	8
Pigs born alive	10.9	10.4
Pigs born dead (%)	5	7
Piglets mummified (%—<4″)	<0.5	1
Piglets mummified (%—>4″)	1	1.5
Piglet		
losses (%)	8	10
defective (%)	<0.5	1
laid on (%)	3	5
low viable (%)	1	2
runt (starvation) (%)	<1	1.5
savaged (%)	<0.5	0.5
scour (%)	<0.5	1
other (%)	2	2
Piglets weaned per litter	10.00	9.6
Litters per sow per year	2.35	2.3
Pigs weaned per sow per year	23.50	22.00
Pigs sold per sow per year	23.00	21.50
Number of boars	5	5
Mean age	21 months	24 months
Age at culling	3 years	>3 years

* Per 100 sows served.

Identification of problems

An essential part of any herd health scheme is problem identification and problem solving. This, with pigs, as with other species, involves a two-fold approach:

1. An initial evaluation of the herd records.
2. A clinical appraisal of the health and welfare of the animals on the farm.

Table 7.8 Average production/disease levels in ten commercial herds over 12 months expressed as means and ranges (from Muirhead 1976, updated to 1990)

	Mean	Range
Total farrowing	4 017	
Total alive	40 404	
Born alive	10.1	9.0–11.3
Dead to total born per cent	6.3	2.8– 7.2
Mummified per cent	0.6	0.1– 2.8
Laid on per cent	4.5	2.2– 7.2
Congenital defects per cent	0.3	0.2– 0.9
Low viability per cent	3.4	1.7– 6.0
Starvation/savage	0.7	0.1– 1.4
Deaths scour per cent	0.9	0.3– 2.0
Joint-ill per cent	1.5	0.8– 5.4
Miscellaneous deaths per cent	1.7	0.4– 4.3
Scoured per cent litters	19	2.6–28.5
Mastitis per cent farrowings	1.6	0.4– 5.3

A pathway leading to the identification of productivity problems has been constructed by Muirhead (1978) and is shown in Figure 7.8.

If an established nationally accepted, recording system is in operation on the farm, and the system uses the standard terminology (see p. 254) then immediately comparisons can be made between the individual herd performance and accepted targets. The PVS would be wise, however, to investigate whether the accepted terms and definitions are being used by the farmer when compiling the production and disease returns. If no recording scheme is in operation then the farmer must be willing to install one and advice from the PVS will be necessary regarding the recording requirements. Unwillingness to record must necessarily make the farmer unsuitable for a herd health scheme. Examination of the analysed records will demonstrate the herd performance and by comparison with accepted targets, problem areas can be identified. However, to identify probable causes of problems and identification of possible remedial action requires a clinical examination of the herd, when both clinical and subclinical disease should be identified. This may also include postmortem examinations, and laboratory tests on samples obtained from postmortems, faeces, blood or skin. The clinical examination will therefore identify causes of impaired productivity revealed by the recording systems and the PVS is then in a position to offer possible solutions.

Identification of animals

It is important that all breeding animals, i.e. boars and sows, are identified. There is no ideal method of identification of pigs, although large flexible plastic

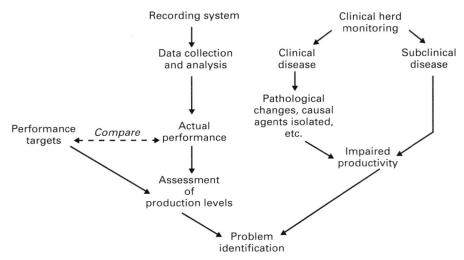

Figure 7.8 Progression pathway leading to problem identification in the pig herd (from Muirhead 1978).

ear tags, with an indelible number, have proved to be satisfactory. Piglets can be identified by ear notching and are sometimes identified relative to their dam. Once weaned, pig identification becomes impractical and the animals are usually identified by pen number, house number or age.

Records

The minimum events and identities that need to be recorded for an effective herd health scheme to operate are shown in Table 7.9. Not only will productivity of the breeding unit be measurable and the parameters identified in Table 7.7 be calculable but growth rates, feed conversion efficiency and margin over feed costs can be calculated; these are required to monitor the economic viability of the unit.

The method of recording will vary considerably between pig farms. Many farms spend an inordinate amount of time on recording, although the advent of computers should reduce this time. The daily diary, as designed by Pigtales Ltd. (Appendix 7.11), provides a useful basis as each member of staff can carry the diary in his or her pocket and enter events and dates as they occur. If a computerized system is in operation this is all that is required and all other reports should be produced from the computer. These are:

1. Individual sow card (Appendix 7.12) on which lifetime and current per-

Table 7.9 Minimum requirements for data recording in a pig herd health scheme

BREEDING
Sow identity
Birth date
Date of entry to herd
Service date(s) and boar(s) used
Boar identity (at service)
Pregnancy diagnosis date
Failure to farrow
Abortion date
Farrowing date
Number piglets born alive
Number piglets born dead
Number piglets born mummified
Total litter weight at birth
Dates routine procedures performed, e.g. iron injections and teeth clipping
Piglet deaths—date and apparent cause of death
Disease incidents for sow
Disease incidents for piglets
Weaning date
Weight at weaning (total litter)
Body condition score of sow at weaning
Sow death date
Sow culling date with reason
Feed consumed by all sows, gilts and boars

WEANING AND GROWER
Pen identification
Date weaned or entered pen
Weight at weaning (of group or pen)
Deaths and cause if known
Medicaments given
Weight at transfer (approx. 30 kg)
Date of transfer
Amounts of food consumed

FATTENING/FINISHING
Pen identity
Weight at transfer
Date of entry
Deaths
Medicaments given
Date of sale
Weight at sale
Total quantity of food consumed
Price received at sale

formance are recorded. These are produced when the sow enters the farrowing house, where they can be updated at farrowing, but should always follow the sow around the unit at the varying stages of the productive cycle.

2. Service records for sows and gilts on which repeat services and abortions are also recorded.
3. Daily records of pigs born (alive, dead and mummified), deaths and weanings.
4. Boar service records and results of service.
5. A monthly stock check of all animals in the farm, classified into the production stages.
6. A monthly herd performance report, calculating the indices shown in Table 7.7.

Pig herd health visit

The objective of the HHV must be to strive continually for increased productivity by managemental, environmental and therapeutic control of disease in order to express the maximum physiological function of the herd (Muirhead 1980).

If the visit is the first in a herd health scheme, most of the time will be occupied in assessing the effectiveness of the recording system: for example, are standard terms and definitions being used? Are all the required data being recorded? Is there duplication of recording and can recording be streamlined? What use is being made of the recording scheme reports and could more effective use be made? And, more importantly, are the results produced in the reports consistent with clinical findings on inspection of the herd; for instance, is the number of pigs in the weaned pig accommodation consistent with the numbers recorded as being weaned? Or, is the number of observed scouring pigs consistent with the records? Or, is the amount of medication supplied to the unit consistent with the number of pigs recorded as requiring therapy?

Using the reports of the recording scheme, the areas of performance that require attention will be identified and a priority list produced. It is impractical to tackle all problems at the outset. The first problem areas that need attention will be those where readily identifiable solutions can be provided and where results are likely to be favourable. Reference to previous clinical disease outbreaks and any postmortem and laboratory reports will also help in determining which are likely to be current problem areas.

It will also be necessary to establish with the owner the frequency of visits required and the method of payment for the scheme. It may be necessary at the outset to make more frequent visits than in a scheme of long standing. Muirhead (1980) suggests the frequency of visits will vary with herd size but produces guidelines which could well be adopted by any PVS considering offering a health scheme for pig herds; these are shown in Table 7.10.

Once the methodology of the herd health scheme has been set out for an individual farm, subsequent visits will follow the routine of pre-visit prep-

Table 7.10 Herd size and suggested frequency and duration of visits for a pig herd
health scheme (from Muirhead 1980)

No. of sows	Visit frequency (weekly)	On-farm hours per year
50–100	6–8	16
150–250	4–6	27
300–400	4	36
450–600	2–4	48
600+	1–2	90

aration, herd clinical examination, record examinations and epidemiology and
remedial activity discussions (Muirhead 1980), as shown in Table 7.11.

Pre-visit preparation

Before each visit the previous visit reports and any on-going laboratory reports
are studied, together with any notes of disease problems that have occurred
since the last visit.

The clinical examination

When conducting a clinical examination of the herd, it is to be recommended
that a consistent approach be developed and adhered to in all visits. This will
generally start with the service area, followed by the dry sows, the farrowing
and suckling pigs, the post-weaned pigs and finally the fattening or finishing
pigs.

Muirhead (1980) has produced a series of checklists (Tables 7.12–7.15)
which can be used to ensure that all production and disease areas are considered.

The clinical examination will reveal conditions that require further investigation and whether further pathological or bacteriological investigations are
required. All pigs found dead on the visit or the previous day should undergo
postmortem examination. If a particular problem involving deaths needs
further investigation, the stockperson must be instructed to present all pigs
that die before the next visit for postmortem examination. Postmortem examinations at a slaughterhouse can also be a valuable aid to determining the extent
of a problem, such as pneumonia, pleurisy or atrophic rhinitis.

The clinical examination will also include inspecting body condition, investigating adequacy of feed levels and welfare, and the suitability of the housing,
particularly on the wear of concrete floors and maintenance of ventilation and
heating systems. Hygiene and effectiveness of the disinfection programmes,

Table 7.11 Standard procedure for a herd health visit (from Muirhead 1980)

1. The pre-visit preparation
   Previous reports
   Laboratory reports
   On-going investigations
   Special topic preparations

2. The clinical examination of the herd

3. The discussion
   Records—significance
   Disease evaluation
   Productivity evaluation
   Epidemiological discussion
   Remedial actions and recommendations

4. The special topic

5. General problems

6. Preparation for next visit

7. The report

Table 7.12 The clinical inspection. A checklist for the reproduction and service area (from Muirhead 1980)

Boar sow ratio
Boar fertility, service problems
Boar usage
Boar condition. Mange, lameness, other diseases
Weaning to service intervals
Return rate and interval of returns
Farrowing rate
Sow stocking density
Sow body condition, trauma stress, lameness
Housing, environment, temperature
Nutrition levels
Oestrus abnormalities
Uterine discharges, mastitis, other diseases
Treatments, hormones

particularly in the farrowing accommodation, and security measures to prevent the introduction of new infectious diseases will also be included in the discussions.

The discussion

Having completed the clinical examination of the herd, the PVS and the

Table 7.13 The clinical inspection. A checklist for the dry sow area (from Muirhead 1980)

Environment, temperature
Stocking densities/stall/tether problems
Feed levels, dung state
Body condition
Udder line, mastitis
Facial changes, occular discharges
Skin diseases, mange
Lameness, leg problems, trauma
Oestrus abnormalities
Discharges, metritis, cystitis
Abortions
Sows not in pig/infertility
Culls and reasons, sudden deaths, pneumonia
Miscellaneous diseases, prolapse
Parasites
Treatments

Table 7.14 The clinical inspection. A checklist for the farrowing and rearing areas (from Muirhead 1980)

Sow body condition
Sows not in pig
Mastitis, metritis, agalactia
Farrowing fever and other diseases
General farrowing, management and bedding
Early or late farrowings
Parturition difficulties, vaginal haematoma
Sudden deaths, prolapse
Litter size, litter scatter
Stillbirths, mummifications
Piglet viability, splay-leg, congenital defects
Neonatal scour, joint/leg infections, starvation
Mortality levels
Growth patterns
Rhinitis (sneezing, ocular discharges, nasal deformity), pneumonia (cough)
Sudden deaths
Skin conditions including teat necrosis
Parasites
Medications in use

farmer or manager retire to the farm office. Hopefully the farmer will have prepared the latest record system reports and identified areas he wishes to discuss. The records are assessed, the problem areas identified and with the impressions of the clinical examination, a discussion will emerge on possible

Table 7.15 The clinical inspection. A checklist for the growing and fattening areas (from Muirhead 1980)

Age at weaning, body-weight and variability in weight
Nutrition, water availability
Evenness of growth
Post weaning enteritis, other enteric disorders
Housing, environment, stocking densities
Insulation, temperature and ventilation
Rhinitis, pneumonia
Skin conditions. Mange
Sudden death
Culls. Lameness, Vices
Days to slaughter
Feed conversion rate
Other diseases
Parasites

---

solutions and recommendations. It must be appreciated that some problems are more easily resolved than others and frequently further investigations will be required, e.g. blood sampling, postmortem or laboratory examinations. This discussion should be a genuine discussion. Opinions of the farmer and the stockpersons should always be valued, in particular if they have ideas as to why a certain problem exists. They will also be able to express an opinion on the viability of any recommendations made. However, stockpersons frequently have 'blind spots' and tactful persuasion may be required to convince them of the value of a specific recommendation, particularly if it involves a change in management procedure or increased workload. One suggestion which is usually accepted is to test the recommendation on a small group of animals or a small number of pens for the stockpersons themselves to assess the results. If the results are favourable adoption of the recommendations in full is more likely to happen.

The special topic

Muirhead (1980) also allocates time at each visit for continuing education of the stockpersons. He selects a special topic before the visit and presents this as an education exercise to all the farm staff. Examples of such topics are: herd security, stock introduction, parasite control, vaccination, fertility, disease levels, boar management, feed costs, liveweight gains and feed conversion, housing conditions, welfare, etc.

The report

Muirhead (1980) described a report form which can be completed on the visit and left with the farmer. This form also provides a checklist. However, when significant recommendations are made this should always be followed by a typewritten report.

To begin with the PVS may wish to restrict his or her activities and advice to disease occurrence and prevention. If the occasion arises where expert advice is required, for example on nutrition, ventilation, building design for effluent disposal, the PVS should be able to identify suitable advisers from the various agricultural advisory agencies that exist.

However, as time progresses, the PVS will understand the interactions of husbandry, health and welfare on production and be able to offer sound advice on most of these subjects.

Pig Health Control Association (PHCA)

The PHCA was founded in the late 1950s at the request of pig farmers. These farmers had already established herds free of enzootic pneumonia and wished to sell stock to others on the basis of regular herd monitoring for freedom from this disease; moreover, they wanted all participating herds to have common veterinary standards, in order to facilitate inter-herd movements of bloodlines. The first control scheme for enzootic pneumonia was launched on 1 January 1959 (Anon 1986b).

The main objective of the PHCA is to establish lists of breeding herds that are free from any of the following six diseases: enzootic pneumonia (EP), swine dysentery (SD), Aujeszky's disease (AD), atrophic rhinitis (AR), mange (MG), and streptococcal meningitis (SM). Follow-up testing and six-monthly veterinary inspections (by the PVS) are carried out to ensure the herd maintains freedom from the disease(s) to which it has PHCA listing.

Very strict regulations regarding introduction of stock, non-use of prescribed medicaments, and the tests that are to be applied to ensure disease freedom are available for each of the six diseases and the farmers must comply with these regulations. Tests for enzootic pneumonia and atrophic rhinitis, for example, must include twice-yearly slaughterhouse inspections of lungs and snouts as well as veterinary certification of freedom from clinical disease. In December 1988, the numbers of herds on the six lists were as shown in Table 7.16.

The PHCA is only applicable to elite herds at the top of the production pyramid. These will be herds which supply breeding stock to multiplying herds and to commercial herds who wish to remain free of one or more of the six diseases. Because of the high standards of testing and the constraints on management practices and movement of animals, it is unlikely to interest the commercial pig producer.

The PHCA does operate closely with the farm's own PVS, who is respon-

Table 7.16 Number of pig herds on PHCA disease-free lists as at December 1988

List	No. herds disease free
Enzootic pneumonia	36
Swine dysentery	49
Aujeszky's disease	47
Atrophic rhinitis	38
Mange	27
Streptococcal meningitis	36

sible for the on-farm examinations and carrying out the relevant tests. However, visits from the PHCA veterinary advisers do take place from time to time.

Pig fattening schemes

A number of UK national pig feed compounders operate schemes whereby they supply weaned pigs (over 30 kg body weight) to farmers with suitable buildings who then manage and feed the pigs for a set fee per pig per week or a fee per kg body weight of pigs produced. The feed compounder is contracted to supply all feed, medicines and veterinary advice. The veterinary advice usually takes the form of a practitioner visit to the respective farms with an adviser from the feed company three or four times a year. The source of the pigs for the fattening schemes is varied; some compounders own breeding units but the majority of pigs are obtained from weaner pools where the sources are multiple. Because of the various sources of these pigs, infectious diseases are common and a major limiting factor in achieving optimum food conversion rates. The buildings used are often less than desirable, frequently being old pig buildings which have had a period of disuse and are suffering from lack of maintenance. Although the intentions are to minimize the effects of disease, there is frequently little that can be done other than to control disease by mass medication. The need for a single source and an 'all in-all out' policy is recognized by some operators of these schemes but it is not yet widespread. The veterinary role in these circumstances is to advise on welfare issues, to reduce the effects of disease by management means where possible (e.g. stocking density) and to prescribe suitable in-feed medication, ensuring recording of medicine use is in operation and medicine withdrawal periods are observed.

Sheep

Sheep have normally been considered the poor relation among farm species as far as the farm animal practitioner is concerned. Many practitioners only encounter their sheep farming clients at lambing time for dystocia correction, Caesarean sections and the occasional disease problem in the lambs. Outbreaks of coccidiosis, parasitic gastroenteritis and pasteurellosis occasionally result in requests for veterinary assistance as do abortion outbreaks. However, much preventive medicine is in fact practised by sheep farmers in the form of vaccination regimes for clostridial disease, pasteurellosis, orf and foot rot, as well as control programmes for internal and external parasites. However, most of this is without veterinary supervision and various surveys, as well as practitioner experience have demonstrated that this lack of veterinary supervision results in inappropriate application of many of the programmes; for instance, over 75% of anthelmintics administered to sheep are probably administered at inappropriate times or at incorrect dosages (Plates 5 and 6).

The economics of sheep production varies enormously around the world. The extensive sheep ranches of Australia, where there are low stocking densities, low value per sheep and shortage of labour, survive with little or no health control input. This is probably because climatic stress and the availability of food are of greater importance than disease control. Disease incidence in such flocks is probably low. However, the situation in northern Europe is much different. The relatively high value of each animal, the profitability of production of lamb carcasses for meat consumption and more intensive stocking densities make the market for flock health control more attractive. However, veterinary input is still low. Perhaps this is due to social reasons; sheep farmers are traditionally less wealthy than dairy producers and are more conservative in their approach. Their conservative attitude also makes it more difficult to institute changes in management practices, which includes paying for veterinary advice. Furthermore, until recently, there has been a distinct lack of teaching of planned flock health and epidemiology of sheep disease in the veterinary schools, certainly in the UK. For this chapter a description or blueprint for a flock health scheme as devised by Clarkson and Faull (1990) will be described. This is similar in approach to those produced by other workers in the UK (Hindson 1982, 1989).

A flock health scheme

Clarkson and Faull's scheme has three components:

1. A written health programme containing recommendations for the control of expected diseases and to improve production.

2. Planned visits (3–6 per annum) to monitor health and production.
3. Reactions to events and advice on new advances during the year, to keep the programme up to date.

The attitude of the farmers (see p. 191) and the enthusiasm and competence of the PVS (see p. 195) will influence the outcome of sheep health schemes just as with schemes for other species.

Health Programme

This programme is in the form of a diary and is tailor made to suit the needs of the farm, following full discussion at the first visit. It is based around the farmer's proposed dates for tupping, housing, lambing and weaning. It also includes dates for some or all of the following depending on needs:

(a) Tupping—including early breeding, synchronization, AI and ram testing.
(b) Condition scoring of ewes.
(c) Vaccination against clostridia, orf, abortion, foot rot, pasteurellosis.
(d) Dosing for copper, cobalt and selenium/vitamin E deficiencies.
(e) Worming for roundworms.
(f) Fluke drenching.
(g) Treatment of coccidiosis.
(h) Tapeworm treatment for dogs.
(i) Feeding and good analysis.

Planned visits

Several visits will be needed in order to assess the application and usefulness of the health programme. In the first year, six visits will usually be necessary, according to the plan as set out in Appendix 7.13. In subsequent years, fewer visits and samples are likely to be required.

Reactions to events

It may be necessary to modify the original health programme from time to time following information obtained during and between the planned visits. Information obtained about some or all of the following will be carefully considered.

(a) Breeds, ages and flock numbers.
(b) Condition of sheep.

(c) Quality and quantity of food.

(d) Housing arrangements.

(e) Lambing arrangements.

(f) Survey of snail habitats and drainage schemes.

(g) Pasture and grazing management.

(h) Clinical disease, e.g. pregnancy toxaemia, abortion, lameness, lamb losses, pneumonia.

(i) Laboratory findings, including postmortem examination of a sufficient number of carcasses to establish the cause of disease.

At the end of each year, the programme will need amendment to incorporate new research, drugs and vaccines in the light of the experience gained during the year and any alterations in the objectives of the farmer.

Clarkson and Faull have designed a set of checklists and forms which any PVS contemplating setting up a flock health scheme may find useful. A farm questionnaire (see Appendix 7.14) is sent to the farm before the first visit to obtain the necessary background information to the farm and its production achievements.

A number of checklists can be used by the PVS during the flock health visit (see Appendices 7.15–7.18). An example of a flock health programme for a flock of 85 ewes, plus 33 ewe lambs, is given in Appendix 7.19. Modification will need to be made to suit the individual farm requirements and disease patterns.

TERMS AND DEFINITIONS OF DAIRY CATTLE REPRODUCTION (MAFF, 1984)

Terms and definitions

Abortion The production of one or more calves between 152 and 270 days after an effective service which are either born dead or survive for less than 24 hours. (**See explanatory note 1 and 5**)

Assumed pregnancy rate The number of cows or heifers served within a defined period not observed to return to oestrus before a specified date expressed as a proportion of the total number of services given over that period. The defined period should finish at least 60 days before the end of the period for which data are available.

Average herd size The average of the number of cows in the herd as counted on 12 or more approximately equally spaced occasions during a year.

Bull An entire male aged 180 days or more.

Bull calf An entire male of less than 180 days of age.

Calving The birth of one or more calves more than 270 days after an effective service. (**See explanatory note 1**)

Calving index The mean calving intervals of all the cows in a herd at a defined point in time calculated retrospectively from their recent calving at that time.

Calving interval The interval in days for an individual cow from one calving to the next.

Calving rate The number of services given to a defined group of cows or heifers or over a specified period which result in a calving expressed as a percentage of the total number of services.

Calving to conception interval The interval in days from calving to the subsequent effective service of a cow.

Calving to first service interval The number of days from calving to the first subsequent service of a cow. (**See explanatory note 10**)

Cow A female after the start of her first lactation.

Cow not to be served A cow which it is not intended to serve again and is destined to be culled.

Cull cow A live cow transferred out of the dairy herd irrespective of the purpose to which she is put subsequently. Cull cows may be separated into two groups; those culled before service and those culled after service. (**See explanatory note 2**)

Culling rate The number of cows calving in a defined period (usually 12 months) which are transferred to live out of the herd before starting another lactation expressed as a percentage of the total number of cows calving in the period.

Dairy herd One or more cows milked,

managed and recorded as a single unit. (**See explanatory note 3**)

Date of conception   The date of the effective service.

Date of service   The date of the first natural mating or artificial insemination during a period of continuous oestrus.

Earliest service date   The date on or after which a cow observed in oestrus would be served as a matter of policy.

Effective service   A service which results in pregnancy.

Embryo   The product of conception (the conceptus) from the date of conception to Day 42 of pregnancy. (**See explanatory note 4**)

Embryo loss   The loss of a conceptus during the first 42 days of pregnancy.

Foetal loss   The loss of a foetus between 43 and 151 days of pregnancy. (**See explanatory note 5**)

Foetus   The developing calf from 43 days of pregnancy to birth.

Heifer   A female aged 180 days or more which has not started her first lactation. (**See explanatory note 6**)

Heifer calf   A female of less than 180 days of age.

Herd size   The number of cows present in the herd on a given date.

In-calf heifer   A heifer which is confirmed in calf.

Inter-service interval   The number of days from one service of a cow to the next in the same lactation. (**See explanatory note 7**)

Maiden heifer   A heifer which has not been served.

Mean calving to conception interval   The average of the individual intervals of a group of cows calving over a defined period.

Mean calving to first service interval   The average of the individual intervals for any defined group of cows.

Non-return rate to first insemination   The number of first inseminations given to a defined group of cows or heifers or over a specified period of time which is not followed by a repeat insemination within a prescribed period, expressed as a percentage of the total number of first inseminations during the period. (**See explanatory note 8**)

Oestrus   The physiological state in which a cow or heifer will stand voluntarily to be mounted.

Oestrous cycle   The regular recurrence of oestrus together with related changes in the genital organs and the reproductive hormones.

Oestrous cycle length   The number of days from the start of one oestrus to the start of the next. The day of the start of oestrus is counted as Day 0.

Overall pregnancy rate   The number of services given to a defined group of cows or heifers or over a specified period which result in a diagnosed pregnancy not less than 42 days after service expressed as a percentage of the total number of services. Services to cull cows should be included. The method of pregnancy diagnosis must be specified. (**See explanatory note 10**)

Percentage culled and died   The number of cows in a herd calving in a defined period (usually 12 months) which are culled or die before starting another lactation expressed as a percentage of the total number of cows calving in the period.

Percentage pregnant of cows served   The number of cows calving in a defined period (usually 12 months) which are diagnosed pregnant not less than 42 days after an effective service expressed as a percentage of the number of cows served. The defined period should be the same as that used to calculate the mean calving to conception interval.

Predicted calving interval   Calving to conception interval + 280 days (mean gestation length) calculated forward from the calving date. The mean predicted calving interval is the predicted calving index.

Pregnancy rate to first service   The number of first services given over a period or to a defined group of cows or heifers which result in a diagnosed pregnancy not less than 42 days after service expressed as a percentage of the number of first services in the period. The method of pregnancy diagnosis must be specified. (**See explanatory note 9**)

Premature calving   The production of one or more calves between 152 and 270 days after an effective service, at least one of which survives for 24 hours or more. (**See explanatory note 1**)

Replacement rate The number of cows or heifers required to replace cows which have left the herd during a defined period (usually 12 months) expressed as a percentage of the average herd size during the same period.

Reproductive efficiency The number of cows becoming pregnant in a 21 day period expressed as a percentage of the number of cows eligible for service at the start of the period.

Served heifer A heifer which has been served or which has received a transferred embryo but which has not been confirmed in calf.

Service One or more natural matings or artificial inseminations during a period of continuous oestrous. (**See explanatory note 11**)

Services per pregnancy The total number of services given to a group of cows or over a defined period divided by the number of services which result in a diagnosed pregnancy not less than 42 days after service. Services to cull cows should be included. The defined period should finish at least 60 days before the end of the period for which data are available. (**See explanatory note 10**)

Stillborn A calf born dead, or found dead after an unobserved calving.

Submission rate The number of cows or heifers served within a 21 day period expressed as a percentage of the number of cows or heifers at or beyond their earliest service date at the start of the 21 day period.

Explanatory notes on terms and definitions

1. Abortion, Premature calving, Calving Where an abortion, premature calving or calving follows embryo transfer, the date of the effective service should be taken to be the date of the first observation of oestrus of the recipient immediately preceding the transfer.

2. Cull cow Although it is realized that live cows are on occasion transferred to other herds for further breeding, these are included to clarify the keeping and interpretation of herd records.

3. Dairy herd Units containing only one cow are included in the definition of a herd in order that they can be accounted for in calculations of mean herd size on a national or regional basis.

4. Embryo The term conceptus used in this definition refers to all the tissues which are the products of conception and therefore includes foetal membranes.

5. Foetal loss/Abortion The loss of a pregnancy before 152 days will not initiate a new fertility record. Cows losing a pregnancy on or after 152 days will start a new fertility record from the date of the abortion as if they had calved normally.

The voiding of a calf at any time before 271 days constitutes an abortion for the purposes of the official brucellosis control schemes and must be reported to the local Divisional Veterinary Officer.

6. Heifer The definition differs from that in colloquial usage where the term continues to be used throughout the first lactation and up to the second calving. Excluding cows in the first lactation avoids confusion when dealing with the total number of animals in milk and is in agreement with the definition used by major recording organizations. When first lactation animals need to be identified the terms 'first calver' or 'first calved cow' should be used.

7. Inter-service intervals These should be allocated to one of the following groups; 2–17 days, 8–24 days, 25–35 days, 36–48 days and 49 or more days. The group of cows or the period over which the services were given must be specified.

8. Non-return rate to insemination Non-return rates to first insemination are used by AI Centres to monitor the fertility of bulls and the performance of inseminators. They are normally assessed at 30–60 days or at 49 days after service. The results are usually some 20 percentage points higher than calving rates.

9. Pregnancy rate to first service The National Group on Reproductive Definitions, USA, recommended that the embryo should be defined as the product of conception up to Day 42. Although pregnancy diagnosis can be carried out before this time the results obtained do not give an accurate prediction of calving because of embryo loss.

10. Pregnancy rates and services per pregnancy Where pregnancy diagnosis is not undertaken evidence of pregnancy such as subsequent calving or abortion is used to calculate these indices retrospectively.

11. Service More than one service at a single oestrus cannot result in more than one pregnancy per cow. Multiple services at a single oestrus must therefore be considered as one service for the purposes of calculating pregnancy rates and services per pregnancy.

TERMS AND DEFINITIONS OF PIG PRODUCTION (MAFF, 1979)

Note: please refer to original source for cross references

Terms and definitions

Animal production recording systems require a precise definition of the various classes of animal that are identified and the periods of time that are measured. There is no comprehensive list of the terms and definitions used in pig recording. Production recording systems have in the past relied on undefined terms and as a result, various classes of pigs are described in different ways. The following list of terms and definitions is recommended for use in manual recording systems and computer-based recording systems (Davies et al. 1983). (With the kind permission of the authors and the Ministry of Agriculture, Food and Fisheries.) Explanatory notes on the terms and definitions appear on pages 256 to 258.

A. The Breeding Herd

Sow Any breeding female that has been served and is on the farm.

Maiden gilt A female transferred to the breeding herd but not yet mated.

Boar A male pig over six months of age and intended for use in the breeding herd.

Sow cull Any live sow removed from the farm.

Boar/sow ratio The ratio of boars to sows as defined in 1 and 3. Any definition must take into account the nonworking boar.

Herd size The average number of sows present in the herd as recorded on 12 or more equally spaced occasions during a year (365 days).

B. Fertility Data

(a) Service One or more completed and recorded matings within the same oestrus period.

(b) Date of service Date of first mating during any one oestrus period (counted as day 0).

First litter sow A female pig between the date of first effective service (a service that results in pregnancy) and the date of the next effective service following successful completion of pregnancy.

(a) Farrowing Production of a litter of one or more live or dead pigs on or after the 110th day of pregnancy (day of service is day 0) (See Note i.)

(b) Farrowing rate The number of sows that farrow to a given number of services expressed as a percentage.

Induction The use of a drug that is capable of inducing farrowing. Usually used from one to three days prior to the expected farrowing date to synchronize the farrowing of a number of sows on the same day.

Conception rate The number of sows that conceive to service expressed as a percentage of these services. Conception is assumed by nonreturn to oestrus 21 days after service or identified by pregnancy diagnosis at about 30 days post service. These measures are not precise and the term *conception rate* is therefore of limited use.

Return to service A sow re-served after a return to service.

Regular return A return to service 18 to 24 days after the date of service. (See Note ii.)

Irregular return A return to service outside the period 18 to 24 days after the date of service. (See Note ii.)

Herd farrowing index The number of farrowings taking place in 365 days divided by the average number of sows in the herd during that period as defined by 6.

Weaning date (sow) The date on which a sow ceases to suckle piglets.

Weaning to service interval The interval between date of weaning and the date of first service (date of weaning = day 0). (See Note iii.)

Empty days Empty days are average number of days between weaning (or gilts' first service) and effective service or removal from the breeding herd. (See Note ix.)

Abortion The observed production of foetuses between service and up to and including the 109th day of pregnancy, and where none of the foetuses survive more than 24 hours. (See Note i.)

Premature farrowing The observed production of foetuses before the 110th day of pregnancy, but where some foetuses survive for more than 24 hours. (See Note i.)

Failure to farrow Sow not farrowed by 120 days after a presumed effective service.

C. Progeny: Preweaning Period

Litter The production of a farrowing.

Number of piglets per litter The total number of piglets born (including stillborn and mummified pigs) per litter.

Liveborn piglets Piglets that are born alive.

Stillborn piglets Piglets found dead behind the sow farrowing (if necessary confirmed by postmortem examination to determine if the piglets have breathed).

Mummified piglets The number of piglets that are born degenerate (discoloured and shrivelled), i.e., they have died some time before farrowing.

Premature pigs Piglets born alive (and surviving for more than 24 hours) before the 110th day of pregnancy. (See Note i.)

Small litter index (sometimes referred to as litter scatter) The percentage of litters born within any specified period in which the number of piglets in any litter (see 23) falls below x, where x is the nearest whole number lower than 1 standard deviation below the mean number of piglets per litter. (See Note iv.)

Live birth weight of litter The total weight of piglets alive at birth or survived first 24 hours. (See Note v.)

Suckler Piglet between birth and weaning.

Suckler (preweaning) mortality The percentage of liveborn piglets that die before weaning.

Fostering The transferal of piglets from one litter to another for management purposes. Fostering-on is the introduction of extra piglets and fostering-off is the removal of pigs from a litter.

Weaning (piglets) The act of permanently removing piglets from the sow.

Age at weaning The number of days from farrowing to weaning (day of farrowing = day 0)

Herd weaning age The average number of days from farrowing to weaning for the herd.

D. Progeny: Postweaning Period

Weaner A weaner is a pig between weaning and either the end of the stay in the weaner accommodation or 30 kg if it is to remain in the same accommodation until slaughter. (As pigs are weaned at vastly differing ages, this definition can cover a wide age range.)

Weaner pig mortality The number of weaners that die expressed as a percentage of the total number of weaners in that group initially.

Feeder/finisher Any pig in the stage of life between the end of the weaner period and slaughter weight or the time of transfer to the breeding herd.

Pigs marketed Pigs marketed alive in any form or transferred to the breeding herd (NOT including sales from the breeding herd).

E. Feeder/Finisher Data

Porker, cutter, baconer, heavy hogs These are classes of finishing pigs that are categorized by weight. Different recording schemes and marketing systems use different weights. (See Note vi.)

Live-weight gain The live-weight gain of the pig when sold less its birth weight. If the birth weight is not available, it is counted as 1 kg.

Days to slaughter The age of a pig at slaughter is the number of days from the date of birth of that pig (day 0) to the date of slaughter of that pig.

Daily live-weight gain The live-weight gain of a pig divided by the number of days between two weighings.

Feed conversion ratio The total weight of dry food consumed by a pig divided by its live-weight gain. (See Note viii.)

Feeder/finisher pig mortality The number of feeder/finishers that die in a group expressed as a percentage of the total numbers of feeder/finishers in that group initially.

Average days to slaughter The average number of days to slaughter for a group of pigs, excluding those that die.

Average weight at slaughter The average live weight at slaughter. (See Note vii.)

Transit death A pig dying in transit on the truck between the end of loading at the farm and the end of unloading at the abattoir or final disembarkation point.

Lairage death A pig dying between the end of unloading at the abattoir and the point of slaughter.

Condemnation A carcass condemned wholly or in part.

Casualty/culls Any pig for which payment is received that is slaughtered on welfare grounds or for persistent slow growth.

Explanatory Notes on the Terms and the Definitions

Gestation length This varies between herds according to breed and other factors, but data held at Weybridge that relate to a large body of accumulated information from British herds give a mean figure $\pm$ 1 standard deviation (S.D.) of 114.5 ± 1.5 days. From this we can say that the 99% tolerance limits are 110 to 119 days.

Oestrus cycle length A review of all available information suggested a mean oestrus cycle length of 21 days $\pm$ 1.5 days (mean length $\pm$ S.D.), and this figure is widely accepted. These figures give 95% tolerance limits of 18 to 24 days, and this is the range that has been used for the calculation of regular and irregular returns (13 and 14).

Weaning-to-service interval This depends on many factors, not the least of which is the length of lactation. Analysis of data from a variety of different sources suggests that for all practical purposes a mean figure of 7.5 ± 2.5 days (mean $\pm$ 1 S.D.) is acceptable. The interval is very variable because a wide range of factors affects it, e.g., the level of nutrition, disease status, management systems, and so on. But this figure is a satisfactory working guide in relation to weaning-to-service interval.

Total litter size It must be clearly recognized that litter size is also affected by a great many factors, including maternal age and breed, and disease status, and that it may vary from country to country. For the purpose of this book, it was felt that some figure that can be regarded as characteristic of the British situation and the variability that occurs between individuals should be given. For British herds the mean figure $\pm$ 1 S.D. for litter size is 10.75 ± 3.0 piglets. It is from this figure that the small litter index (28) is calculated, i.e., for the above figures the small litter index is the percentage of litters that contain less than seven pigs.

Piglet birth weight Some indication of the mean and variability of normal piglet birth weights may be useful, and data obtained from Weybridge and other sources give the following:

$$\text{Mean} \pm 1 \text{ S.D.} = 1250\,g \pm 250\,g$$

From this, the 95% tolerance limits are 750 to 1750 g.

Values for slaughter pigs The Cambridge Pig Management Recording Scheme (Agricultural Economics Unit, Department of Land Economy, University of Cambridge), The Farmers Weekly, and the M.L.C. Economics Department use the following sets of values for slaughter pigs:

	Cambridge kg. (Live Weight)	F.W. kg. (Live Weight)	M.L.C. kg. (Dead Weight)
Porker	50–75	40–67	Up to 50
Cutter	75–105	68–82	50–81
Baconer	80–100	83–101	59–77
Heavy hog	105+	102+	82+

Herd values for slaughter pigs Many herds do not operate under a system of production that identifies individual slaughter pigs nor do they operate on a batch system. This precludes the use of the preceding definition. However, it is possible on a herd basis to estimate figures for the data given above, and the method used by the MLC in their pig herd recording scheme is shown at the top of the opposite page.

Feed conversion ratio On the farm, feed conversion ratio (FCR) estimates are required either for groups of pigs or for the whole finishing herd. If this is to be done accurately for any given period, it is necessary to record the weight of the food in stock at the beginning of the period, the weight of food entering stock during the period, and the weight of food in stock at the end of the period.

Similarly, it is necessary to know the weight of pigs in the group at the beginning and end of the period in question and the weight of pigs entering or leaving the group during the period. This means that all pigs entering and leaving the group need to be weighed and that all the pigs in the group also are weighed at the beginning and end of the recording period. This is a demanding task, and on most farms it is not attempted more than twice a year.

In assessing pig feed conversion efficiency as indicated by FCR, notes should be taken of the nutritive density of the diet.

Empty days The number of empty days gives an indication of the regularity or rhythm of a herd's breeding performance and is independent of weaning age. The merit of this particular index is that it is easy to collect and gives a continuous indication of the regularity of breeding within the herd.

Information required is taken from the service book. A typical example in the simplest form contains the information shown at the bottom of the opposite page.

Planned animal health and production in swine herds

1. Average weight of pigs sold

$$= \frac{\text{Total wt. of sales} + \text{total wt. of transfers}}{\text{No. of sales} + \text{no. of transfers}}$$

2. Average weight of pigs on entry

$$= \frac{\text{Total wt. of purchases} + \text{total wt. of transfers in}}{\text{No. of purchases} + \text{no. of transfers in}}$$

3. Total weight gain

= Total wt. of sales + total wt. of transfers out + end of period total wt. − (total wt. of purchases + total wt. of transfer in + start of period total wt.)

4. Per cent mortality

$$= \frac{\text{Deaths} \times 100}{\text{No. of sales} + \text{transfers out} + \text{deaths}}$$

5. Feed conversion ratio $= \dfrac{\text{Total wt. of feed consumed}}{\text{Total wt. gain}}$

6. Daily live-weight gain $= \dfrac{\text{Av. wt. gain/pig}}{\text{Av. no. of days in herd}}$

7. Average weight gain $=$ Av. wt. of pigs sold $-$ av. wt. of pigs entering

8. Average days in herd $= \dfrac{\text{Av. no. of pigs in feeding herd} \times 30.4}{\text{Av. no. of sales and transfers out per month}}$

EXAMPLE OF AN ACTION LIST FORM FOR COWS TO BE PRESENTED AT A HERD HEALTH VISIT

VET LIST	Date		

REASON PDS	Service date	Result	COMMENTS

Not served by 70 days	Date calved	Findings	Treatment

Others (Irregular cycles, whites, retained afterbirth, re-examines)

Reason	History	Treatment

EXAMPLE OF A HERD REPRODUCTIVE PERFORMANCE ANALYSIS (DAISY)

HERD REPRODUCTIVE PERFORMANCE ANALYSIS

Cows calving between 1JUL88 and 31MAR89

JUL88-MAR89
All these figures refer to cows calving in the month in question

	JUL88-MAR89 for herd	Target	JUL	AUG	SEP	OCT	NOV	DEC	JAN	FEB	MAR	COMMENTS
Number calved												
Heifers	49		0	48	0	0	1	0	0	0	0	
Cows	144		6	67	31	19	10	11	0	0	0	
Total	193		6	115	31	19	11	11	0	0	0	
Per cent	100											
Cumulative Per cent			3	59	16	9	5	5	0	0	0	
			3	62	78	88	94	100	100	100	100	
Number served since calving	182		6	111	31	15	10	9	0	0	0	See A5,A9
Per cent of calved	94	95	100	96	100	78	90	81	0	0	0	
Calving-1st serve(days) Average	70	65	96	76	61	56	57	55	0	0	0	
Num cows under 40 days	3	0	0	0	2	1	0	0	0	0	0	
Num cows over 100 days	9	0	3	5	0	1	0	0	0	0	0	
1st service 24day submission rate	85	95	83	85	83	93	80	88	0	0	0	See P2
First service preg rate %	58	55	50	65	54	53	40	22	0	0	0	See P2
Number conceiving	157		6	102	27	12	6	4	0	0	0	
Per cent of served	86	95	100	91	87	80	60	44	0	0	0	
Per cent of calved	81	90	100	88	87	63	54	36	0	0	0	
Num in calf-unknown serve	0	0	0	0	0	0	0	0	0	0	0	
Num not yet PD positive	21		0	6	3	4	3	5	0	0	0	See A3,A4,A5
Calving-conception(days) Average	88	85	124	93	77	75	60	63	0	0	0	
Days open average	103		124	104	95	106	94	101	0	0	0	
Num cows under 40 days	1	0	0	0	1	0	0	0	0	0	0	
Num cows over 120 days	24	<13	3	19	1	1	0	0	0	0	0	
Num serves/conception	1.5	1.6	2.0	1.6	1.5	1.4	1.3	1.5	0.0	0.0	0.0	See P2
Number dried off	0		0	0	0	0	0	0	0	0	0	
Average lactation in days	0	300	0	0	0	0	0	0	0	0	0	
Number recalved	0		0	0	0	0	0	0	0	0	0	
Average dry period	0	56	0	0	0	0	0	0	0	0	0	
Average calving interval	368	365	404	373	357	355	340	343	0	0	0	
Number culled Total Num sold or died	15		0	7	1	3	2	2	0	0	0	
Per cent culled of calved	7	20	0	6	3	15	18	18	0	0	0	
Num sold poor fertility	4	<9	0	2	0	1	0	1	0	0	0	
Number still to recalve or cull	178		6	108	30	16	9	9	0	0	0	See A7,A9

END OF REPORT

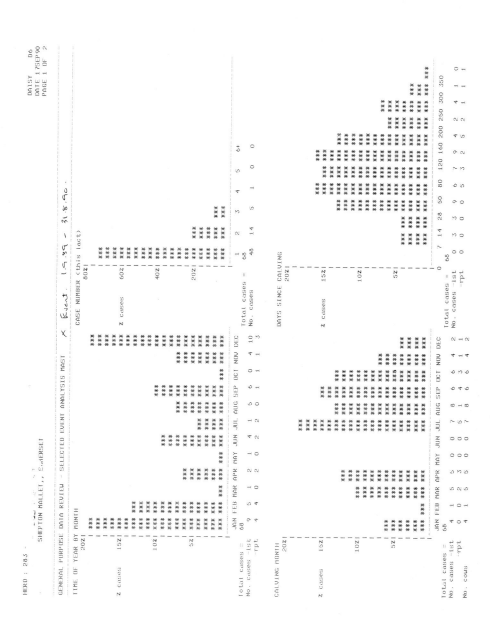

DAISY   D6
DATE 17SEP'90
PAGE 2 OF 2

HERD : 283 -

SHEPTON MALLET, SOMERSET

GENERAL PURPOSE DATA REVIEW - SELECTED EVENT ANALYSIS MAST

LACTATION NUMBER

% cases

	1	2	3	4	5	6	7	8+
Total cases =	68							
No. cases -1st	0	1	2	4	11	6	1	8
-rpt	2	1	2	4	11	1	0	8
No. cows	2	11	4	5	11	6	1	8

GROUP (at time of event)

% cases

	1	2
Total cases =	68	
No. cases -1st	40	8
-rpt	15	5
Av. cow days	207	59

EXAMPLE OF A MASTITIS INVESTIGATION CHECKLIST

Mastitis investigation checklist

Name: _____ Date _____/_____/_____
Address: _____
_____

Reason for visit: High SCC / TBC / Clinicals / Routine

Background information:

No. of cows in herd: _____   No. dry: _____
12 month RHA SCC: TBC range;
_____ mastitis cases in last _____ months from _____ cows.
Mastitis rate: _____ cases per 100 cows per annum.
Replacements: all homebred / in-calf-calved down heifers / cows
NMR individual cow cell counts available: yes / no
Culling policy: Clinical cases / SCC / Conformation / None

Bulk tank analysis:

TBC   SCC   Coliform Count
Str ag / dysg / uberis / faecalis / Staph aureus / Coli / Bacillus

Housing and yards:

No of cubicles: Loose housing
Cubicle design and length   (7′ 3″ × 4′)
Bedding: straw / shavings / sawdust / paper / other
Condition of housing:
Calving facilities: wind exposure: yes / no
Well drained yard free from stagnant water: yes / no

Premilking procedures:

Condition of cows entering the parlour: good / average / poor
Willingness of cows entering parlour: good / average / poor

Long tails / hairy udders
Washing: dry wipe / predipping / hose / udder cloth
Predipping: yes / no
Drying: none / individual paper towels / cloth
Stripping of cows: all / some / none

Milking procedure:

Do all milkers wear gloves: yes / no
Mastitis identification: stripping / detectors / visual / filters
Are mastitis detectors checked: no / some / none
Units attached within one minute of preparation: yes / no
Cows milked out rapidly: yes / no (3 to 5 minutes)
Magic water / undermilking / overmilking
Liner slip / unit fall-off / stray voltage / ACR function
Throughput: _____ cows / hour with _____ milkers
Hygiene during milking: good / average / poor
Vacuum shut-off prior to unit removal: yes / no / ACRs
Teat dipping / spraying. RTU dip / diluted correctly / storage
Dip type: iodine / chlorhexidine / hypochlorite / other
Teats dipped all year round: yes / no
Teat lesions: No / black spot / Prolapse / BHM / PseudoCP
Milking order: fresh / highs / low

Clinical mastitis:

Proper records kept: yes / no
Treatment regime: full course (3 tubes) / Part course / 2nd choice
Teats disinfected before infusion: yes / no
Treated cows properly identified: yes / no
Mastitis milk into: dump bucket / recorder vessel / separate cluster
Recorder vessel rinsed between milkings: yes / no
Clusters sterilised between cows: yes / no

Dry Cow Therapy:

Type of preparation used: None / SCDC / SPMC / LeoRed / other
Blanket treatment of herd: yes / no
Abrupt / gradual drying off. Cows starved: yes / no
Cows dried by calving date and/or yield (5 ltrs/day):   yes / no

Wash-up routine:

	MORNING	AFTERNOON
Rinse:	none/cold/warm	none/cold/warm
Main wash	hot/cold	hot/cold
Temperature:		
Circ time:		
Chemical:		
Concn:		
Volume:		
Final Rinse:	none/cold	none/cold
Boiler capacity: _____ litres for _____ units (10 ltrs/unit)		
Temperature of hot water:	F/C	

Milking Parlour:

Type: Age:
General condition of plant: satisfactory / needs attention
Vacuum level: _____ fluctuating _____ ″Hg. Gauge reads _____ ″Hg.
Pulsation rate: per minute.   Pulsation ratio:
Last test date: by MMB / dealer. Checked every _____ months
Liners changed every _____ months or after _____ milkings

Recommendations:

1.
2.
3.
4.
5.
6.
7.
8.
9.
10.

Reproduced by kind permission of P W Edmondson.

EXAMPLE OF A MASTITIS ADVISORY VISIT REPORT

A N Farmer
Brookfield Farm,
Ambridge

Report on the Mastitis Advisory visit of 11/12/1990

Target levels: Rolling herd cell count under 300 000/ml,
TBC levels under 10 000/ml,
Mastitis rate under 30 cases per 100 cows per year.

Listed below are my recommendations to improve your mastitis management:

Milking Routine:

– Milkers should wear gloves to reduce the spread of infection from cow to cow on hands.

– Cows should be dry wiped using disposable paper towels, unless they are dirty in which case they should be washed and dried. Washing but not drying cows will increase the number of environmental bacteria entering the bulk tank, reducing milk quality. There will also be an increased risk of environmental mastitis.

– Under no circumstances should an udder cloth be used as this will spread infection from cow to cow.

– Early identification and treatment of mastitis will result in a more rapid response to therapy, will reduce the risk of infection spreading to the rest of the herd, and will help maintain milk quality by ensuring that mastitis milk, which would increase the TBC levels, does not enter the bulk tank.

– Cows should be stripped before milking. This has three advantages: it removes any bacteria from the teat that may have entered since the last milking thus reducing the chance of infection; it allows for the early identification and treatment of mastitis; and finally it stimulates the udder which results in a faster milk-out.

– Once cows are milked out units should be removed, shutting off the vacuum prior to removal. Overmilking and/or pulling off clusters, can lead to teat-end prolapse allowing bacteria easy entry to the udder and an increase in the mastitis incidence.

– Teats should be dipped once the unit is removed. Iodine is the dip of choice and is far more effective than other preparations. It has the added advantage in that it stains teats and so the efficiency of dipping can easily be visually assessed. Dipping is more effective than teat spraying as it gives a more uniform coating of the teat, and less dip per cow is used.

– In order to maximize the benefits of teat dipping, it is important to coat each teat after every milking throughout the year. Seasonal teat dipping is ineffective.

Clinical Mastitis:

– Once a cow has been identified with mastitis she should receive a full course of treatment to ensure that all bacteria are eliminated from the udder, even if the milk appears normal. If this is not carried out, bacteria may remain in the udder, mastitis could recur at a later date, during which time infection may have spread to other cows in the herd.

– Mastitis cows should be milked into a dump bucket. Milking these cows through recorder jars, even if rinsed out after milking, may lead to an antibiotic failure.

– A solution of hypochlorite should be sucked through the cluster after milking to minimize the risk of passing on infection to the next cow milked. The ideal situation is to have a separate cluster for milking mastitis cows, but even this must be disinfected between uses.

– These cows must be carefully identified to ensure that contaminated milk does not enter the bulk tank and cause an antibiotic failure. The permitted level of antibiotic residues in milk has been halved to 0.005 IU/ml since October 1990.

– Teats should be dipped BEFORE AND AFTER tubing any cow with either a milking or dry cow preparation. This will reduce the risk of introducing infection on the end of the tube, and is especially important with dry tubes when the animal will not be milked for some time.

– If a clinical case does not respond to three tubes, then change to the next tube of choice.

– All cases of clinical mastitis should be recorded so that problem cows can be culled. Cows with three or more cases should be culled as they will be uneconomic irrespective of milk yield, and will also act as a reservoir of infection to the rest of the herd.

– A sample for bacteriological examination should be taken from one clinical case per month.

Dry Cow Therapy:

– Dry cow therapy has two aims: firstly, to remove any subclinical infection present at the end of lactation, and secondly, to help prevent the establishment of new infections in the dry period.

– Cows should be dried off according to the expected calving date or if the yield is below 5 litres per day. Once cows have been dried off they should be fed a restricted diet for three or four days to halt milk production.

– Drying off dates must be recorded as you are obliged to keep these under medicine recording regulations. This information is important in checking that cows to be sold are free from any residues.

General Management:

– Cubicles should be bedded daily with plenty of a suitable bedding material such as chopped straw. One bale of straw per 10 cows should be allocated for bedding each day. Materials such as wood shavings or sawdust are not suitable as they become rapidly contaminated with organic matter and can increase the likelihood of environmental mastitis.

– Calving facilities should be well maintained, and cleaned out when possible between calvings. If this is not possible then they must be well bedded down between calvings in order to minimize the risk of coliform mastitis.

– Ensure there are sufficient cubicles for the cows in your herd because cows that lie in the passageways are more prone to infection with environmental organisms.

EXAMPLE OF BLOOD TEST RESULTS FROM THE DAIRY HERD HEALTH AND PRODUCTIVITY SERVICE
(Kelly et al. 1988)

Dairy Herd Health & Productivity Service
BLOOD TEST RESULTS

NAME: J BLOGS **CODE:** 710/008/2

Blood Sample Date 18/02/87
Milk Record Date 30/01/87
CDF Herd N

Butter Fat 4.04g/100g
Solids Not Fat 8.49g/100g
Protein 3.23g/100g

Name		Early	Mid	Dry	DM	ME	DCP	pH	D	NH₃N
Forage 1	SILAGE	25.0	25.0	25.0	0.24	10.2	104	4.3	64	12.0
Forage 2										
Forage 3										
Conc 1	MILKW16	See cow data below								
Conc 2	MILKM18	4.0	4.0	0.0						
Conc 3	SBP	1.5	1.5	1.5						
Conc 4	DRAFF	6.0	6.0	6.0						

Constant fed amounts and feed analysis

COW DATA

	EARLY LACTATION GROUP							Mean	MID LACTATION GROUP					Mean	DRY GROUP					Mean
Cow number	27	62	50	79	55	51	20		80	69	66	53	10		95	9	100	98	92	
Days calved	27	30	24	17	36	15	42	27	106	105	91	131	83	103	-31	-22	-47	-13	-4	-23
Approx Wght	740	670	708	550	560	560	708	642	608	650	608	738	550	630	688	670	648	818	800	724
Condition	3.0	2.0	3.0	1.0	1.0	3.0	2.5	2.2	2.0	2.0	2.0	3.0	3.0	2.4	3.0	2.5	2.5	2.5	3.0	2.7
Milk Yield	35.0	42.0	33.0	37.0	37.0	37.0	38.0	37.0	38.0	31.0	32.0	27.0	28.0	31.2	0.0	0.0	0.0	0.0	0.0	0.0
Exp Yield	35.0	42.0	35.0	37.0	37.0	37.0	38.0	37.3	34.0	29.0	30.0	25.0	27.0	29.0	0.0	0.0	0.0	0.0	0.0	0.0
Lact Number	4	4	9	2	2	3	5	4	5	3	5	7	2	4	4	2	2	2	4	2
Variable Feeds																				
MILKW16	6.6	8.0	7.0	8.3	8.3	8.3	8.6	7.9	8.6	6.3	6.6	5.6	5.3	6.5	0.0	0.0	0.0	0.0	0.0	0.0

BLOOD RESULTS

Butyrate	10.9	4.8	5.5	7.4	4.6	5.9	7.8	6.7	4.5	6.8	7.4	8.1	7.7	6.9	3.8	5.5	4.2	6.4	8.8	5.7
Glucose	57.0	65.7	58.7	67.9	76.4	65.1	61.4	64.6	61.9	46.1	64.1	72.5	67.4	62.4	70.3	61.2	67.4	61.5	67.7	65.6
Urea	23.0	26.5	22.0	24.5	25.0	22.0	22.0	23.6	20.0	21.0	24.5	20.0	22.0	21.5	21.0	19.0	20.0	17.0	12.0	17.8
Albumin	3.4	3.7	3.4	3.9	3.6	4.0	3.8	3.7	3.5	4.0	4.0	3.7	4.0	3.8	3.5	4.2	3.7	3.7	3.9	3.8
Globulin	4.1	4.5	5.5	4.2	4.8	3.9	4.1	4.4	4.8	4.0	4.2	4.8	4.0	4.4	4.7	3.8	4.4	4.6	4.0	4.3
Albu : Glob	0.8	0.8	0.6	0.9	0.7	1.0	0.9	0.8	0.7	1.0	0.9	0.8	1.0	0.9	0.7	1.1	0.8	0.8	1.0	0.9
Magnesium	2.4	2.6	2.3	2.4	2.4	2.5	2.5	2.4	2.5	2.4	2.1	2.5	2.5	2.4	2.4	2.3	2.5	2.1	2.2	2.3
Phosphate	5.4	8.4	5.4	5.8	7.4	5.8	7.4	6.5	6.0	6.8	5.5	5.4	6.1	6.0	6.2	6.0	5.8	4.9	5.6	5.7

FEED DATA

FED TOTAL DM	18.1	19.4	18.5	19.6	19.6	19.6	19.6	19.2	19.9	17.9	18.1	17.3	17.0	18.0	8.9	8.9	8.9	8.9	8.9	8.9
Theor'cal DM	21.4	21.6	20.0	16.8	19.1	16.8	23.2	19.8	21.0	20.5	19.8	21.6	17.7	20.1	9.7	9.4	9.2	10.6	9.8	9.7
Fed Conc DM	12.1	13.4	12.5	13.6	13.6	13.6	13.9	13.2	13.9	11.9	12.1	11.3	11.0	12.0	2.9	2.9	2.9	2.9	2.9	2.9
Prot Conc DM	12.1	13.4	12.5	12.6	13.6	12.6	13.9	13.0	13.9	11.9	12.1	11.3	11.0	12.0	2.9	2.9	2.9	2.9	2.9	2.9
Fed F'age DM	6.0	6.0	6.0	6.0	6.0	6.0	6.0	6.0	6.0	6.0	6.0	6.0	6.0	6.0	6.0	6.0	6.0	6.0	6.0	6.0
ProtF'age DM	9.2	8.2	7.4	4.2	5.4	4.2	9.3	6.8	7.1	8.6	7.6	10.3	6.6	8.0	6.7	6.5	6.2	7.6	6.9	6.8
Conc/F'ageDM	1.3	1.6	1.7	3.2	2.5	3.3	1.5	2.2	2.0	1.4	1.6	1.1	1.6	1.5	0.4	0.4	0.5	0.4	0.4	0.4

REQUIRED ME	257	287	244	250	251	251	269	258	260	228	229	215	203	227	86	86	80	101	102	91
Fed Conc ME	160	177	165	180	180	180	184	175	184	157	160	149	145	159	36	36	36	36	36	36
Exp F'age ME	96	110	78	69	70	70	85	82	76	71	68	66	58	67	50	50	44	65	65	54
ProbF'age ME	93	84	76	42	55	42	95	69	72	88	78	105	68	82	68	66	63	78	70	69
Fed Total ME	221	238	226	241	241	241	245	236	245	218	221	210	206	220	97	97	97	97	97	97
ProtTotal ME	254	261	241	210	236	209	279	241	256	245	238	254	213	241	104	102	100	114	106	105
INDEX OF ME	98	91	99	83	94	83	103	93	107	107	103	118	104	106	120	118	124	112	104	115

REQUIRED DCP	2315	2665	2192	2339	2343	2343	2464	2380	2419	2057	2092	1878	1848	2058	635	626	476	696	688	624
FedTotal DCP	2507	2684	2557	2723	2723	2723	2761	2668	2761	2468	2507	2380	2341	2491	1087	1087	1087	1087	1087	1087
ProtTotalDCP	2841	2920	2711	2379	2667	2374	3106	2714	2877	2742	2678	2834	2414	2709	1163	1142	1116	1259	1182	1172
PrtDCP/PrbME	11.1	11.2	11.2	11.3	11.3	11.3	11.1	11.2	11.2	11.2	11.2	11.1	11.3	11.2	11.1	11.1	11.1	11.0	11.1	11.1

EXAMPLE OF A QUARTERLY HERD HEALTH REPORT FROM THE DAIRY HERD HEALTH AND PRODUCTIVITY SERVICE
(Kelly et al. 1988)

Dairy Herd Health & Productivity Service

QUARTERLY HERD HEALTH REPORT FOR
PERIOD ENDING DEC 1986

NAME:

FARM CODE:

		LAST QUARTER	THIS QUARTER	SAME QUARTER LAST YEAR	12 MONTHS ENDED DEC 1986		
Average number of cows of milking age in herd		151	147	137	142		**COMMENTS**
Number of cows sold because of	Yield	0	0	0	0	0.0 %	
	Infertility	3	1	1	11	7.7 %	
	Mastitis	2	0	0	7	4.9 %	
	Lameness	6	0	0	8	5.6 %	
	Age	0	0	1	4	2.8 %	
	Other	1	2	1	4	2.8 %	
	Total	12	3	3	34	23.9 %	
Number of cows treated for	Fertility	8	8	6	72	50.6 %	
	Mastitis	16	19	14	54	37.9 %	
	Digestive Upset	0	0	0	0	0.0 %	
	Hypomagnesaemia	0	0	0	0	0.0 %	
	Hypocalcaemia	0	5	0	10	7.0 %	
	Ketosis	0	0	0	1	0.7 %	
	Lameness	5	19	29	74	52.0 %	
	Other	0	0	0	2	1.4 %	
Average mastitis cell count ('000 cells/ml)		197	138	175	173		
Number of cows served by AI	First Time	36	43	44	134		
	Second Time	14	17	23	56		
	Third Time	4	5	7	24		
	Fourth Time +	6	3	1	23		
Number of cows served by bull	First Time	0	1	0	1		
	Second Time	0	2	0	2		
	Third Time	1	0	0	1		
	Fourth Time +	0	3	0	3		
Percentage of cows of milking age in herd receiving a first service (target 100+)		–	–	–	95 %		
30 Day first service non-return rate % (target 70-80)		55	58	43	57		
Pregnancy Diagnosis	Milk + ve	0	0	0	0		
	Milk - ve	0	0	0	0		
	Vet + ve	40	20	0	102		
	Vet - ve	2	1	0	10		
Negative rate of milk tests % (target less than 15)		0	0	0	0		
Pregnancy rate of cows examined by vet % (target 95 +)		95	95	0	91		

EXAMPLE OF A MLC PRODUCTION REPORT FOR A PIG BREEDING HERD

PIGPLAN

Recording and Costing

BREEDING HERD REPORT
1-MONTHLY REPORTING

PERIOD ENDED : 3^ JUN 1991
MEMBER NUMBER : 14142

NAME : A BOAR
ADDRESS : SOW LANE
HOG TOWN
HAMPSHIRE

	CURRENT YEAR			PREVIOUS YEAR			MLC TOP THIRD COMPOUND YEAR END 30/06/91	MLC AVERAGE COMPOUND YEAR END 30/06/91
	Period ended 31/01/91 (3 MONTHS)	Period ended 31/04/91 (6 MONTHS)	Year ended 30/06/91	Period ended 31/06/90 (3 MONTHS)	Period ended 30/06/90 (6 MONTHS)	Year ended 30/06/90		
HERD STRUCTURE								
1. Av. no of sows and gilts in the herd	335	340	337	337	341	336	406	335
2. Av. no of unserved gilts	11	15	17	20	21	19	33	24
3. Av. no of productive sows (LAEEED +)	324	325 *	330 *	317	327 *	335 *	373	282
4. Av. no of sows and gilts per boar	29	30	20	21	21	20	19	19
SOW PERFORMANCE FACTORS								
5. Percentage breeding sow replacements	9.0	17.6	40.4	10.1	19.4	44.3	39.9	40.2
6. Percentage breeding sow sales and deaths	13.1	33.5	41.5	11.6	24.3	44.3	38.5	33.9
7. Percentage breeding sow deaths	2.7	4.1	6.5	0.9	1.5	3.6	3.4	4.3
8. Percentage successful services		83.5	80.0		83.7	83.0	86.7	85.4
9. Av. no of litters per sow and gilt per year	2.43	2.42 *	2.36	2.42	2.55 *	2.37 *	2.37	2.27
10. Av. no of pigs reared per sow and gilt per year	22.7	22.2 *	22.5	24.3	22.9 *	22.8 *	23.8	21.5
11. Qty. of sow and boar feed per sow and gilt per year (t)	1.239	1.197	1.167	1.336	1.279	1.219	1.223	1.234
12. Cost of sow and boar feed per sow and gilt per year (£)	209.18	196.63	189.23	214.19	235.45	224.95	178.71	179.30
13. Cost per tonne of sow and boar feed (£)	167.97	164.14	162.03	160.30	183.98	182.03	146.35	145.48
LITTER PERFORMANCE FACTORS								
14. Av. no of pigs born per litter ALIVE	10.45	10.39	10.87	11.16	10.77	10.79	11.12	10.66
15. DEAD	0.66	0.75	0.85	1.05	0.97	0.97	0.82	0.82
16. TOTAL	11.11	11.13	11.72	12.21	11.74	11.76	11.94	11.48
17. Av. no of pigs reared per litter	9.35	9.44	9.50	10.07	9.73	9.65	10.03	9.46
PIG PERFORMANCE FACTORS								
18. Percentage mortality of pigs born alive	10.5	13.2	12.7	9.8	9.7	10.6	9.8	11.2
19. Total qty. of feed per pig reared (Kg)	57	56	56	58	59	56	56	63
20. Total feed cost per pig reared (£)	9.94	9.37	9.40	9.74	11.01	10.26	8.25	9.22
21. Qty. of piglet feed per pig reared (Kg)	0.9	0.7	0.6	0.7	0.6	0.4	0.2	0.2
22. Cost of piglet feed per pig reared (£)	0.44	0.34	0.29	0.35	0.29	0.21	0.10	0.11
23. Cost per tonne of piglet feed (£)	515.15	505.90	501.76	484.65	483.39	484.83	502.89	484.04
24. Av. weight of pigs weaned (Kg)	6.2	6.4	6.5	6.0	7.4	6.8	5.9	6.0
25. Overall cost per tonne of feed (£)	173.11	168.21	155.66	164.20	187.00	184.38	147.53	146.67
26. Av. weaning age (days)	23	22	25	22	22	22	22	23

SAMPLE PAGE FROM POCKET DIARY FOR
FARM RECORDING AS DESIGNED BY
PIGTALES LTD.

PIGTALES		N⍛ 000893

DATE: ○ 14. 10. 82	COMPLETED BY: PGT.	
IDENTITY	EVENT	DETAIL
96	X₁	6 LR
97	X₁	7 LW
○ 16	FW	12L 1s
101	FW	9L 3s
○ 16	-1	To 101
16	PL	1 died L
96	X₂	6 LR
○ 17	RT	116
25	INDUCED.	

EXAMPLE OF AN INDIVIDUAL SOW RECORDING CARD

SOW NUMBER   3910   LITTER SIRE   388

DATE SERVED   06/08/90   DATE DUE   29/11/90   RETURNS 0

DATE FARROWED   28/11   NO. BORN ALIVE   10   DEAD   1

DATE WEANED   22/12   NO. WEANED   9   (Poor/Small/Average/Good)

0 Overlay   __ 1 Non-viable __ 2 Scour   __ 3 Destroyed   __ 4 Trembles   __

5 Starved   __ 6 Unknown   __ 7 Chilled   __ 8 Savaged   __ 9 Diseased   __

CONDITION SCORE __ 2 ____   COMMENT _____ 10/27/11

PARITY	FARROWED	ALIVE	DEAD	WEANED	DIED	AGE	SIZE	SCORE	I.F.P.	INDEX	S.I.
1	22/08/88	12	0	11	1	28	A	2	150	2.44	5
2	28/02/89	14	0	11	1	29	A	2	190	1.92	47
3	16/09/89	13	1	10	1	32	A	2	200	1.83	56
4	14/02/90	15	0	11	2	21	A	2	151	2.42	4
5	04/07/90	14	3	6	5	28	A	2	140	2.61	4

LIFETIME YIELD : LIVE PIGLETS 29.9/YEAR, WEANED PIGLETS 21.5
LAST 2 LITTERS   36.4   21.3
Age at 1st conception : 30 weeks
29/09/87 MB 301   06/04/88 Parvo   28/02/89 -2
03/04/89 p.m.   23/05/89 RT 03/04/89 (360) 16/09/89 -2
14/02/90 -2   12/03/90 p.m.   04/07/90 -3
06/08/90 p.m.

PLAN OF VISITS TO PRODUCE AND MONITOR A SHEEP HEALTH PROGRAMME
(Clarkson and Faull, 1990)

	Date of visit (approx)	Jobs (some or all)	Time (approx) (for 500–1000 ewe flock)
VISIT 1*	Two months before tupping	1 Rams (all): Condition score, check fertility and feet. Ensure that the farmer/shepherd is able to condition score rams and ewes 2 Ewes (100 selected) Condition score, cull (teeth, age, udders) 3 Store lambs (a selection): Condition score 4 Take samples of blood and faeces for copper, B12, selenium, fluke and worms and abortion profile (Toxoplasma and Enzootic) 5 Check hay or silage and take samples for fibre, protein and energy estimates 6 Inspect pasture, examine for snail habitats 7 Check and discuss Farm Questionnaire (sent and hopefully returned in advance) 8 Discuss 'clean grazing' 9 Discuss farmer's objectives and possible targets for production	3 hours

* Prepare draft programme following this visit and receipt of laboratory results

VISIT 2	Approx 1 month later	Discuss draft programme with farmer and finalise programme	1 hour
VISIT 3★	6 weeks before lambing	Condition score 100 ewes Advise about feeding (including trace elements) Treat clinical cases	1 hour
VISIT 4	2 weeks before lambing	Condition score 100 ewes Advise about housing facilities, colostrum, lambing and recording Treat clinical cases	1 hour
VISIT 5★	At peak lambing time	Clinical events Recording of lambs Advise about hypothermia and starvation, *E. coli*, coccidia and worming	1 hour
VISIT 6	12 weeks after lambing	Check growth rates	1 hour
		Total	8 hours

Notes

When more than one flock is involved with widely different lambing dates, more than 6 visits will be necessary, although it is probable that some can be combined. In addition to the 6 planned visits, advice will be available by phone.

★ Visits in subsequent years

Possible charges

First Year (October 1989 prices)

1 For 6 visits	8 hours @ £30 per hour	£240.00
2 Laboratory services eg.	12 bloods for mineral trace element profile	£70.00
	12 faeces for fluke	£36.00
	12 faeces for round worm eggs	£42.00
	12 separate necropsies	£120.00
	2 food analyses	£40.00

These tests need not be applied routinely and may be reduced due to information obtained from clinical records from the farm.

EXAMPLE OF A FARM QUESTIONNAIRE SENT IN ADVANCE OF THE FIRST FLOCK HEALTH VISIT
(Clarkson and Faull, 1990)

Farm questionnaire

(Sent in advance of visit 1 with a request to be returned 7 days before the visit. The questionnaire will be completed in June–August, depending on tupping dates)

Date	Farmer's name
	Address
	Telephone
Veterinary surgeon (for sheep consultant only)	Address
	Telephone
General information	total area (ha)
	total grassland
	silage
	hay
	roots
	home produced oats/barley for sheep
	other stock beside sheep
	labour available
	tenant owner
	is there a large scale map of farm available?

Flock information

Total number of ewes _____

Total number of flocks _____

(A flock is a group of sheep with an identity! ie. lambing date, pedigree, special purpose. If a group of sheep has a planned lambing date a month or more apart, treat as a separate flock.) Since a sheep year normally commences at tupping (Summer/ Autumn) and concludes with lamb sales about 12 months later, the information requested should refer to the ewes and their lamb crop.

	Flock 1	Flock 2	Flock 3
Breed of ewe			
Number of ewes excluding ewe lambs			
Ewe lambs number			
age at tupping			
Breed of rams			
Number of rams			
Tupping date			
Lambing date			
Shearing date			
Dipping date			
Weaning date			
Housing date			
Wintered away dates			
Ewe feeding what			
when			
how much			
Dock/castrate			

how _____ _____ _____

when _____ _____ _____

Where lambed

Is clean grazing available at turnout ie. not grazed by sheep the
year before _____ _____ _____

Is clean grazing available in July
ie. not grazed by sheep this year _____ _____ _____

Lamb sales
   where _____ _____ _____

   _____ _____ _____

   when _____ _____ _____

Purpose of flock _____ _____ _____

Special practices
(eg. synchronisation, AI,
scanning) _____ _____ _____
Ewes purchased
   age _____ _____ _____

   source _____ _____ _____
Percentage of flock lambed over
4 week period _____ _____ _____

Example of a farm questionnaire sent in advance of the first flock health visit

Disease control

	With what	To what	When
Vaccination			
Clostridia			
Pasteurella			
Foot rot			
Orf			
Any others			
Mineral			
Copper			
Cobalt			
Selenium			
Parasites			
Worms			
Fluke			
Coccidia			
Others			
Footbathing			
Condition scoring			
Tape-worm dosing to dogs			
Clinical problems encountered			
Ewes			

Lambs

_____ _____ _____

_____ _____ _____

_____ _____ _____

Laboratory reports

_____ _____ _____

_____ _____ _____

_____ _____ _____

What do you think is your most
important problem?

_____ _____ _____

_____ _____ _____

_____ _____ _____

_____ _____ _____

_____ _____ _____

_____ _____ _____

_____ _____ _____

_____ _____ _____

Production figures

Lambs	Flock 1	Flock 2	Flock 3
Number of lambs			
Born alive			
Born dead			
Dying in first 7 days			
Sold for slaughter before weaning			
Weaned			
Sold for slaughter after weaning			
Sold as stores			
Retained as stores			
Retained for breeding			

Lambs sold for slaughter

Month	Number	Average edcw in kg	Average price (state whether including variable premium)

Ewes	Number	When	Why
Died			
Culled			
Sold			
Purchased			

SHEEP FARM VISIT CHECK LIST—FARM/FARMER
(Clarkson and Faull, 1990)

It is useful to have a checklist, particularly for the first visit, along the following lines

	Observations
(1) Geography	
(2) Geology	
(3) Climate	
(4) Possibilities for	Ticks Fluke
(5) Economic position	Income from sheep Income from other sources Gross margin/ewe Gross margin/ha
(6) Drugs and instruments (have a good look around)	

(7) Disease control
measures
(what's wrong with
them?)

_____

(8) Welfare/care of sick

_____

(9) Labour/dogs
(particularly availability
of labour at lambing
time)

_____

(10) Use of   Vets
                              ADAS
                              Commercial reps
                              ATB

_____

SHEEP FARM VISIT CHECK LIST—THE SHEEP
(Clarkson and Faull, 1990)

	Observations
(1) General look at each flock/age group	Number of flocks
	Variety of breeds
	Extensive/intensive
	General condition
	Lameness
	Coughing
	Dirty tails
	Wool break
(2) Examine (handle) (a) 10% (or minimum of 50) ewes of each flock/age group	Condition score
	Teeth/age
	Blood sample (if necessary)
	(i) Abortion 'profile', ie. EAE/Toxoplasma
	(ii) Deficiencies
	Faecal sample (if necessary and from appropriate animals)
	(i) Fluke
	(ii) Worms

	(iii) Coccidia
(b) Clinical cases	Very thin
	Very lame
	Very sick
	Very nervous/depressed
	Very 'moth-eaten'
	Very dirty-tailed
	Tail end lambs
(c) Rams (all)	Condition score
	Feet
	Genitalia
	Faeces
(3) Abortions	Samples
(4) Suitable carcases	For PME

SHEEP FARM VISIT CHECK LIST—THE FOOD
(Clarkson and Faull, 1990)

Observations

(1) Stocking rate (ewes/ha)

(2) Quantity and quality of grazing

(3) Reclamation/ fertilization

(4) History of deficiency diseases

(5) Mineral supplementation (food and dosing)

(6) Stored roughage   quantity/quality
    (hay, silage)

_____

(7) Concentrates   menu and quantity per ewe/day

_____

(8) Storage of concentrates
    (and cats!)

_____

(9) Rack and trough space/
    ewe

_____

(10) Colostrum (source and
     quantity)

_____

_____

SHEEP FARM VISIT CHECK LIST—THE SHELTER
(Clarkson and Faull, 1990)

	Observations
(1) State of repair	
(2) Size/space/stocking density (ewes/sq m)	
(3) Atmosphere	
(4) Bedding	
(5) Water supply	
(6) Lighting	

(7) Trough space/ewe

_____

(8) Lambing pens   Numbers
Cleanliness
Heating
Risks
Lambing and revival kit
Drugs

_____

(9) The sheep   Puffing/blowing/coughing
'Sweating' (if not shorn)
Cleanliness
Lameness

_____

(10) Isolation facilities
eg. abortions/sick)

_____

_____

AN EXAMPLE OF A HEALTH PROGRAMME
(Clarkson and Faull, 1990)

MONTH	VISIT	FLOCK 85 ewes	FLOCK 33 ewe lambs
SEPTEMBER	VISIT 1	**check ewes and rams** condition score feed feet footbath Footvax culling **ewes** blocks with monensin 10th TUP	
OCTOBER			**check ewes and rams** condition score feed feet footbath Footvax culling **ewes** blocks with monensin 5th TUP
NOVEMBER		**ewes** Footvax footbath	
DECEMBER	VISIT 2	**ewes** house shear footbath worm condition score	**ewes** Footvax footbath
JANUARY	VISIT 3	**ewes and rams** Heptavac P condition score lambing kit pens	**ewes** house shear footbath worm condition score
FEBRUARY	VISIT 4	**LAMBING** **lambs** decoquinate in creep feed from 2 weeks	
MARCH			**ewes** Heptavac P condition score lambing kit pens
	VISIT 5	**TURN OUT** **ewes** Footvax	**LAMBING TURN OUT** **lambs** decoquinate in creep feed from 2 weeks ewes Footvax
APRIL			
		3 WEEKS **ewes** worm	**3 WEEKS** **ewes** worm
MAY	VISIT 6	**3 WEEKS** **ewes and lambs** worm	**3 WEEKS** **ewes and lambs**
JUNE		**3 WEEKS** **lambs** worm Heptavac P Footvax	
JULY		**WEAN**	**lambs** Heptavac P Footvax **WEAN**
AUGUST		**lambs** Heptavac P	**lambs** Heptavac P Footvax

PROBLEMS OF FEEDING AND HOUSING: THEIR DIAGNOSIS AND CONTROL

A J F WEBSTER MA, Vet MB, PhD, MRCVS

Diagnosis of feeding problems
Energy
Protein
Allergens, toxins and anti-nutrient factors
Disorders of mineral and vitamin metabolism
Oral satisfaction
Diagnosis of housing problems

Proper feeding and housing constitute the major part of good husbandry. Since husbandry may itself be defined as animal science tempered with tender loving care, the word 'proper' implies both a scientific approach to the biological principles that determine health and efficiency of production and a compassionate concern to provide animals with a reasonable quality of life. Thus the act of feeding becomes more than just the act of acquiring nutrients; it is also a very satisfactory way for an animal to pass the time. Similarly, our view of housing cannot be restricted to physical criteria such as air temperature, hygiene and output per unit area. For many farm livestock the house, or cage within the house, represents the totality of their experience of the environment—which prompts the question 'if this is all, is it enough?'

Farm animal nutrition and housing are big subjects, each meriting at least one textbook. The latest editions of two very good books, both entitled *Animal Nutrition*, by McDonald et al. (1988) and by Maynard and Loosli (1979), keep up-to-date with this subject in a European and North American context respectively. For general principles of housing in Europe I would recommend the work by Sainsbury and Sainsbury (1988), *Livestock Health and Housing*. I also strongly recommend Curtis (1983), *Environmental Management in Animal Agriculture*, not just for its North American perspective but as a thoroughly good read. This chapter assumes a reasonable knowledge of the principles of nutrition and environmental management and concentrates on the systematic approach to diagnosis and control of those problems of productivity, health and welfare in farm animals which may be attributed, wholly or in part, to disorders of feeding or housing.

Diagnosis of feeding problems

The science of nutrition relates the metabolic requirements of an animal to the food it eats by expressing both in terms of a common currency, namely nutrients. Disorders of nutrition and metabolism arise when the intake of one or more nutrients fails to meet the animal's requirement for the maintenance of life or its physiological potential for growth or lactation. The broader implications of this truism are illustrated by Figure 8.1. Nutrients are categorized,

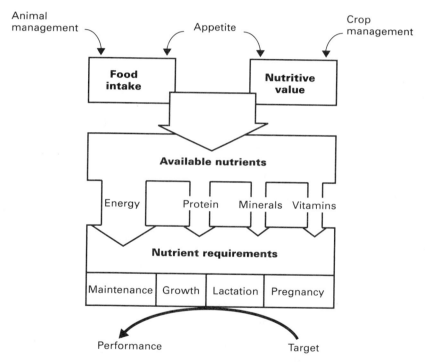

Figure 8.1 Factors affecting nutrient supply and requirement (from Webster 1987).

at this stage, simply under four headings—energy, protein, minerals and vitamins. The supply of available (or absorbed) nutrients is determined by food intake (kg dry matter (DM)/day) and the nutritive value of the food. In the case of energy this is conventionally defined by digestible energy (DE) or metabolizable energy (ME) (McDonald et al. 1988). I shall hereafter refer to ME only. ME intake is expressed in megajoules (MJ) ME/day and the energy value of feeds is defined by the ME concentration per unit dry matter (M/D; units = MJ/kg). Available protein for simple-stomached species is conventionally defined by digestible crude protein (DCP; g/kg DM). Most modern protein systems for ruminants distinguish between the requirements of rumen microbes for rumen degradable protein (RDP) and the requirement of the host animal for truly absorbed amino acid nitrogen (TAAN) or metabolizable protein (MP) (Webster 1987). The availability of minerals and vitamins should also be taken into account when assessing nutrient requirements but this is beyond the scope of this chapter (see Agricultural Research Council 1980, 1982; Underwood 1980).

Evaluation of a feeding system and diagnosis of any associated problems should be based on a comparison between estimated supply of available nutrients and requirements for maintenance, growth, lactation, etc. (Figure 8.1).

The first task for the nutritional consultant therefore is to compare actual and target performance. Targets for growth rates in pigs, for example, may be obtained from records of breeding companies or annual reports of the Meat and Livestock Commission (MLC). Targets for lactation can similarly be taken from National Milk Records provided by the Milk Marketing Board (MMB). If performance fails to meet the target one proceeds to compare supply and requirement for the various nutrients in sequence to discover where supply is failing to meet demand and whether this is due to a failure in quantity or quality of food eaten.

Before proceeding to discuss the major nutrients in more detail, I wish to emphasize five important points which have general application.

1. The concept of dietary requirement is very useful for the formulation and evaluation of rations. It should not, however, be interpreted too rigidly since it implies that nutrients are used with a fixed efficiency up to the point where requirement is met, and are 'wasted' thereafter. In real life it is more common to observe a curvilinear response to increase in a specific nutrient subject to the law of diminishing returns (e.g. increasing milk yield in response to increasing protein intake in dairy cattle). In this case nutrient requirement would be calculated on the basis of existing milk yield in the first instance to assess the adequacy of the diet. To improve efficiency it is then necessary to measure the marginal response of the cows to a change in the quantity or quality of diet and assess the response in the light of criteria such as feed costs, milk prices and quotas. A lactating dairy cow does not therefore have an absolute requirement for nutrients. Instead there is a level of feeding which produces an optimal response when all biological and economic factors are taken into account.

2. Requirements for protein, expressed as dietary concentration, range approximately between 100 and 200 g/kg DM, major minerals from 1 to

40 g/kg, and requirements for trace elements and vitamins are usually expressed in mg or μg/kg. Thus over 80% of available nutrients are used for energy metabolism, less than 20% for protein metabolism and only 1–2% for the whole of mineral and vitamin metabolism. In quantitative terms it is most important to control energy supply with precision, with protein a poor second and the rest of the field out of sight. The corollary to this is that far more cases of nutritional deficiency can be attributed to lack of the major unit, energy, than to trace elements such as copper or selenium.

3. All the information available on performance, food intake, nutritive value, etc. will be subject to some degree of uncertainty. However, measurements of performance, such as weight gain or milk yield, are often far more accurate than estimates of food intake and nutritive value, especially in the case of ruminants eating unmeasurable amounts of silage of uncertain quality. If the estimate of nutrient supply fails to match requirement for a known level of performance (e.g. 35 kg milk/day from a dairy cow) the error can usually be attributed to the supply side. Modern, elaborate, computer-based feeding systems for animals give an impression of precision that may, on occasions, be spurious. The diagnostician should place more faith in simple but real measurements of animal performance than sophisticated but speculative outputs from a computerized feed plan.

4. The supply and metabolism of available nutrients is a highly dynamic process and is better evaluated in terms of inputs and outputs than by measurements of the status quo. The 'Metabolic Profile' (Payne and Payne 1987) attempts to diagnose disorders of nutrition and metabolism from 'snap-shot' measurements of the concentration of metabolites in blood. These can be of value, particularly if taken while an animal is in the process of adapting to a change in nutrient requirement (e.g. dairy cows in early lactation; Blowey 1985). However, after it has adjusted performance downwards to the rate permitted by the first limiting nutrient, the metabolic profile may well appear normal. This is, I admit, oversimplistic. There are many specific cases where persistent changes in the concentration of a specific metabolite can aid in diagnosis of a nutritional problem. However, the metabolic profile is not an effective substitute for a proper evaluation of nutrient supply and demand.

5. When performance is restricted by lack of one or more specific nutrients, recovery is impossible unless the deficiency is remedied. Nutritional disorders differ therefore from infectious diseases where the natural history is (usually) progression towards recovery or death. Thus, the successful treatment of a nutritional disorder provides a more reliable confirmation of the original diagnosis than can be claimed in many cases of infectious disease.

Energy

Because most food is eaten to provide energy, it is economically far more important to balance energy supply to target performance than (say) phosphorus, where one can err on the side of generosity without incurring bankruptcy. Energy supply (ME; MJ/day) may be regulated either by feeding a fixed ration in which ME concentration (M/D; MJ/kg) is known (more or less) or by adjusting M/D so that spontaneous DM intake provides the required daily amount of ME. As an example of the first approach, a dry sow may be fed a fixed ration, 2 kg DM/day, of a diet with a known, high M/D of 13 MJ/kg to meet a maintenance energy requirement of 26 MJ ME/day. Within the limited context of energy supply this is entirely satisfactory, although the diet may be deficient in other nutrients and may fall far short of her spontaneous desire to eat, particularly if she has nothing better to do (Lawrence et al. 1988).

As an example of the second approach, consider a Friesian dairy cow yielding 28 kg milk/day with an ME requirement of 200 MJ/day. She may be fed ad lib a complete, mixed diet with an estimated M/D of 11.5 MJ/kg on the assumption that she will eat 17.4 kg DM/day (200/11.5). The uncertainties attached to this double assumption as to food quality and intake are large. An individual cow (or group of cows) may fail to sustain 28 kg milk/day on this ration because:

(i) M/D has been overestimated.
(ii) DM intake is less than expected.
(iii) The cow is directing less nutrients to milk production and more to maintenance and/or body gain than predicted.

All these questions need to be considered in diagnosis. The subject is too complicated to develop here (see Webster 1987) but it is important to note that unsatisfactory dry matter intake in ruminants does not necessarily imply that the food does not taste good. The ruminant with a high production potential, such as the high-yielding cow or fast-growing lamb, has a metabolic demand for nutrients that exceeds the digestive capacity of the rumen, especially when eating diets such as silage which ferment (and therefore leave the rumen) slowly. Whereas the dry sow given 2 kg/day of highly digestible food may be replete with nutrients but hungry for food, the high-yielding dairy cow on a predominantly roughage ration may be hungry for nutrients but full up. Neither situation is ideal when viewed in the context of welfare.

Energy allowances for maintenance

The ME requirement of an animal for maintenance is determined by its size, physiological state, spontaneous activity and the thermal environment to which it is exposed. Comprehensive textbooks of nutrition such as the Agricultural Research Council publications on the nutrient requirements of pigs (Agricultural Research Council 1982) and ruminants (Agricultural Research Council 1980) are available for those seeking high precision (if not accuracy). As a first approximation, however, one may set the ME *allowance* for maintenance (ME_m) of all farm mammals and birds at 450–500 kJ ME/kg weight$^{0.75}$ per day in circumstances where activity is minimal and the animals are neither stressed by heat nor cold (Webster 1989a). The exponent 0.75 converts body weight (kg) to 'metabolic body size' (Kleiber 1961), an extraordinarily powerful concept which confers proportionality between species or individuals within species on estimates of heat production, nutrient requirements, and effectively all other physiological or metabolic rates (e.g. growth rate, cardiac output, protein synthesis). In the present context one can state simply that the maintenance allowance of all farm animals at rest in a thermoneutral environment when divided by metabolic body size (W, kg$^{0.75}$) is approximately the same.

I illustrate this concept for my students with an exotic parable, 'the twenty-five loaves and one large elephant.'

There was a man who purchased an elephant (weight 2 tonnes) hoping one day that it would carry him to a far off land. Meantime, the elephant did very little and would eat only loaves of fresh bread (0.5 kg/loaf). 'How shall I feed him?' the man bemoaned.

Kleiber (had he been there) would have reasoned:

(i) Body weight = 200 kg, thus $W^{0.75}$ = 300 kg
(ii) M_m = 0.5 MJ/kg$^{0.75}$/day = 150 MJ ME/day
(iii) ME concentration in fresh bread = 12 MJ/kg
(iv) Bread requirement = 150/12 = 12.5 kg/day = 25 loaves/day

Nagy (1987) has estimated ME_m for free-ranging wild ruminants to be approximately 700 kJ/kg$^{0.75}$/day. Some of the difference between this value and that for housed farm animals may be attributed to thermal stress but most can be attributed to the extra activity of animals on range. One of the prime objectives of intensive housing is to reduce feed costs by reducing activity. Sometimes this fails. Cronin et al (1985) demonstrated that the development of prolonged stereotypic behaviour in some tethered sows increased ME_m by 36% so that it became significantly greater than that of animals in the more enriched environment of a straw yard. Stereotypies such as 'weaving' in horses are also known to cause loss of condition.

An adult animal may fail to maintain body weight and condition on a ration that is calculated to provide ME requirement for maintenance because:

(i) The energy cost of spontaneous and enforced activity has been under-estimated.

(ii) It is exposed to cold stress (see below).

(iii) The quality (digestibility) of the diet is lower than predicted so that the animal has not been given, or cannot eat, enough for maintenance.

(iv) Digestibility is impaired, e.g. by parasitic roundworms.

(v) Metabolic rate is increased, e.g. by infection or neoplasia.

Air temperature and maintenance requirement of housed animals

Mammals and birds maintain homeothermy by balancing metabolic heat production (H_p) against heat loss to the environment by sensible means (H_n)—i.e. convection, conduction, radiation—and by evaporation of moisture from the skin surface and respiratory tract (H_e). Sensible heat loss (H_n) is related to the temperature gradient from the body core to the air ($Tr - Ta$) and passes through two layers of insulation in series: tissue insulation (I_t) and external insulation (I_e) provided by the coat of hair, wool or feather. Thus:

$$H_p = H_n + H_e \text{ where } H_n = \frac{(Tr - Ta)}{(I_t + I_e)}$$

Tissue insulation is regulated by constricting or dilating blood vessels convecting heat to the skin surface. External insulation increases with increasing depth of coat or plumage and is reduced by wind and precipitation (for details see Monteith and Mount 1974). Evaporative heat loss is controlled more or less effectively in different species by regulating the secretion of sweat or by thermal panting—rapid, shallow breathing which increases evaporative loss from the upper respiratory tract without altering ventilation.

Patterns of heat exchange in farm animals divide neatly into two groups (Figure 8.2) (Webster 1983). Group I, exemplified by pigs and poultry, are species where H_p and H_n are related almost linearly to air temperature and H_e is almost constant. Pigs and poultry have almost no capacity to sweat and limited capacity to regulate H_e by thermal panting. Maintenance of homeothermy in most naturally occurring environments involves adjustments to H_p in order to keep body temperature *up* to the regulated level (Figure 8.2). In severely cold environments this involves shivering but in more normal circumstances the increase in H_p can be achieved simply and without stress by an

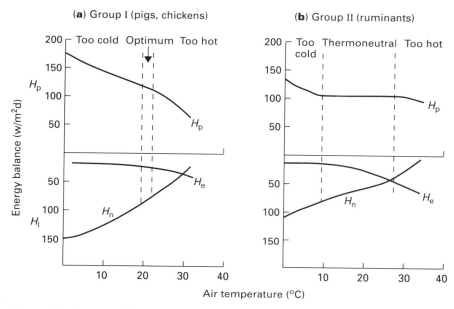

Figure 8.2 Patterns of heat exchange in farm animals. (a) Group I, e.g. pigs and chickens, animals which maintain homeothermy primarily by regulating H_p. (b) Group II, e.g. horses and ruminants, animals who maintain homeothermy primarily by regulating H_e (from Webster 1983).

increase in food intake. A hen free-ranging among the scattered grain in a dry, sheltered farmyard is not cold but her food intake and H_p will be about 30% greater than that of a hen in a battery cage at the optimal temperature of 21°C. Intensive housing for pigs and poultry has evolved to minimize H_p, and therefore food costs, by keeping air temperature as high as possible. The recommended air temperature in an intensive poultry unit is not necessarily the temperature preferred by the birds but the temperature for optimal productivity and is just below the threshold for heat stress.

This point is illustrated by Figure 8.3, which shows the sharp decline in output as air temperature exceeds 21°C (Emmans and Charles 1977). Figure 8.2 resolves the apparent paradox whereby species which are kept at the highest air temperatures (pigs and poultry) are most susceptible to death from heat stress, e.g. during transport. Both the fact that they are kept at high temperatures and susceptible to high heat loss can be attributed to their limited capacity to regulate H_e. In cool environments homeothermy can be maintained at some metabolic costs but no risk to life by increasing H_p; in acute heat stress, their inability to increase H_e leads rapidly to hyperthermia.

Group II includes ruminants and horses, which have an excellent ability to regulate H_e, horses largely by sweating, sheep by thermal panting, cattle half-

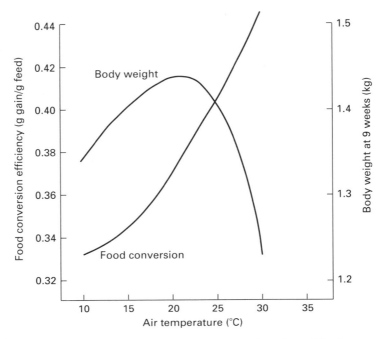

Figure 8.3 Effect of air temperature on growth rate to 9 weeks and food conversion efficiency (kg gain/kg food) in broiler chickens (from Webster 1983).

and-half (Monteith and Mount 1974). This creates a wide thermoneutral zone wherein the animals maintain homeothermy at negligible metabolic cost by regulating H_e to keep body temperature *down* to the regulated level.

Most farm animals spend most of their time earning their living by the production of milk, eggs, meat, wool or labour and should be fed accordingly. Species-specific requirements for energy and other nutrients to meet specific targets for growth, lactation, etc. are given in standard textbooks on nutrition and will not be reproduced here. I shall outline only some general principles as they apply to product quality, animal health and welfare. Table 8.1 uses the concept of metabolic size to compare intakes of ME (kJ/kg $W^{0.75}$ per day) in different species engaged in work of various forms. Generally speaking, ME intakes in farm species most intensively selected and managed for rapid growth (pigs and poultry) are 2–2½ times maintenance, and their energy expenditure (H_p) is similar to that of animals at maintenance on free range. Lactation in the high-yielding cow (35 l/day) or sow with 12 piglets requires an ME intake at least three times maintenance and an energy expenditure far greater than that associated with all but the most extreme forms of heavy manual labour (passerine birds feeding their young or similarly frenetic cyclists in the Tour de France).

Table 8.1 Intake (ME) and expenditure (H) of energy (kJ/kg $W^{0.75}$ per day) by man and animals during growth lactation and different forms of labour

| Work and species | Energy exchange (kJ/kg $W^{0.75}$ per day) | | Reference |
	ME	H	
Labour			
Man, clerk	520	520	Garry et al. 1955
miner	625	625	
cyclist (Tour	985	1510	Westerterp et al.
de France)			1986
Herbivores, on range	700	700	
Passerine birds,			Nagy 1987
feeding young	1580	1580	
Growth			
Pig (20 kg)	1200	800	Kirkwood and
Broiler fowl (2 kg)	1000	600	Webster (1984)
Lactation			
Dairy cow (35 l/day	1860	1020	
Sow (12 piglets)	1680	900	Webster 1987
Woman (one child)	720	590	

Growth

The main determinant of appetite in the growing animal is its capacity for lean tissue growth, which imposes a demand for nutrients that the animal will attempt to meet if the quantity and quality of available food permit. The capacity for lean tissue growth is determined by properties of the animal— genotype, sex and stage of maturity. Control of nutrient supply can only be used to manipulate lean tissue growth up to this limit. It cannot exceed it. Fat deposition, on the other hand, is strongly influenced both by phenotype and nutrient supply. Since one gram of fat contains approximately eight times as much energy as one gram of pure lean (protein plus associated water), it is policy to keep meat animals as lean as possible not only to meet consumer demand but to maximize food conversion efficiency. Selection for lean tissue growth rate and carcass quality (low fat) has been more successful in pigs and poultry than with ruminants (within this limited definition of success) for three main reasons (Webster 1989a):

(i) Shorter generation interval.
(ii) Higher nutritive value of food.
(iii) Relatively low costs of maintaining breeding generation permitting animals to be slaughtered at a lower proportion of mature weight.

Most intensive pig and poultry units operate close to the phenotypic potential of the animals for lean tissue growth. If a particular strain of pig has been selected to deposit large quantities of fat relative to lean during growth (e.g. the Saddleback breeds selected for traits more suited to the breeding sow kept out of doors) nutrient intake must be restricted to ensure optimal carcass composition. If a strain is selected intensively for extremely low fat concentration (e.g. Piétrain) then both lean tissue growth rate and appetite tend to fall. Entire male pigs have a greater capacity for lean tissue growth than castrate males by virtue of the anabolic properties of their sex hormones. There are very few circumstances in intensive pig units where castration is necessary. It is certainly compatible neither with pig welfare nor efficient food conversion. When anabolic steroids were administered to growing females and castrate males the effect was to achieve a rate of lean tissue growth similar to that of the intact male. However, growth hormone can increase lean tissue growth rate in pigs and direct nutrients away from fat in all 'three' sexes (males, females and castrates) (Serjsen et al. 1989).

Intensive selection of pigs for growth and carcass quality has created some problems of health and welfare. Animals with low backfat have a reduced tissue insulation so increased sensitivity to cold stress. This matters less to the young, growing animal eating large amounts of food than the sow on a maintenance ration whether outdoors or installed on concrete. Thin animals are also more prone to bruising and abrasions.

It is also possible to design animals, whether by conventional breeding or genetic engineering, that grow fast and convert food efficiently but suffer the chronically painful consequences of abnormal skeletal development. The most dramatic example of this has perhaps been pigs crippled by the transgenic insertion of human growth hormone (Pursel et al. 1990). This was recognized to be a mistake and has not been carried forward into commercial practice. A much more serious problem has arisen within intensive systems for production of broiler chickens, where by 'conventional' manipulation of phenotype, nutrition and housing we have created severe and crippling disorders of bones and joints (Duff 1988). It may be possible to control this by reduction of lighting to restrict food intake in the first two weeks of life but this slows down the turnover of birds. Thus, crippling abnormalities of bone development have become institutionalized within commercial broiler production.

Growth in ruminants is generally a more leisurely process, since nutrient supply normally limits both the genetic potential of the individual and the response to selection for faster growth. The digestion of high-fibre diets, such as grass and forage, by fermentation in the rumen produces substrates for growth at a slower rate than the gut of, for example, a pig fed a high-cereal diet. Volatile fatty acids absorbed from the ruminant gut are also utilized less efficiently than simple sugars absorbed by the pig or chicken. This nutritional constraint on the speed of growth is, on balance, beneficial to health and welfare, i.e. the animal population benefits from not being driven flat out. It is significant that the greatest problems of digestive, metabolic and infectious disease in growing cattle are recorded in feedlot animals fed high-cereal diets (Martin et al. 1981) and veal calves (van der Mei 1987). In both cases there is clear evidence from statistical epidemiology to link both metabolic and infectious disease to high intakes of dietary energy.

Lactation

Table 8.1 revealed that lactation is the most energetically demanding of all forms of animal production. The sow may only experience two 3-week periods of lactation each year interspersed by the lesser demands of pregnancy. The modern dairy cow, on the other hand, is either producing high quantities of milk or is heavily pregnant for almost the whole of her adult life. Most of the common veterinary problems of the dairy cow can be linked to the high demands placed on her capacity to digest and metabolize food to support the needs of lactation (Figure 8.4). Direct associations include ruminal acidosis,

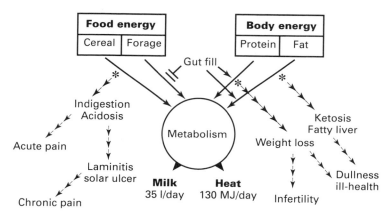

Figure 8.4 The 'overworked cow'—metabolic stresses in early lactation (from Webster 1987).

abomasal displacement, ketosis and the fatty liver syndrome, emaciation and infertility. Indirect, but statistically significant, links have also been made with lameness and environmental mastitis (Blood and Radostits 1989). The dairy cow can be compared to a highly tuned racing car being driven to its limit, and it is hardly surprising that the majority of animals are culled by the end of their fourth lactation, not in the interests of genetic improvement but because they have broken down with infertility, lameness or mastitis.

Recombinant bovine growth hormone (or bovine somatotrophin—BST) will stimulate the high-yielding cow to even greater production at almost any stage of lactation so long as sufficient nutrients are available for milk synthesis—

BST does not give something for nothing. Normally the increase of 10–15% in milk yield is supported initially by the cow 'milking off her back'; food intake catches up with the increase in demand for nutrients after a delay of approximately three weeks (Serjsen et al. 1989). As indicated earlier, it is 'normal' for the high-yielding cow to be simultaneously hungry for nutrients and full up with undigested food. BST increases the hunger and thus the tolerance limit for rumen distension.

Most of the nutrition-linked problems of the dairy cow occur in the first 100 days of lactation. Administration of BST to dairy cows after 100 days of lactation (or when they are confirmed to be back in calf) does not appear to have significant effects on health. Administration before 100 days can reduce fertility. On strictly mechanistic grounds, it is reasonable to argue that BST can be administered to cows in such a way as to increase production without significantly affecting health. However, on grounds of ethics (or politics, which is the practical expression of ethics) it is less easy to justify a process which involves giving cows regular injections simply to produce more milk per head when it is already known that most of their problems of health and welfare can already be attributed to production disease.

Increases of 10–15% in milk yield, comparable to those obtainable from BST, can be achieved by milking cows three times, rather than twice, daily. The increased demand on the processes of digestion and metabolism will be the same in both cases. However, the reduction in distension of the udder may well reduce the incidence of mastitis and hindfoot lameness. One of the most abnormal things we do to the high-yielding dairy cow is to milk her only twice a day. The fully computerized milking parlour which the cow can enter free-choice (more or less) four to six times daily could improve productivity and welfare by spreading concentrate feeding into smaller portions, reducing udder distension and reducing queueing time in collecting yards. One of the great drawbacks of conventional thrice-daily milking systems is that neither the cows nor the herdsmen get enough rest.

Protein

Crude protein (6.25 × N) is, as its name implies, a non-specific expression which describes all the organic nitrogen in a sample of food or body tissue. True protein, i.e. complete molecules made up of chains of amino acids, constitutes by far the greatest proportion of organic N in the body. Other contributors include the nucleic acids DNA and RNA, which contain N in the form of purines and pyrimidines. However, there is no absolute dietary requirement for purines and pyrimidines since they can by synthesized within the body using N from amino acids.

Thus the only absolute requirement for dietary protein is to provide essential amino acids as building blocks for body proteins (plus nucleic acids, peptide hormones, etc.). Protein supplied in excess of this requirement will be deaminated and used as a source of energy.

In simple-stomached animals the true digestibility or availability of most dietary proteins is close to 85%. The efficiency of utilization of available protein is not a fixed value but depends on the balance between supply and demand of individual amino acids. The rates of synthesis and degradation of some proteins can be very high; for instance, in the liver or gut epithelium, protein turnover time can be less than 24 hours. However, about 25% of amino acids involved in protein turnover are recycled. Thus at maintenance, protein requirement is small relative to ME (which cannot be recycled). Typical diets formulated to support maintenance or maintenance plus work (e.g. a horse in training) contain only 12–13% protein and this is generous.

In pregnancy, growth and lactation there is net synthesis of protein. Thus as growth rate or milk yield increase, amino acid requirement increases not only in absolute terms but when expressed as a concentration relative to dietary DM or ME. Thus diets for young piglets or high-yielding dairy cows may contain 18–22% protein.

If protein is supplied in excess of requirement the efficiency of utilization will decline as amino acids are catabolized to provide energy. In theory each amino acid will be used for (e.g.) growth at a fixed efficiency until requirement is met, whereupon efficiency will decline abruptly to zero. The efficiency of protein utilization is only at its peak when the supply of all amino acids is below requirement. As supply of each essential amino acid meets requirement its efficiency of utilization falls to zero. The cumulative effect is to create the classical diminishing response curve obtained from practical feeding trials (Figure 8.5a).

Estimates of essential amino acid requirements for synthesis of tissue protein (i.e. growth), milk and egg production are given in Table 8.2 (Fuller 1987) which indicates that in strictly quantitative terms the amino acids required in greatest quantities for growth are arginine, lysine, leucine and phenylalanine plus tyrosine. The quality or *biological value* of a protein is determined by how closely its amino acid composition meets requirement. Milk and egg proteins (casein and egg albumen) have a high biological value for growth, not surprisingly because that is what nature (i.e. evolution) designed them for. The protein values of some typical animal feeds are expressed in Table 8.3 in terms of total protein concentration and concentration of individual amino acids relative to an ideal protein (milk casein). Barley and maize, the most common energy foods for non-ruminants, are especially deficient in lysine, which becomes therefore the first limiting amino acid for (e.g.) growing pigs on cereal

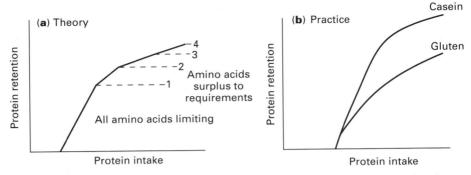

Figure 8.5 Efficiency of utilization of dietary protein. (a) Theoretical pattern showing how efficiency declines as supply of successive essential amino acids exceeds requirement. (b) Efficiency of utilization of casein and gluten.

Table 8.2 Amino acid requirements for net synthesis of protein in body tissues, milk and eggs (from Fuller 1987)

	Amino acid requirement (mg/g protein synthesized)		
	Tissues	Milk	Eggs
Lysine	68	76	67
Phenylalanine + tyrosine	65	85	90
Leucine	68	86	82
Isoleucine	35	41	50
Methionine + cystine	29	33	57
Threonine	37	42	46
Valine	47	54	62
Histidine	26	28	23
Arginine	69	42	61
Tryptophan	16	13	17

diets. Fish meal is nearly as good as casein as a source of lysine and threonine and especially rich in the sulphur-containing amino acids methionine and cystine. Soyabean and field bean meal are both well balanced with respect to amino acids which explains why soyabean meal is such a popular source of vegetable protein and why field beans would be if they were easier to grow and harvest.

Figure 8.5b illustrates the practical consequences of feeding protein of very high or very low biological value. Casein is utilized with high efficiency to provide protein retention until it approaches the animal's genetic potential for

Table 8.3 Crude protein concentration and amino acid proportions expressed relative to casein in some typical feeds

| | Crude protein (mg/g) | Amino acid proportions relative to casein | | | |
		Lysine	Histidine	Methionine + cystine	Threonine
Barley	110	0.50	0.65	1.59	0.95
Maize	88	0.32	0.71	1.05	1.10
Soyabean meal	500	0.87	0.66	1.16	0.95
Field bean meal	284	0.90	0.79	0.71	1.04
Rapeseed meal	396	0.68	0.81	0.71	1.10
Fish meal	657	0.97	0.56	1.33	0.94

Note: the underlined values are those where the proportion of an essential amino acid is less than 0.75 of the 'ideal' protein casein.

growth. Increments of cereal gluten are used with low and diminishing efficiency and protein retention does not approach the genetic potential of the tissues because the supply of essential amino acids is seriously out of balance with requirement. Growth rate is restricted by an absolute deficiency in one or more limiting amino acids (e.g. lysine) while other amino acids are catabolized because they are present in relative excess.

The values for growth and milk production in Table 8.2 relate to simple-stomached animals but can be applied with reasonable confidence to ruminants since, downstream of the rumen, the protein chemistry of the cow is much like that of the pig. However, the main source of available amino acids to the tissues of the ruminant is microbial protein leaving the rumen and digested in the abomasum. Rumen microbes require some preformed amino acids but can derive most of their nitrogen from ammonia, produced by degradation of dietary protein or simpler (and cheaper) sources of non-protein nitrogen such as urea. The rate of microbial synthesis is regulated by the supply both of rumen degradable crude protein (RDP) and fermentable energy (Webster 1987). In most normal diets where carbohydrate forms the main source of ME, an optimal balance can be achieved when:

RDP = 8–9 g/MJ ME.

A dairy cow may be fed a ration with an ME concentration of 11.5 MJ ME/kg DM and protein which is 75% degradable in the rumen. In these circumstances the crude protein concentration necessary to achieve an RDP:ME ratio of 9.0 would be:

9/0.75 × 11.5 = 138 g CP/kg DM

Most lactating cows are fed a ration containing at least 16.0 g/kg CP overall. If this extra protein was presented as RDP it would be degraded to ammonia and lost. It is therefore essential to ensure that sufficient of the protein in the concentrate mixture is in the form of undegradable dietary protein (UDP) which escapes the action of rumen microbes and undergoes acid digestion to amino acids which supplement those supplied from microbial protein.

As indicated earlier, the greater the rate of growth or milk production the greater the requirement for amino acids with respect to energy. There is a slight tendency for the yield of microbial protein to increase with respect to yield of ME as volatile fatty acids (i.e. from 8 to 9 g microbial protein:MJ ME) as food intake increases but this falls far short of the relative increase with increasing productivity in amino acid requirement. In formulating diets for high-producing ruminants (high milk yields or rapid growth) it is therefore necessary to ensure a proper balance between RDP to feed the microbes and UDP to provide supplementary amino acids. In theory the protein nutrition of ruminants should be described, as it is for poultry, according to the supply of each of the essential amino acids. At present this is unrealistic, mainly due to uncertainty in predicting microbial protein yield. Moreover, the biological value of microbial protein is high, which reduces the sensitivity of the animal's response to changes in the amino acid composition of the UDP. There may sometimes be problems with feeds such as maize gluten and distillers' grains which are fed to ruminants in large quantities primarily as an excellent source of digestible fibre. These feeds are also rich in UDP but the protein has a low biological value and may give a disappointing response when incorporated in a diet that is marginal for protein.

Protein deficiency

Protein deficiency is unlikely to occur in adult non-ruminant farm animals at maintenance or engaged in work. In young animals a deficiency in one or more specific amino acids attributable to an absolute deficiency in protein or low biological value will reduce lean tissue growth rate. This may be associated with a low appetite or, if appetite is maintained, a tendency to grow slowly but lay down fat. In the lactating cow a primary deficiency in metabolizable protein will reduce milk yield. If ME is not limiting, the cow will repartition energy from milk to body fat. When dairy cattle are in good condition but yields are disappointing the supply of metabolizable protein must be a prime suspect.

If, in any ruminant, the supply of RDP is deficient with respect to fermentable energy (less than 8 g RDP/MJ ME) then microbial protein synthesis will be impaired. This, in turn, will reduce fermentation rate, increase retention time in the rumen and so impair appetite. Ruminants at maintenance on poor quality fibrous foods (e.g. on winter hill pastures in the UK or during the dry season in the tropics) can therefore be restricted in their ability to eat fibre for energy by a lack of RDP. This is why non-protein N is an essential constituent of feedblocks for outwintered cattle and sheep.

Excess protein

There is no good reason to suppose that feeding protein in excess to young, healthy pigs or poultry will do them any harm; it would simply be a waste of money. In ruminants, the situation is less straightforward. Excess RDP can, in extreme cases, lead to urea or ammonia toxicity (Blood and Radostits 1989). Less extreme excesses of protein (especially RDP) have been implicated in cases of laminitis in dairy cattle although the case is unproven. My current, tentative view is that laminitis of dietary origin in cattle is always associated with a disorder of carbohydrate fermentation leading to ruminal acidosis; high RDP may exacerbate the condition but is unlikely to be the primary cause (Webster 1987).

It is not, however, uncommon for the dairy cow to be fed a very high metabolizable protein ration in order to maximize milk yield. If, in these circumstances, the cow cannot eat enough to meet her energy requirement, milk yield may be sustained for some weeks but she will lose condition rapidly and may become infertile or more susceptible to infection or injury.

Allergens, toxins and anti-nutrient factors

Many plant proteins, or partially digested fragments of plant proteins, can be harmful to farm animals. These include:

1. Protease inhibitors: present in all seeds but potentially dangerous in uncooked high-protein beans (soya, lima, kidney beans, etc.).
2. Lectins or haemogglutinin: present in uncooked oil seeds, soyabeans, etc. These may cause inflammation of intestinal epithelium and haemorrhage.
3. Goitrogens: anti-thyroid substances present in the green plant and especially the seeds of brassicas, e.g. kale, oilseed rape.
4. Allergens: nearly all plant proteins are recognized by the immune system as antigenic. In most cases recognition proceeds to tolerance. In some circumstances they may induce severe hypersensitivity, e.g. villous atrophy in the small intestine leading to profuse diarrhoea.

In addition to these intrinsic hazards, high-protein feeds present an especially favourable substrate for fungal attack and so may become contaminated with mycotoxins. These problems are all well known to the food industry, which tests for mycotoxins and treats protein-rich feeds with heat or solvents as appropriate to destroy or remove toxins and anti-nutrient factors.

The problem of food allergens is not fully under control because it is not fully understood. Hypersensitivity reactions to plant proteins have been recorded in young calves on liquid diets containing improperly treated soya rather than milk casein, and in post-weaning pigs suddenly faced with large quantities of plant proteins rather than mother's milk. This problem can be especially severe if they have previously eaten a very small quantity of creep feed, enough to induce hypersensitivity but not enough to induce tolerance (Newby et al. 1985). Allergy to food proteins should always be included as a possibility within the differential diagnosis of scouring problems in animals being weaned off mother's milk onto liquid or dry feed.

Disorders of mineral and vitamin metabolism

There is not space in this chapter to consider specific disorders of mineral and vitamin metabolism in detail (see Underwood 1980; McDonald et al. 1988). There are, however, some questions of general relevance to the differential diagnosis. As with all nutrients, the central question is 'how well does intake match requirement?' Mineral and vitamin requirements for healthy cattle, pigs and poultry are described comprehensively in nationally approved publications of nutrient requirements (e.g. Agricultural Research Council 1980, 1982; National Research Council 1988). In accepting these publications as the best available evidence I would only add that there may be circumstances when minerals or vitamins fed in excess of requirement may have a growth-promoting or therapeutic effect. The growth-promoting effect of copper in pig diets may be ascribed in part to its antibacterial effect within the gut (Visek 1978). Vitamins such as biotin or vitamin A may also have therapeutic or prophylactic effects when fed in excess of 'requirement' to an animal that is in less than perfect health.

The only problem I wish to address in this section is the control of mineral and vitamin intake. Although nearly all edible organic matter can provide energy and most natural protein sources provide all the essential amino acids (more or less efficiently) there is no single food source that is *not* deficient in one or more minerals or vitamins; for example, milk, the 'ideal food' is deficient in iron and vitamin D. In the natural state most farm animals, including grazing animals, tend to select a reasonable wide mixture of feed sources and seek access to natural sources of minerals. There is considerable controversy as to the extent that animals may display 'mineral wisdom', i.e. the ability to recognize a mineral deficiency and seek to remedy it. Wild ruminants appear to recognize a state of sodium deficiency and identify by smell a source of salt at a distance of many miles. However, ruminants do not appear to respond to experimentally induced deficiencies of calcium, magnesium or phosphorus by an increase in spontaneous intake of that mineral, or of minerals in general (Forbes 1986). This conflicts with some clinical impressions and it may be that the definitive experiment has yet to be done. However, when groups of animals at pasture are given free access to mineral licks, intakes range from zero to amounts grossly in excess of requirement. This suggests that farm animals cannot be relied upon to control their own dietary intake of minerals and vitamins.

Intensively housed pigs and poultry tend to be fed rations carefully formulated to provide all essential nutrients. Primary mineral deficiencies are unlikely to occur unless a mistake has been made. Osteoporosis in laying hens in battery cages is due primarily to enforced inertia rather than to a deficiency of dietary calcium (Wokac 1987).

In practice, animals most susceptible to primary deficiencies are those which obtain all or nearly all their nutrients from grass supplemented only by rather erratic uptake from mineral licks.

Acute mineral deficiency

To understand the aetiology and control of acute conditions of cattle such as hypocalcaemia ('milk fever') and hypomagnesaemia ('grass staggers') it is necessary to understand the dynamic nature of the exchanges of these cations between the main compartments of the body. Figure 8.6 illustrates calcium exchanges in a dry cow and a cow in early lactation. Over 99% of body calcium (Ca) is contained within the mineralized skeleton. Only about 12 g is freely available in the extracellular fluid (ECF) pool. The dry cow eats 30 g Ca/day and excretes 29 g/day in faeces; 5 g/day is absorbed from the gut and 4 g/day returned to it. This exchange, amounting to 40% of free Ca per day, is under hormonal control. At the onset of lactation, 30 g Ca may be secreted into the milk per day, 2.5 times the amount in the free pool. To accommodate this loss there is a massive increase in uptake of Ca from the gut and a much smaller increase in uptake of Ca from the skeleton. Factors known to predispose to milk fever such as increasing age and the paradoxical effect of high Ca:P ratio diets can be interpreted as a failure to move Ca sufficiently rapidly between body compartments rather than to a deficiency of Ca in the diet. It follows that Ca concentrations in blood cannot be used to predict susceptibility to milk fever.

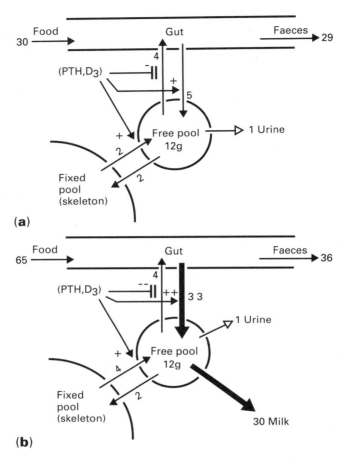

Figure 8.6 Exchanges of calcium (g/day) (a) in a dry cow (b) in early lactation. (PTH = parathyroid hormone, D_3 = vitamin D_3 cholecalciferol (from Webster 1987).

Acute hypomagnesaemia can be similarly explained in terms of magnesium (Mg) exchanges between body compartments. The quantity of freely exchangeable Mg in the ECF of a cow is only about 3 g whereas 6–8 g/day may be exchanged between ECF and the lumen of the gut. There appears to be little or no hormonal control of this exchange. Although serum magnesium concentration is under precise homeostatic control, low serum concentrations do suggest a predisposition to peracute hypomagnesaemia, which can be overcome by dietary supplements (Payne and Payne 1987). However, the acute condition is typically precipitated by stress, such as stormy weather, which reduces or may even reverse net uptake of Mg from the gut and so rapidly drains the small (3 g) pool of freely exchangeable Mg (Webster 1987). The problem of erratic mineral intake is compounded in the case of Mg by its unpalatable taste. As a general rule I would never rely on any free-choice system to meet the Mg requirements of cattle at risk. Indeed, I normally recommend farmers to adopt a 'belt and braces' approach to Mg supplementation using two of the following options: Mg-enriched concentrates or drinking water, Mg in mineral licks or feedblocks, rumen boluses or pasture dressing.

Chronic deficiencies of trace elements

Diseases associated with deficiencies of the trace elements, such as the classic triad of copper, cobalt and selenium deficiency in growing ruminants, are all, of course, quite specific in a biochemical sense, but have sufficient features in common to permit a standard approach to diagnosis.

1. Trace elements are usually slowly excreted and can be stored in the body. There may be an interval of weeks or months between the onset of a dietary deficiency and the development of clinical signs (unlike magnesium where an acute deficiency can develop within hours of an interruption to Mg absorption from the gut). Many trace elements (e.g. copper, selenium, fluorine) can also be toxic if stored to excess.

2. A grazing animal may acquire trace elements from both food and water in amounts related to concentrations in soil. All three may be worthy of analysis. In the UK regionals (and local) differences in concentrations of copper and selenium in grass and soil are well documented. There are, however, logical reasons to conclude that there has been a general decline in the supply of trace elements from heavily fertilized pastures, for a variety of reasons, not least being the overall increase in yield of dry matter achieved by supplementation with the minerals N, P and K alone.

3. The availability of trace elements in pastures (or compound feeds) may be markedly affected by the presence of other elements (e.g. sulphur, molybdenum, zinc and cadmium can all reduce the availability of copper). The presence of adequate amounts of a specific element in the diet does not exclude the possibility of a conditioned deficiency.

4. Although there are many specific clinical signs (e.g. 'spectacles' in copper deficiency), these may only develop after the condition has been in progress for some weeks. Early signs of trace element deficiencies may be very non-specific, like reduced weight gain and food intake. Other signs, like infertility, may not be specific to the element itself but secondary consequences of a general loss of body condition. A clear dietary history may therefore be more useful than clinical signs in achieving early diagnosis of, say, copper or selenium deficiency in a herd of beef cattle.

5. As a general rule, chronic deficiencies of trace elements do produce

significant biochemical changes in blood and other tissues which can be used for diagnosis (Payne and Payne 1987).

6. Trace element deficiencies do not get better unless that deficiency is restored, which means that treatment can help to confirm the diagnosis.

Vitamin deficiencies

Once again I shall not describe vitamin requirements or the clinical consequences of specific vitamin deficiencies, but consider only those circumstances which may impair vitamin supply.

1. Vitamins A, D and E are fat soluble and can be stored in body tissues. However, most animals are born with very low reserves. Colostrum provides the main source of (especially) Vitamin A, which has a protective role against diseases of mucous membranes. The vitamin status of young calves is therefore highly dependent on their access to colostrum. Moreover, when cows have been deprived of precursors of vitamin A, such as carotene in green grass, the vitamin A supply in colostrum may be inadequate to protect their calves against the consequences of enteritis and pneumonia.

2. Most vitamins have a relatively short 'shelf-life' after incorporation into compound feeds. Deficiencies may occur if feeds have been kept too long in storage.

3. Because fat-soluble vitamins are stored in the body it is both logical and reliable to administer them by injection when necessary.

4. Although deficiencies of vitamins cause ill-health, it does not follow that vitamin intake in excess of requirement will promote good health. There are, however, circumstances where vitamins fed in excess of requirement can be of benefit. Biotin clearly can improve and restore the quality of hoof horn in horses and pigs (Kempson et al. 1989). 'Excess' vitamin E (tocopherols) *may* help to avoid muscle damage in exercising horses (Maylin et al. 1980). In both cases it can be argued that requirement is unusually high.

5. It is generally accepted that ruminants do not have a specific requirement for B vitamins because they are synthesized in the rumen. However, several claims have been made recently that B vitamins may improve appetite, food conversion and performance in dairy cattle—most of these claims originate from North America (e.g. Mathison 1984). The diet of a high-yielding North American Holstein cow contains a large amount of maize starch and other materials which may escape fermentation and undergo digestion in the abomasum and duodenum. In these circumstances the supply of B vitamins may be less than in the case of a cow on a

typically European diet where a higher proportion of organic matter is fermented in the rumen. There may also be circumstances where the horse has an absolute requirement for B vitamins. Absorption from the hind gut of the horse is not well understood, but uptake of B vitamins must be less efficient when they are synthesized in the hind gut rather than in the rumen.

Oral satisfaction

I implied earlier that the provision of adequate nutrients should not be equated with oral satisfaction. A dry sow which consumes its maintenance ration in two minutes may well, during the next 23 hours 58 minutes, become progressively bored, hungry and bad-tempered. When sows are housed in groups this will exacerbate their innate tendencies towards aggression and fights may occur, especially at critical points, such as the access to electronically controlled feeders. One of the main (and valid) reasons for confining sows in individual stalls was to confer security. However, imprisonment of the entire population cannot be considered an acceptable solution to the vices of a few. When we speak of humane alternatives to the sow stalls we are probably using the wrong word since 'humane' implies goodness by human standards. What we must develop, in this case, is a system that is 'pig friendly' and the only way to discover this is to ask the pig. There have been two approaches to this. One is to observe the behaviour of animals in wild or feral conditions then attempt to reproduce those conditions on commercial farms (Wood-Gush 1988). The second is to ask animals specific questions about what they want in life (food, space, bedding, the company of conspecifics, etc.) and what price they are prepared to pay for it (Dawkins 1983b). Dawkins' application of economic theory to the assessment of what matters in the life of a farm animal is, in my view, more useful than the Wood-Gush approach of defining what is natural.

Within the specific context of oral satisfaction, evidence is accumulating to suggest that if 80–90% of nutrient requirement is provided in such a way that it can be consumed easily and rapidly, then animals are prepared to forage (or otherwise work) for several hours to acquire relatively little food (say 10% of requirement) by way of reward. Lawrence et al. (1988) have shown that this amount of work is similar whether the ration initially fed to the animals is below or considerably in excess of requirement. This suggests that they are motivated by the desire for oral satisfaction rather than hunger *per se*. Foraging for relatively modest rewards may therefore not only provide farm animals with considerable oral satisfaction but also keep them out of mischief. Intensive husbandry systems for dry sows, laying hens and veal calves are those which currently attract most criticism on welfare grounds. All three can be enhanced by providing the opportunity for constructive foraging.

Diagnosis of housing problems

There are many good reasons for housing farm animals. These include:

1. Protection of the animals from the effects of weather, predators, rustlers, etc.
2. Protection of the land from the effects of the animals, e.g. overgrazing, poaching.
3. Better utilization of conserved feed via control of intake, reduced waste, reduced energy expenditure by animals.
4. Convenience—easier management of feeding, breeding and routine preventive medicine.
5. Economics—increasing income by increasing the number of stock that can be carried on a fixed area of land or managed by a fixed number of people.

Inevitably the economic imperative has proved dominant. The costs of livestock farming are conventionally divided into *variable costs*, mostly for feed and replacement animals, and so-called because they vary according to the productive output of the farm; and *fixed costs*, mostly for land, labour, housing and machinery. Fixed costs are, of course, not fixed at all; they increase with inflation, but they are largely independent of productive output.

The intensification of livestock production may be viewed as an attempt to increase income with respect to fixed costs. As is inevitable in a market-led, competitive economy, some have succeeded at the expense of others. Success in intensive farming has been achieved largely by selling cheaper, i.e. increasing the quantity of produce sold relative to fixed costs so permitting a reduction in net profit per animal. This benefits the consumer but when consumption is static the uncontrolled effect of the free market is to force producers to the biological limits of intensification in order to remain competitive. Here is a simple example: when the first producer discovered that he could cram five laying hens into a battery cage designed for four, other producers had to follow suit or go out of business.

Much public criticism of the principle of intensive housing is neither constructive nor fair since it fails to recognize the economic constraints on farming systems. The suggestion that animals should be turned out doors to live a 'natural' life can only be tolerated from one who is him or herself prepared to live in a cave. On the other hand, the argument that optimal productivity is a sufficient criterion of welfare—'if they weren't happy they wouldn't grow so fast'—cannot be sustained when faced with production diseases such as the orthopaedic problems in broilers (Duff 1988) and bone weakness in laying hens (Wokac 1987).

There are three parties involved in the business of livestock farming—the producer, the consumer and the animal. The producer and consumer are well able to define and regulate their own needs. It is the business of the veterinary surgeon and others directly involved in farm animal welfare to represent the third party and this can best be done by objective analysis of the quality of the environment as perceived by the animal. The essential question is not whether the environment is 'natural' but what features, if any, cause suffering either because they are painful or aversive or because they frustrate the animal's need to achieve certain goals. Having decided what 'matters' we next have to ask how much it matters.

Several years ago I proposed that any animal in the care of man should be permitted a basic five freedoms (Webster 1984). These are:

1. Freedom from malnutrition
2. Freedom from thermal and physical discomfort.
3. Freedom from injury and disease.
4. Freedom to express most normal patterns of behaviour.
5. Freedom from fear and stress.

The expression 'five freedoms' as applied to animals came originally from the Brambell Committee (Brambell 1965) but their definition, in my opinion, was inadequate because it related only to maintenance behaviour (standing up, lying down, turning round, grooming and stretching limbs). My broader definition can provide a logical structure for the preliminary analysis of any husbandry system in terms of health and welfare. The provision of proper nutrition was discussed in the first section of this chapter. The application of freedoms 2–5 to the evaluation of alternative husbandry systems for dry sows is illustrated by Table 8.4 (Webster 1989b). Of course, each item merits more explanation than appears in the table, but it does avoid the trap of evaluating systems in terms of productivity alone (a fault of some producers) or behaviour

Table 8.4 Evaluation of alternative accommodation for dry sows (Plate 1a)

	Paddocks and arks	Individual stalls (no bedding)	Covered straw yards
Thermal comfort	Very variable	Fair to poor	Good
Physical comfort	Variable	Bad	Good
Injury	Slight	Feet, 'bed sores'	Fighting
Hygiene	Fair to poor	Usually good	Fair to poor
Disease	Some parasitism; control difficult	Usually good	parasitism; control easy
Abnormal behaviour	Slight	Severe	Slight

alone (a fault of many welfarists). It recognizes at the outset that all systems have to be a compromise.

The expression 'controlled environment' features prominently in most text-books on housing. Rather like Brambell's original five freedoms it is usually given too narrow a meaning, i.e. regulation of air temperature in an animal house. Man starts to control the environment of farm animals when he erects a fence. Generally speaking, the more intensive the system the more control of the environment passes from animal to man; the sow on a short tether in a confinement stall can do practically nothing constructive to regulate the quality of her immediate environment. As humans assume greater control they need not only to understand with ever greater precision what are the environmental needs of their animals but also to understand that denying animals the oppor-tunity to work to provide their own needs may constitute a source of severe frustration.

The remainder of this chapter will expand on the analytical approach out-lined within the five freedoms to the evaluation of the housing environment and the diagnosis of problems related to comfort, health and behavioural satisfaction.

Thermal comfort

Freedom from the stresses of heat and cold is achieved when an animal is constantly within a thermoneutral environment as defined already by Figure 8.2. A more comprehensive picture of recommended air temperatures within livestock buildings is provided by Figure 8.7. The solid lines indicate ideal air temperatures for optimal productivity in a well-designed building where con-vective heat loss is not increased by draughts or conductive loss increased by poorly insulated lying areas. The difference in thermoneutral range between, on the one hand, pigs and poultry and, on the other, ruminants is striking. As indicated earlier, battery hens are kept strictly at 21°C because it pays to do so but it would be unrealistic to contend that animals should never, on welfare

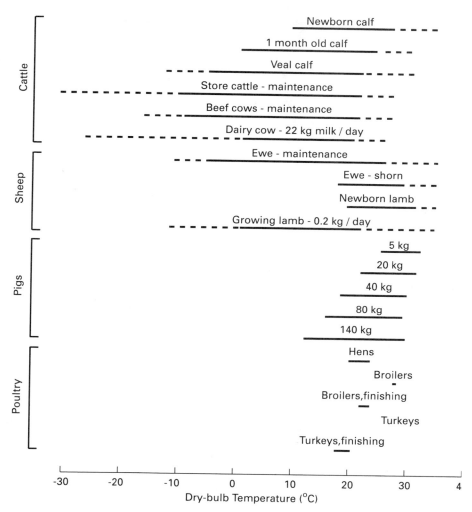

Figure 8.7 Recommended air temperatures within livestock buildings based on measured values for upper and lower critical temperature and on production trials (from Wathes et al. 1983).

grounds, be exposed to the sensations of heat or cold. Indeed ruminants, in particular, acclimatize extremely well to moderate intensities of heat and cold, the effect being to shift the thermoneutral zone to the extent of the dotted lines in Figure 8.7.

The precise control of air temperature in intensive houses for pigs and poultry is usually achieved without recourse to additional heating. Animals are held at a high stocking density in insulated buildings so as to generate heat at a high rate. For example, in a house containing 10 000 broilers each weighing

2 kg, animal heat is generated at a rate exceeding 100 kilowatts! Heat loss is regulated by control of ventilation. A thermostat set at the desired temperature either controls the number (or speed) of fans, or the size of openings within the building. This latter process is called automatic controlled natural ventilation (ACNV). The design of ventilation systems for pig and poultry houses is outside the scope of this chapter (see Sainsbury and Sainsbury 1988).

The control of air temperature solely by ventilation has its limitations. When outdoor temperatures are very low, fans regulated by a thermostat may operate rarely if at all, thereby permitting the concentration of airborne micro-organisms and pollutant gases to increase to levels dangerous for the animals and stockpersons. When outdoor temperatures are very high, environmental control through ventilation alone cannot avoid heat stress.

In intensive units for pigs and poultry, direct problems of thermal discomfort occur most commonly on hot summer days, and heat stress can be rapidly fatal for reasons illustrated in Figure 8.2. Faced by the problem of hundreds of thousands of heat-stressed pigs or poultry in a building the only options are to increase heat loss by evaporation or forced convection. Evaporative cooling is, in theory, the more effective approach, partly because of the large amount of heat required to evaporate water (2.48 kJ/g) and partly because it is not essential to wet the animals directly. A pig that emerges from a pool of water or mud cools rapidly by direct evaporation of heat from the skin surface. (Incidentally mud is more efficient than clean water because it sticks and so a far greater proportion is actually evaporated.) However, the simple act of sprinkling or 'fogging' moisture into the air of a building will cool the air by evaporation, provided, of course, that ambient relative humidity is below 100%.

Slight increases in air movement at the skin surface can greatly increase heat loss. For example, an increase from 0.2 to 2.0 m/s is perceived by a young calf as equivalent to reducing air temperature by 8°C (Webster 1984). Air speeds of 2 m/s are not uncommon in draughty animal houses. A draught may be defined simplistically but accurately as too much air movement in the wrong place. On a cold winter's day, if air movement at animal height can be sensed by the human skin (more than 0.5 m/s) it is probably too much.

Animals may also experience cold stress if floors are wet or poorly insulated. The effect of floor type on the lower critical temperature of an adult sow is illustrated by Figure 8.8. A bed of straw or similar litter is splendidly warm, but only when dry. Lying in wet litter is bad enough but heat loss is actually increased after the animal stands up and the accumulated moisture starts to evaporate from the skin and coat. In strictly thermal terms, lying on a dry concrete slatted floor (or expanded metal) is equivalent to standing up in still air conditions. A solid concrete floor can, however, feel very cold to a sow lying in an individual stall (Figure 8.8). The thermal conductivity of concrete is high. This can be reduced by incorporating insulating material within the top layer of concrete, but insulation laid under 3 cm of concrete screed is largely

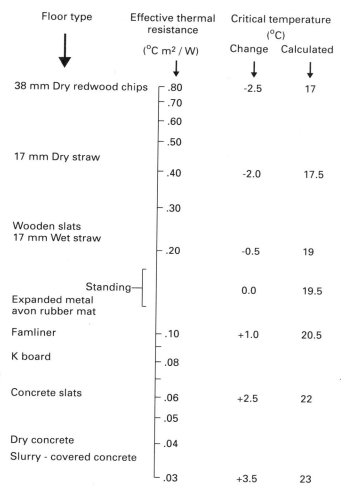

Figure 8.8 Effect of floor type on the lower critical temperature of a 45 kg pig (data from Bruce 1979).

ineffective because a high proportion of heat loss from the animal is conducted *sideways* and subsequently lost to air (Bruce 1979).

The thermal state of a group of animals (hot, comfortable or cold) can be judged from behavioural and physiological signs such as posture (limbs huddled or spread out), piloerection of hair or feathers, respiration rate and shivering. In ruminants, which use thermal panting as a major contributor to thermal regulation both during heat stress and within the thermoneutral zone, respiration rates between 25 and 60 per minute may be considered very comfortable. Above 60/minute the environment may be too warm. Respiration rates of 18–20/minute in a sheep or ox suggest that the animal is cold but do not indicate how cold. Unless the animal is clearly perceived to be shivering by sight or touch the stress of cold may be deemed unimportant on grounds of health or welfare.

Physical comfort

The surface upon which a farm animal stands, walks, excretes and lies down to rest must variously be dry, hygienic and easily cleaned, yielding to the body but firm to the foot, non-abrasive but non-slip. There is probably no single surface that meets all these specifications—not even a field of young grass— and it may be futile to contemplate one. It is better to consider resting areas and thoroughfares in animal houses as separate entities having different properties.

Table 8.5 A ranking of the properties of the resting area according to the needs of different farm animals

	Dryness	Hygiene	'Give'	Warmth	Security*
Poultry					
Broilers	+++	+	0	+	(+)
Layers	++	+	0	0	(++)
Pigs					
Weaners	++	++	+	+	+
Dry sows	++	+	++	++	++
Cattle					
Calves	+++	++	+	+	+
Beef, fatteners	+	0	++	0	+
Dairy cows	++	+++	++	0	++
Neonates (general)	+++	+++	+/0	+++	(+++)

* Pluses in brackets in the 'Security' column indicate that security is important but usually achieved by other means.

Optimal conditions for the resting area tend to be species-specific. Table 8.5 assesses the needs of different farm animals for a resting area according to the following properties: dryness, hygiene, warmth, 'give' (in the sense that a mattress has 'give') and security. Poultry (broilers and layers) do not need a bed as such, which is why I have avoided the word in favour of the more pedantic expression 'resting area'. In the natural state they perch (and sleep) in branches. These are dry underfoot (which is good for the feet) but the properties of warmth and 'give' are unimportant. In the wild state, security is paramount. In intensive units a perch may confer an atavistic sense of security but fail to confer protection against attack from other hens.

The resting area for a dry sow should possess all the properties of a good bed. I have given warmth a higher ranking for sows than weaners to reinforce my concern for the dry sow lying on dry concrete in an individual stall. Weaners certainly require warmth but can huddle. The heavy dry sow also needs, but often fails to get, a bed with 'give'. Equally she requires security from the real threat of aggression from other sows. The sow stall provides this in a crude and unsubtle way.

The cubicle or free-stall provides a secure resting area for dairy cows. Care is usually taken to ensure that cubicles are dry and hygienic to minimize the risk of environmental mastitis involving the ubiquitous organism *Escherichia coli*. There is less general concern to provide a bed with suitable 'give' because there is no obvious economic advantage. However, there is overwhelming evidence that cows prefer to lie, and lie for longer, on sprung rubber mats or in deep straw than on an unyielding surface, which is hardly surprising given their weight and the design of their limbs.

The criteria listed in Table 8.5 raise serious doubts about the welfare of large animals such as finishing beef cattle housed entirely on concrete slats. At high stocking densities (to ensure that dung is tramped through) slats are acceptably dry, warm and hygienic. The feet of cattle are normally good but they would undoubtedly prefer a bed with more 'give', and young bulls in particular are not secure from risk of injury during encounters of an aggressive or sexual kind. On the other hand, finishing cattle kept in an inadequately strawed yard can be wet, filthy and suffer severe foot problems. Both systems suffer from the fallacy of assuming that a single floor surface can provide for all an animal's needs.

The newborn animal requires in abundance the properties of dryness, warmth, hygiene and security. A bed with 'give' may not be particularly important but the surfaces of many floors can damage the delicate skin of the newborn animal. The incidence of scabby knees in piglets on concrete or expanded metal floors is so high that it might be called normal, but this is not to say that it is acceptable.

Hygiene and infectious disease

It is an article of faith that animal houses should be designed and managed to ensure good hygiene and so minimize the risk of infectious disease. Such faith, however, is seldom exposed to analysis; thus a veterinary surgeon may state with confidence that 'the pneumonia is due to bad housing', whereas he would never dream of saying, with equal vacuity, 'the disease is due to a germ'.

In analysing what housing may or may not achieve in the control of hygiene and infectious disease, it is necessary first to distinguish two simple, but relevant categories.

Simple, pathogen-host diseases are those where exposure of a susceptible (non-immune) individual to a sufficient dose of a specific pathogen (virus, bacterium, etc.) is itself sufficient to cause disease. Such pathogen-specific diseases range from the great epidemics, like foot-and-mouth, to sporadic conditions like the clostridial diseases of sheep. The enormous difference in morbidity between foot-and-mouth and tetanus, for example, is determined by what happens to the organism in the environment rather than in the animal. Diseases such as these, which rigidly conform to Koch's postulates, can be controlled either by eradication of the pathogen (e.g. foot-and-mouth) or by vaccination (clostridial diseases). The same can be said of the major respiratory disease of poultry (Newcastle disease, infectious bronchitis). When there is an effective vaccine against the primary pathogen, poultry remain free of respiratory disease in housing conditions that would be considered intolerable, say, for young calves.

Complex, pathogen-host-environment diseases may be defined as those which are induced by interactions between potential pathogens, the host animal and the environment. These include the most common conditions of intensively housed animals, diarrhoea and pneumonia, associated with a multiplicity of organisms which may be found almost anywhere in the environment or indeed on the outer and inner surfaces of the animal. Staphylococci may be present on the skin, salmonellae in the gut and *Pasteurella haemolytica* in the respiratory tract without necessarily inducing disease or indeed conferring protective immunity. For such environmental diseases infection may be said to be the natural state and disease the consequence of disturbance to the equilibrium between potential pathogen, host and the environment.

In practice, therefore, control of simple pathogen-host diseases is likely to involve vaccination or a degree of hygiene guaranteed to eliminate the organism from the environment altogether. Improvements to housing may well reduce the severity of secondary infections but are unlikely to affect morbidity from the primary pathogen. However, improvements to housing design may control an environmental disease such as calf pneumonia more effectively (and cheaply) than administration of most current vaccines because the number of immunologically distinct potential pathogens is so large. It is equally important therefore to reject the absolutism of the immunologists who claim that all infectious disease can be prevented by vaccines as it is to reject that of the holists who claim that a disease such as tetanus can be prevented by grazing sheep on 'organic' grass.

Effects of the environment within an animal house on the incidence and severity of infectious disease may be analysed as follows:

1. Effect within building—release, survival and spread of:

   (a) pathogens, primary and secondary;
   (b) pollutants, gaseous and particulate.

2. Effect at interface between animal and environment:

   (a) presentation of pathogens and pollutants to vulnerable epithelial sur-
      faces;

   (b) clearance (mechanical and immunological) of pathogens and pollutants
      from epithelial surfaces.

3. Effect on systemic resistance of animal:

   (a) immune competence;
   (b) non-specific defences.

To illustrate these general principles, let us examine how housing and husbandry may affect the incidence and severity of the ubiquitous environmental diseases, diarrhoea and pneumonia.

Environmental disease—enteritis

Consider an outbreak of enterotoxaemia associated with *Salmonella typhimurium* in a group of 30 young calves purchased from market at about 10 days of age and placed at once into individual, solid-sided pens, each with their own buckets. The pens have been steam-cleaned, disinfected with a phenolic solution and left empty for two weeks. In short, hygiene appears to be good. All calves appear to be in good health on arrival but rectal swabs reveal four animals positive for *S. typhimurium* 204c, resistant to most common antibiotics. Two days later, two of the salmonella-positive calves fall sick and during the next 10 days the disease spreads to 12 more calves, apparently at random among the pens. Four of these calves die. Two of the calves that were salmonella-positive on arrival remain healthy. In another group of calves within the same air space, group-housed and sharing access to milk replacer from a teat dispenser, two calves become sick but recover rapidly.

Now the complexity of the interactions between host, pathogen and the environment is such that this is only one of a wide range of possible consequences of the situation on day 1. It can, however, serve to illustrate the questions that need to be asked in attempting to interpret the epidemic.

How did the infection arise? Given the initial standards of hygiene, and the absence of disease previously, it may be assumed that infection was brought in by the calves, not necessarily only those which swabbed positive on day 1.

How did the infection spread? The use of individual, solid-sided pens with individual buckets practically eliminates the possibility of spread by direct contagion. Moreover, the disease has spread at random rather than from pen to pen. It could have been carried from calf to calf by the stockperson but in this case airborne transmission seems more likely. Wathes et al. (1988) have demonstrated that salmonellosis can be transmitted between calves (and mice) as effectively by inhalation of aerosols as by oral dosing.

Why did only some calves become sick? The calves will undoubtedly have differed in the amount of specific and non-specific immunity acquired from colostrum. However, this seems an unlikely explanation for the fact that the disease spread presumably by the airborne route to two of the group-reared calves but failed to develop further despite the maximum opportunity for contagion at and around the common teat. We have no reason to assume any difference, initially, between the two groups in systemic resistance. Whether organisms were acquired initially by inhalation or ingestion, they will eventually have been swallowed. However, when calves drink more slowly and more frequently from a teat dispenser the bacteria are more likely to be killed in the acid medium of the abomasum (Webster 1984).

I must re-emphasize that this is only one possible sequence of events and does not constitute an advertisement for group housing. Epidemiological surveys of enteric disease in calves (Waltner-Toews et al. 1986; Van der Mei 1987) reveal little difference in incidence between groups and individual pens suggesting that the advantages of isolation v. 'natural' feeding tend to cancel one another out unless group-housed animals are overstocked (see below).

Each outbreak of enteric disease in housed animals may provoke different answers (and therefore different remedies) but the basic questions remain the same. In this example, the possibility that systemic resistance may have been affected by an environmental stress such as cold can be discounted for reasons illustrated by Figure 8.7. On the other hand, cold stress can precipitate enteric disease in post-weaning piglets in two ways: by reducing systemic immune resistance and by increasing food intake thus encouraging incomplete digestion and increasing the presentation of enterotoxigenic *E. coli* to the epithelial surface of the small intestine (Wathes et al. 1989).

Environmental disease—pneumonia

At least seventeen distinct species of virus and bacterium have been isolated from cases of calf pneumonia (Thomas 1978) with, of course, much variation in virulence and antigen type within these species. Multiple vaccines against, for instance, respiratory syncytial virus, parainfluenza 3 virus, etc. can control calf pneumonia in some cases but offer no guarantees (Howard et al. 1987).

In normal circumstances, the young calf, whether reared artificially or suckled by its mother, is certain to inhale several species of microorganism that *can* cause pneumonia. Progression from exposure to infection and disease can be visualized in terms of a dynamic balance between the rate at which potential pathogens are presented to the lung and their rate of clearance. This, the 'Inverse Micawber Hypothesis', states, 'incoming pathogens 20 per minute, capacity for clearance 21 per minute, result—good health; incoming pathogens 20 per minute, capacity for clearance 19 per minute, result—pneumonia.'

As indicated above, the challenge presented to the lung by inhaled pathogens, allergens and pollutants needs to be considered in two stages—events inside the house and events inside the respiratory tract. The factors that determine the concentration of respirable particles within an animal house are illustrated in Figure 8.9.

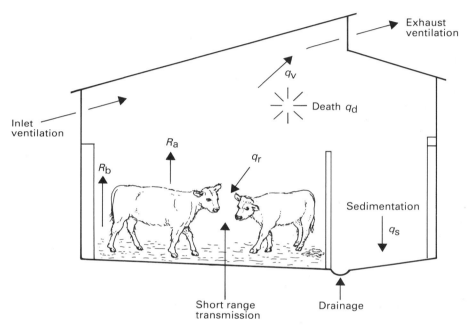

Figure 8.9 Pathways for release (R_a and R_b), transmission and clearance (q_v, q_d, q_s, q_r) of microorganisms within the air of an animal building (from Webster 1984).

The concentration, C (n/cm³), of any particle in the air of an animal house is determined by its rate of release from animals, R_a, and the rest of the building, R_b, (n/cm³/h). Clearance of particles is principally by ventilation, q_v, and death *in situ*, q_d. The units of clearance are h^{-1}. Clearance by ventilation is therefore defined by ventilation rate in air changes per hour. The relative importance of q_v and q_d depends on the nature of the challenge. Conditions such as chronic obstructive pulmonary disease (COPD or 'heaves') in horses associated with the inhalation of fungal spores, depend largely on the balance between R_b and ventilation, q_v, since the spores in dusty hay and straw are equally antigenic whether dead or alive (Webster et al. 1987). Ventilation is also the primary route for clearance of pollutant gases and nuisance dusts.

The situation with regard to infectious agents is more complex. Most of the organisms that can be recovered from the air and grown on appropriate culture media are non-pathogenic, although if present in sufficient numbers they may contain enough endotoxin to damage the surface of the lung. Very small numbers of respiratory pathogens can be recovered from air samples even when the building contains many animals that are sneezing or coughing. This is because most pathogens die within seconds or minutes of aerosolization. For an organism such as *Pasteurella haemolytica* survival after 1 minute may be only 1% (Donaldson 1978). This means that death *in situ* (q_d) is a far more important mode of clearance than ventilation (q_v). Figure 8.10 illustrates the effects of

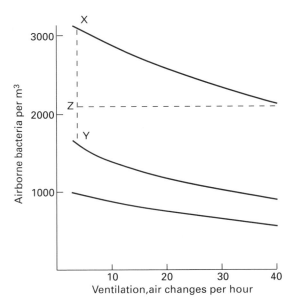

Figure 8.10 Effect of space allowance (m per animal) and ventilation rate (air changes per hour) on the concentration of airborne bacteria in a calf house when q_d accounts for 90% of total clearance. The intervals XY and XZ indicate effects of increasing ventilation space allowance from 5 to 10 m³/calf (XY) and increasing ventilation rate from 4 to 40 air changes per hour (XZ) respectively (from Webster 1984).

changing ventilation, q_v, and stocking rate, R_a, on the concentration, C, of live bacteria in the air of a calf house when q_d is 50. Increasing air space per calf from 5 to 10 m³ halves C, since the animals are the main source of the organisms. Increasing q_v from 4 to 40 h^{-1} only reduces C by 60%.

In this example, a tenfold increase in ventilation is only two-thirds as effective as halving stocking density in reducing the challenge from infectious organisms. For any specific pathogen the exact balance between q_d and q_v depends, of course, on its survival characteristics in different conditions of temperature and humidity. In practice, however, one can say with assurance that when respiratory infection is present in an animal house, 'improvements' to ventilation cannot compensate for the effects of overstocking. When the practice of group-rearing unweaned (and veal) calves became popular in the early 1980s, many producers experienced an increased incidence of calf pneumonia. Some of this may have been due to increased infection by contagion or short-range transmission. However, many farmers had taken advantage of the space created by removing individual pens to increase stocking density by at least 50%. When they reverted to the original allocation of air space per calf, the problem of pneumonia reverted to manageable proportions.

After inhalation, particles deposit in the respiratory tract at sites determined largely by their size. Particles 5 μm in diameter deposit mainly in the nose and upper airway. Particles less than 2 μm in diameter, which include the bacteria and viruses unless transported on something larger like a skin squame, deposit either in the alveoli or terminal bronchioles. Particles depositing in the bronchioles are cleared mechanically by the mucociliary escalator within a few hours unless the bronchial cilia have been destroyed by previous viral infection (Agnew et al. 1986).

Living organisms that enter the alveoli are taken into macrophages and killed so long as the macrophages are not overwhelmed by numbers or compromised by pollutants (Gilmour et al. 1989). To restate the Inverse Micawber Hypothesis in rather more detail, infection occurs when the rate of presentation of living organisms to the lung surface exceeds their clearance by mechanical and immunological means either because of the magnitude of the challenge or because the clearance mechanisms have been impaired.

Effects of housing design on the inhaled dose of pathogen and pollutants can be defined with some confidence. Effects of environmental stresses on clearance mechanisms are less clear. The predilection sites for enzootic pneumonia in the calf and pig are the right apical lobes of the lung. Since these are the first to branch from the trachea I used to assume that they received the greatest dose of particulates and other pollutants. However, recent studies by Davies (1991) have shown that when calves are at rest, most inspired particles (thus most air) enter the diaphragmatic lobes, which are seldom affected by pneumonia except in the most severe cases. This suggests that the apical lobes may be predilection sites for pneumonia not because their defence mechanisms are impaired by pollutants but due to relatively poor conditions of ventilation and perfusion which create a favourable environment for the multiplication of pathogens which may have initially entered the lung either in inspired air or by movement down the bronchial tree against the action of the mucociliary escalator. It is certainly more logical to ascribe the regional distribution of pneumonic lesions to regional differences in ventilation and perfusion than to regional differences in immune mechanisms.

If this is so, then optimal housing design for young calves at risk of contracting enzootic pneumonia involves attention to more than just stocking density and ventilation. Practical experience reveals that cold stress *per se* does not predispose calves to pneumonia, which is more common in cool, damp conditions than when the air is cold and dry. Such conditions can prolong survival of pathogens so increasing the challenge and may induce calves to lie for long periods with slow, shallow breathing giving rise to conditions of partial anoxia in the apical lobes that may favour the multiplication of pathogens such as *Pasteurella haemolytica*.

Systems where batches of active calves are reared before and after weaning in groups in spacious, naturally ventilated accommodation that merely provides shelter from wind and rain and does not attempt to elevate temperature above that outdoors, tend to be associated with a low incidence and severity of pneumonia. I have previously attributed this simply to clean air, i.e. a low pathogen challenge (Webster 1984). The greater activity of such animals may also help to protect their lungs.

Once again, this is not the place for a detailed exposition of environmental requirements to minimize respiratory infections in farm animals but to suggest a series of general questions that may be applied to the evaluation of the environment in relation to a problem of pneumonia in housed animals.

1. How severe is the pathogen challenge? This is determined by overall stocking density, numbers of sick animals and recovered carriers, and close proximity of infected animals in other buildings. It is *not* particularly affected by ventilation except via indirect effects on humidity.
2. How severe is the challenge from inhaled pollutants which may compromise the defences of the lung? These can be reduced by controlling sources of dusts (in fodder, bedding, etc.) and by ensuring minimum ventilation rates of at least 4–6 air changes per hour (Webster 1989b).
3. What factors may have compromised resistance to infection? Here, of course, the immune status of the animal, itself determined by supply of colostrum and specific antibodies therein, is of paramount importance. However, there is good epidemiological evidence to link calf pneumonia to non-specific stresses such as concurrent infection or abrupt weaning but not to the stress of cold (Waltner-Toews et al. 1986).

Behavioural satisfaction

I have stressed throughout this chapter my belief that husbandry systems should be based on the premise that farm animals are sentient beings who need more from life than food, comfort and freedom from disease. There is now clear evidence that animals are strongly motivated to work for the good things in life and frustrated by systems which deny them the opportunity to make a constructive contribution to meeting their own needs. Dawkins (1983) has applied economic demand theory to measure the relative strength of motivation of hens to work for a nest box (high) and dustbath (low). Research of this sort, designed to discover how much things matter in the life of an animal, is time-consuming and slow but should in time provide a sound scientific foundation for legislation designed to ensure improved minimal standards within systems of housing and husbandry. Meantime, the good stockperson can devise for his or her animals things to do that are interesting, rewarding, inexpensive, unthreatening and safe.

A chain or rubber tyre hanging in a pig pen is interesting and inexpensive but not particularly rewarding. A feeding system for sows that scatters pellets onto deep straw so that some fall through and can be hunted for hours is interesting, rewarding, inexpensive and improves safety by reducing aggression. Increasing the bulk in the main ration may provide the satisfaction of a fuller stomach but will occupy less time than encouraging the sow to forage in straw and may prove more expensive than a commercial compound feed. The simple provision of social contact, achieved for example by legislation which bans battery cages for hens or individual pens for sows or veal calves, may be unrewarding and unsafe because of increased disease or injury resulting from the aggressive intentions of others. Allowing hens to range free in an open field can provoke fear from threats, real or imagined (hawks or helicopters). A free-range unit for hens cannot be considered humane unless it can ensure the birds are at all times close to bushes or artificial substitutes that provide cover from attack from the sky and a perch to escape attack from the ground.

How can the stockperson or veterinary surgeon diagnose frustration or the absence of behavioural satisfaction in the individual animal? In an extensive or enhanced environment where there is plenty for an animal to do, any departure from normal behaviour may be interpreted as a sign of ill-health or distress. However, in intensive systems most natural behaviour becomes pointless (e.g. foraging) or impossible (wing-flapping in a battery cage). Thus apathy or listlessness cannot be distinguished from 'normal' behaviour except perhaps at feeding time.

Attempts to diagnose the 'stress' of confinement tend to be based on analysis of blood samples for stress-related hormones like cortisol or opioid-like peptides, or on the development of stereotypies—compulsive, persistent performance of apparently purposeless behaviour, such as bar chewing in sows or weaving in horses (Fraser and Broom 1990). So-called objective indices of stress like plasma cortisol can be useful in diagnosis but they are non-specific and bleeding itself *may* introduce a further confounding stress. The very presence of stereotypic behaviour can be taken as evidence for a barren environment but, despite much research, we do not yet understand what happens to an animal's mind as its behaviour becomes progressively stereotypic. It does appear that the perception of the environment becomes progressively abnormal but we do not know whether the compulsive, pointless activity constitutes a mechanism to reduce frustration by reducing (or increasing) arousal or is itself a measure of active frustration (Dantzer 1986).

When examining a row of sows in confinement stalls one cannot be sure which animals are more distressed, those performing stereotypies or those doing nothing. However, there is good evidence from studies with zoo animals that stereotypies can be reduced or eliminated by giving animals more to do. Indeed, the publication *Animals and Ethics* (Carpenter 1980) suggests 'Diligent human care for the welfare of such animals as are confined in a few advanced zoological parks can act as a touchstone for the welfare standards of the managed (farm) animal.' This recommendation may be a little ambitious but it does raise a point of principle that transcends science. If a husbandry system is such that a farmer can take pride in showing it off to the public then it is probably acceptable to the animals as well. If the farmer is concerned that the public may not understand the system he is probably revealing his own doubts, usually justified by the expression 'I have to do things this way to remain competitive'. There is now an increasing awareness among both farmers and consumers that if we are to improve quality of life on the farm, for animals and for their human keepers, we need new legislation to enforce welfare standards that will permit farmers to recover their pride without being driven to poverty.

9 ROLE OF ANIMAL WELFARE SOCIETIES NATIONALLY AND INTERNATIONALLY

H C ROWSELL PhD, DVM

The international scene
Eurogroup for animal welfare
Animal welfare and the veterinarian
Transportation of animals
Animal welfare in the 1990s
The animal rights movement
The dark side of the animal rights movement
Conclusions

Thirty years ago, the writing of a chapter outlining the role of animal welfare societies, both nationally and internationally, would have been a relatively straightforward task. It would, for example, have required a standard definition of what constituted animal welfare, listing the various animal welfare societies and their specific objectives and philosophy, and the means of achieving them through activities, publications and programmes.

Even though the changing moral status of animals will be one of the most visible issues confronting us in the 1990s (Loew 1990), it might prove beneficial to examine the history of animal use and protection in order to better understand present trends.

Perhaps the first legislation to forbid cruelty to animals was adopted by the General Court of Massachusetts in 1641. This legislation stated that 'No man shall exercise any tyranny or cruelty towards any brute creatures which are usually kept for man's use' (Traystman 1990).

In 1822, Martin's Act was enacted in England to provide protection to farm animals, and on 16 June 1824, the Society for the Prevention of Cruelty to Animals (SPCA) was founded under the direction of its first secretary, the Reverend Arthur Broome (French 1975), to ensure that Martin's Act was followed (Traystman 1990).

Some 16 years later, Queen Victoria recognized the importance of this society and endorsed it by allowing it to use the term 'Royal'; thus, it became the Royal Society for the Prevention of Cruelty to Animals (RSPCA) (Henshaw 1989). A service of 'thanksgiving and dedication' was held in Westminster Abbey on 4 October 1990 to mark the Society's 150th Anniversary (Anon 1990b). Its aim has been the advancement of animal welfare based on the premise that all unnecessary suffering should be curtailed. The growth of the RSPCA in the UK led to the formation of other RSPCAs in what was then the British Empire, and these continue to be highly respected wherever they exist.

The American Society for the Prevention of Cruelty to Animals (ASPCA) was founded in 1866 by Henry Burgh. Its primary *raison d'être* was the protection of beasts of burden, namely horses, in the Atlantic seaboard states of the USA; however, it now cites abolition of animal use in research, trapping and ranching as an aim. It was followed by the establishment of the American Humane Association (AHA: PO Box 1266, Denver, CO 80201-1266, USA), which later spawned the Humane Society of the United States (HSUS: 2100 L Street NW, Washington, DC 20037, USA). All of these were considered respectable animal welfare organizations.

One of the first animal-related US laws was the 28-hour law of 1873, which said that animals could not be transported for more than 28 hours at a time. Many years later, the Humane Slaughter Act 1958 assured that animals must be slaughtered by humane means, and the Laboratory Animal Welfare Act 1966 was passed in order to reassure pet owners who were concerned that their dogs and cats were being sold to laboratories for research purposes.

In Canada, even predating its confederation in 1867, laws for the protection of animals were passed in the City of Halifax in 1822. The laws called for a fine 'not exceeding three pounds or less than five shillings' on conviction. Amendments in the years 1824, 1825 and 1840 stipulated that the punishment for 'maliciously, unlawfully and wilfully killing, maiming, wounding, etc., animals' would be 'such public punishment by imprisonment or public whipping as such courts shall, in their discretion, adjudge' (Anon. 1969).

The Nova Scotia Society for Prevention of Cruelty to Animals (NSSPCA) was founded in 1876, and incorporated in 1877. In 1909 the name changed to its present form, dropping the word 'animals', and women and children were included in the Society's jurisdiction (Anon. 1969).

The Montreal-based Canadian SPCA was established in 1869. Although the name suggests that this a national association, the CSPCA has not extended its influence and its work beyond the Province of Quebec and, indeed, for many years limited its interests to the City of Montreal.

In all other nine provinces of Canada, SPCAs have been established, again based on the concept of prevention of unnecessary suffering and thus cruelty, similar to the original aim of the RSPCA, which has been emulated by organizations worldwide. There was no national animal welfare organization in Canada until the Canadian Federation of Humane Societies (CFHS) was established in 1957. It now represents 112 member societies and branches across the country, with 200 000 members.

It is difficult to state with any accuracy the precise influence that these national and international SPCAs have had on livestock animal welfare legislation. There is, however, no doubt that one of their primary roles was fostering and encouraging an interest and a concern on the part of the general public, which in turn was reflected by the governments of the day. They had considerable input and influence in the framework of various pieces of animal welfare legislation, leaving the legal language to the legislators.

Many of the founding members of the early SPCAs were strident animal welfarists who spoke out with fervour and conviction for the animals which 'could not speak for themselves'. In the 19th century and until the mid-20th century, the animal welfare societies had historically established criteria for the needs of animals and crusaded for their welfare.

Initially, the concerns related to horses, particularly those used as transporters or in agriculture. However, in the 20th century, the societies' interests turned more and more to companion animals, such as dogs and cats. This was to be expected because of the increased urbanization. The SPCAs were literally pushed into animal control situations, responsible for the millions of stray and unwanted dogs and cats, many of which must be euthanized—in the USA some 10–15 million (Franklin Loew quoted in Yaukey 1991). Such animals created problems in the urban environment, for example through bites, the spread of disease such as rabies, and spread of both external and internal parasites (Hubbert et al. 1975). Although today's societies continue their ongoing basic interest in dogs and cats, their interest in agricultural animals continues to be limited by both their human and financial resources. However, the Canadian Federation of Humane Societies (1988) recently published a survey of surface livestock transportation in Canada, aided financially by the Animal Welfare Foundation of Canada (AWFC).

The international scene

Although the RSPCA influenced the establishment of SPCAs throughout the world, these latter organizations did not speak to an international audience, but remained either national or local voices for animal welfare. The RSPCA, however, recognized that there was an international problem in that unnecessary suffering had to be prevented among those animals transported from country to country, or where there was no local organization to work against cruelty to animals. The issues were many; examples include slaughter practices, stray dogs, and animals in entertainment such as bull fighting.

The RSPCA attempted to work in the international field, but recognized that, philosophically and practically, its efforts should remain within Great Britain. Therefore, it was through its influence that the International Society for the Protection of Animals (ISPA) was founded. This Society, with headquarters in London and staffed initially by individuals trained by the RSPCA, developed field offices in Europe, Africa, India and North America. Although stray dogs were a matter of concern, much of ISPA's effort went towards the welfare of livestock, both in transportation and in assurance of humane slaughter techniques. ISPA's participation in animal welfare and its work overshadowed the activities of the World Federation for the Protection of Animals (WFPA) based in Zurich, Switzerland. This organization had its primary role in the European theatre, although it used the designation of a 'world' society.

The WFPA took some initiatives in animal control, outlining animal welfare legislation in Western Europe and the former Eastern Bloc countries, at that time behind the 'iron curtain'. With the establishment of the European parliament in Strasburg, France, as part of the European Community, WFPA attempted to influence governments and animal protection legislation through the establishment of local branches. However, although these initiatives had some effect, a lack of resources and active field efforts limited their productivity.

Through an increased interest in the international field, the Humane Society of the United States (HSUS) became one of the prime instigators of the movement to meld WFPA with the International Society for the Protection of Animals (ISPA). The necessary documentation to effect the merger was orchestrated by M Madden, a HSUS lawyer. Both he and John Hoyt, who later became HSUS President, effectively brought together the two international organizations to form the World Society for the Protection of Animals (WSPA). This organization maintained and extended the field offices of ISPA, utilizing its former head office in London as headquarters. John Hoyt later became the President of WSPA.

WSPA representatives took part in programmes in various countries to influence such matters as slaughter practices and the killing of unwanted dogs, the influence being exerted through literature produced by WSPA for distribution in various languages to various countries throughout the world. The WSPA's main efforts were concentrated on the same issues with which ISPA had effectively dealt, albeit more strongly opposing the Canadian seal hunt and trapping.

However, the coming of age of the European Economic Community (EEC) and European Parliament surpassed the expectations and the abilities of WSPA to oversee animal welfare issues in Europe. Thus grew the Eurogroup for Animal Welfare, with WSPA as one of the members. One WSPA initiative, taken many years ago, was a presentation to the Council of Europe of a seven-point plan for conventions to improve the welfare of animals. In 1990, five of these animal protection conventions had been drawn up, including one on farm animals ratified in 1976, and one on slaughter, finalized in 1979 (Anon. 1990a).

Eurogroup for animal welfare

Animal welfare societies, for the most part, do not present a single unified voice, having policies that are specific to their own mandates. While on occasion, overtures of unification of purpose and policy with other animal welfare organizations are made, active co-operation is rarely practised and is often impossible. This is particularly true of organizations that serve as local voices on specific animal issues. Thus, given this diversity of effort, it is not difficult to understand why animal welfare issues, and especially livestock animal welfare, have not taken precedence over other issues in the legislatures of the world.

The Eurogroup for Animal Welfare (EAW) was established in 1980 as the result of an initiative taken by the RSPCA, which recognized the importance of European legislation, particularly in the area of farm animals.

A consortium of national animal welfare organizations, its objectives are to identify areas of concern in the treatment of animals and to lobby for the introduction and enforcement of legislation at a European level. Eurogroup acts as a two-way channel of communication between animal welfare organizations in the EEC, on the one hand, and the institutions of the EEC (the Council Ministers, the Commission, the European Parliament and the Economic and Social Committee) and the Council of Europe on the other. This organization also is responsible for maintaining links with animal welfare organizations outside the EEC. It is interesting to note that while the Eurogroup, working from a Brussels office, is responsible for liaison with animal welfare organizations and for administration, its policies are determined by its 13 Member States representing one animal welfare organization in each of the 12 EEC Member States, along with WSPA.

Some initiatives of the Eurogroup include the introduction and enforcement of minimum standards for intensive rearing of veal calves and pigs, tighter controls over the transport of animals, protection of animals which are to be slaughtered, as well as other animal issues such as the harmonization of EEC legislation on the manufacture, sale and use of the leghold trap, minimum standards for the welfare of animals in zoological collections, and a continuation of the EEC import ban on pelts from hooded and harp seal pups.

The Eurogroup recognized initially the need to bring together, in a friendly, co-operative relationship, the leading animal welfare organizations of the European Community as well as, over the long term, the encouragement of humane treatment of animals, which is dependent upon public awareness and a recognition of human responsibility towards all living animals. More recently, their efforts have also incorporated environmental concerns as they relate to the welfare of animals.

337

The membership of the Eurogroup includes: the Association Nationale des Sociétés de Protection Animale (Belgium); Foreningen Til Dyrenes Beskyttelsei Danmark (Denmark); Deutscher Teirschutzbund e V (Germany); Conseil national de la protection animale (France); Hellenic Animal Welfare Society (Greece); Irish Society for the Prevention of Cruelty to Animals (Ireland); Associazione Italiana Difesa Animali (Italy); Ligue nationale pour la protection des animaux (Luxemburg); Nederlandse Vereniging tot Bescherming van Dieren (The Netherlands); Liga Portuguesa dos Direitos do Animal (Portugal); Federaçión Espanalo de Sociedades de Animales y Plantas (Spain); Royal Society for the Prevention of Cruelty to Animals (Great Britain); Royal Society for the Protection of Animals, the European Section (Eurogroup for Animal Welfare 1988).

This Eurogroup for Animal Welfare will continue to exert a significant influence on animal welfare and represents what is probably the most effective lobby for animal welfare legislation in the world. Its influence will be felt as Europe moves, in 1992, to the establishment of a single market within a common border.

Animal welfare and the veterinarian

Historically, veterinarians have been asked to render professional judgement concerning pain and distress in animals by animal welfare societies who did not feel they had the competence or the legal standing for such decisions. This alliance of veterinarians with animal welfare societies has resulted, on occasion, in veterinarians' election as officers of the society. In some cases, veterinarians are responsible for veterinary divisions within the societies themselves. Additionally, those who pursue veterinary medicine as a career are most intimately involved in animal welfare. How else could one describe the contributions of the veterinary surgeon to the diagnosis, treatment and prevention of disease, prevention of pain and suffering, the prolongation of life and the promotion of animal welfare and well-being. Veterinarians in livestock practices and in regulatory services consider that they are helping the livestock industry to be economically sound or, in the case of the regulatory veterinarian, to eradicate disease and prevent zoonoses.

Animal welfare is described by Broom (1986) as an animal's 'state as regards its attempts to cope with its environment'. Blood and Studdert (1988) define it as 'maintaining appropriate standards of accommodation, feeding and general care, the prevention and treatment of disease'.

Fraser (1989) notes that animal well-being encompasses 'both the physical and psychological. These normally coexist. Physical well-being is manifested by a state of clinical health. Psychological well-being is reflected, in turn, in behavioural well-being. The latter is evident in the presence of normal behaviour and the absence of substantially abnormal behaviour.'

The World Veterinary Association (WVA) states that animal ethology 'puts the emphasis on knowledge which is scientifically based. Its aim is to clarify a) needs that can be filled, and b) harm that can be avoided' (Anon. 1991b).

Originating from various sources in applied ethology, the report of the Brambell Commission in 1965, described the farm animal's 'Five Freedoms' as the ability to easily 'turn around, groom itself, get up, lie down, and stretch its limbs' (Brambell 1965). However, in 1990 the WVA developed its own Five Freedoms, which apply to all species (Anon. 1991b):

  (i) freedom from hunger and thirst
 (ii) freedom from physical discomfort and pain
(iii) freedom from injury and disease
 (iv) freedom from fear and distress
  (v) freedom to conform to essential behaviour patterns

Most veterinarians do not become involved in discussions of the numerous animal issues which, through the years, have been addressed by the animal welfare societies. In the 1990s these animal issues have become myriad and have gained significant attention and public interest through the media, which realize that animal-based stories have a high viewer or reader appeal.

The result has been that the general public has bestowed upon the veterinarian the mantle of responsibility for providing leadership in all issues relating to animal welfare and well-being (Rowsell 1991b). The veterinary profession in most countries, particularly those with a history of established animal welfare societies, has demonstrated a willingness to accept this significant responsibility. While it is undeniable that the animal welfare societies have drawn attention to the animal welfare issues and lobbied the regulators and members of the elected governments in this regard, it has been the veterinary profession that has played a significant role in preparing the related terms and regulations. Most veterinary associations worldwide have taken an increased interest in ensuring that their profession is recognized as being concerned with animal welfare in their respective countries.

Possibly the first veterinary association to tangibly demonstrate an interest in animal welfare was the British Veterinary Association (BVA), which in 1984 established the BVA Animal Welfare Foundation (Address: 7 Mansfield St., London, England W1M 0AT). In 1986, this foundation established the first Chair in Animal Welfare in the Veterinary School of the University of Cambridge. Thus began the BVA's commitment to the pursuit of scientific study and education in relation to animal welfare. The overall purpose of the foundation is 'to further the veterinary surgeon's natural concern for the health and welfare of animals' in striving to relieve animal suffering, which is undeniably the major animal welfare issue and which formed the basis for the establishment of the RSPCA in the mid-19th century (Bennett 1991).

Research projects receiving funding from the BVA Animal Welfare Foundation in 1991 included a behavioural assessment of the function of stereotypic behaviour, a study of the control/elimination of foot rot in sheep, an assessment of immune responses as indicators of welfare in cattle, and the study of feeding and housing of sows. This research is coupled to educational initiatives in relation to the welfare of horses, ponies and donkeys, funding a student in Applied Animal Behaviour and Animal Welfare, publishing the Pig Veterinary Society's Casualty Pig Booklet, and organizing the Pain in Practice road shows and various symposia (Bennett 1991). The 10th BVA Animal Welfare Foundation Symposium, held in June 1991, was entitled 'Animal Welfare Implications of Alternatives to Intensive Farming Systems'. Although the Chair in Animal Welfare created by the Foundation remains the only such Chair sponsored by a veterinary association, others have encouraged various universities to establish such Chairs. Other veterinary associations have established animal welfare committees within their specific associations.

The American Veterinary Medical Association's (AVMA) Animal Welfare Committee in 1989 defined animal welfare as encompassing 'all aspects of animal well-being, including proper housing, management, nutrition, disease prevention and treatment, responsible care, humane handling, and when necessary, humane euthanasia' (Boyce 1990). This committee also attempted to define 'animal rights', stating that it did not agree with the present common use of the term because it was incompatible with the responsible use of animals for human purposes, such as food, clothing, companionship and research (Boyce 1990). However, the AVMA Board did not approve these initiatives.

In Canada in 1968 the Canadian Veterinary Medical Association (CVMA) established a Humane Practices Committee. This produced a number of position statements, subsequently approved by the CVMA Council and membership, which covered the use of elastrators, dehorning, use of animals in rodeos, etc. In 1990, the name of the committee was changed to the CVMA Animal Welfare Committee to relate its function to today's terminology. Its present chairman, Dr Alan Longair, believes the farm animal welfare issue to be 'one of the most prominent issues of this decade' (Anon. 1991g). In so saying, he echoes animal activist Henry Spira, who greatly influenced reduction of animal use in testing, but who calls farm animal well-being 'the emerging issue of the nineties' (Spira 1991).

The concern for farm animal welfare is also being shown in the European Community, for Wilkins (1989) has noted that the attitudes in the UK, Holland, Denmark and Germany tend to be moving very strongly towards an awareness of the need for greater protection of farm animals, although this does not yet appear to be the case in Belgium, France, Greece, Italy, Spain and Portugal. It is interesting to note that, in Belgium, there had been a government initiative to set up a Council for the Welfare of Animals in 1986. There are two animal welfare federations in Belgium, the larger being Association nationale des sociétiés de protection animale (ANSPA). This is the society which is listed as a member of the Eurogroup for Animal Welfare; however, its main concern is cats and dogs, with little involvement in farm animals. The other federation in Belgium is the Conseil nationale pour la protection animale (CNPA). This society is closely involved with the Belgian Veterinary Association and thus plays a significant role in the discussions concerning farm animal welfare. Both of these federations now sit on the Council for the Welfare of Animals, which is concerned with farm animals.

In The Netherlands, the leading animal welfare society has close links with veterinarians in the Ministry of Agriculture and thus there is consultation on legislation concerning farm animal welfare. Coupled to this, the society maintains extremely good liaison with the veterinary profession.

In Germany, there is close co-operation between the major federation of animal welfare organizations, the Deutscher Tierschutzbund, and some veterinary advisers, as well as contact with veterinarians in the Ministry of Agriculture.

Since 1971, in Sweden, plans for construction or remodelling of buildings used to house farm animals must be scrutinized and approved from the animal health and welfare point of view by officially appointed veterinarians, before the building can be used (see Chapter 2). A special scientific unit at the Veterinary Faculties Department of Animal Hygiene in Uppsala gives Swedish veterinarians further advice on complicated cases or on request. Similarly, in Switzerland, new methods and equipment must be tested from the animal health and welfare point of view.

Veterinary associations in Australia played a significant part in the 1989 Australian Senate Select Committee's report on animal issues and welfare. Practices used in livestock production were thoroughly reviewed and documented.

The Society for Veterinary Ethology (SVE), established in England in 1966, soon became an international society, and was the forerunner in discussing the importance of understanding behaviour of livestock. Interestingly, a joint SVE/RSPCA symposium, 'Stress in Farm Animals', held in London on 25–26 May 1973, marked the first time the RSPCA had co-sponsored a scientific symposium (Napier 1974). Unfortunately, veterinary involvement has been reduced, and it has now been named the International Society for Applied Ethology (ISAE). As a result, one of the founding officers of the SVE, Professor Andrew Fraser, Memorial University of Newfoundland, at the World Veterinary Congress in Rio de Janeiro in August 1991, recommended the establishment of a World Association of Veterinary Ethologists.

The World Veterinary Association (WVA) has had an Animal Protection Committee for almost 20 years. In 1988, this committee was replaced by an Animal Welfare Committee. This came as a result of a resolution passed at the World Veterinary Congress, held in Montreal in 1987, calling upon the WVA to address the issues of animal welfare as a professional responsibility, and to have animal welfare as a subject for all future World Veterinary Congresses.

In May 1990, the Animal Welfare Committee drafted a 'World Veterinary Association Policy Statement on Animal Welfare/Well-being and Ethology'. This policy statement discussed animal welfare under the following headings: (a) animal ethology and welfare; (b) freedoms of animals; (c) animal welfare in veterinary education; (d) animal experimentation; (e) transport and slaughter of animals; (f) conservation of wildlife; and (g) welfare legislation.

This policy statement was followed by an addendum which stated: 'The animal owning public welcomes the guidance of the veterinary profession in connection with all aspects of animal well-being.'

At the 24th World Veterinary Congress in Rio de Janeiro, Brazil, 18–23 August 1991, the opening plenary session was entitled 'The Veterinarian and Animal Welfare'. Following this, a symposium was held on issues in animal welfare as well as three separate sessions where oral presentations addressed these aspects.

Also in the international field, the World Society for the Protection of Animals (WSPA) in 1990 re-established its Scientific Advisory Panel (SAP). Chaired by Professor C R W Spedding also Chairman of the Farm Animal Welfare Council of the Ministry of Agriculture, Fisheries and Food, the panel includes experts on various aspects of the biological and agricultural sciences.

Transportation of animals

Transportation is undoubtedly a most stressful event for most animals, including farm animals. The International Air Transport Association (IATA), recognizing this, established as one of its standing boards the IATA Live Animals Board, which publishes annually the IATA Live Animals Regulations (International Air Transport Association 1991). Its principal objective is the assurance of the welfare of the animal in transit through the publishing of requirements for transportation of animals as well as the requirements for containers used in the transport of animals to ensure their comfort, security and safety. A veterinarian sits as a permanent member of the Board, while other veterinarians are encouraged to attend as observers on behalf of a number of associations, such as the Eurogroup for Animal Welfare (EAW), the

International Council for Laboratory Animal Science (ICLAS), the Canadian Council on Animal Care (CCAC), as well as veterinarians from national departments of agriculture worldwide. The US-based Animal Transportation Association (AATA) comprises an international membership which disseminates information and encourages uniform national and international regulations.

Animal welfare in the 1990s

In the foregoing discussion the activities of a number of animal welfare societies have been described. However, it is not possible to enumerate all the many societies that historically have played a part in livestock animal welfare. Nonetheless, since the 1960s, the numbers of participants in animal welfare and animal issues have increased so significantly that it would be a gargantuan (if not impossible) task to attempt to deal even superficially with the names, purposes and contributions or lack thereof of the panoramic mosaic of animal welfare/animal rights/animal liberation groups. Just 15 years ago, promotion of animal welfare was primarily the responsibility of the humane societies. Today, there are some 7000 animal 'protection' groups in the USA, with a combined membership of 10 million and total budget of some $50 million (Cowley et al. 1988). Additionally, scholars say that 'more has been written in the last 12 years on animal issues than has been written the previous 3000' (Cowley et al. 1988).

The present plethora of animal rights societies is the result of dissatisfaction with the conservative animal protection societies, and the sense that these societies were not making progress rapidly enough (Ryder 1989). Ryder characterizes Frances Power Cobbe as 'the most doughty and effective anti-vivisectionist of the nineteenth-century'. Dissatisfied with the conservative, incremental regulatory approach to vivisection favoured by the RSPCA, she decided to pursue an abolitionist agenda. This led her to form, in November 1875, the Victoria Street Society, later to be renamed the National Anti-Vivisection Society (NAVS), which she ably led for more than two decades, only to find herself and her allies out-voted in the NAVS elections of 1898, whereupon she formed the British Union for the Abolition of Vivisection (BUAV) (Lansbury 1985).

A number of organizations have decided that no longer is it suitable to discuss the animal issues with those involved in the 'exploitation' of animals whether it be farm animals, animals in entertainment, animals in research or wildlife. The Toronto Humane Society (THS), for example, was roundly criticized for a ban on membership for pet breeders, rodeo participants, slaughterhouse workers, animal researchers and trappers and the spouses of these individuals. Regarding the trapping, the THS has been branded racist, as many of Canada's aboriginals make their living in this manner (Valpy 1991). Faced with the loss of financial support from the City of Toronto for animal control services, the THS has since had to revise these requirements (Hurst 1991).

It has been said that some of the impetus for the splintering of animal rights societies from the mainstream animal welfare societies is related to the surge of feminism in the 1960s and 1970s. Women dominate the animal rights movement, with membership percentages in the various organizations in the USA varying from 70 to 100% (Greanville and Moss 1985). Most are well educated, with 80% holding business and professional positions. Although most of the 'traditional' animal welfare societies are controlled by a board of male directors and have mainly male staff, in the animal rights (AR) movement, women activists are making inroads (Greanville and Moss 1985). It is also said that a 'feminization' or nurturing attitude is being attributed to the present leadership, both male and female (Clifton 1990).

There is no doubt that in the 19th century and the first part of the 20th century the oppression of women was likened to the oppressive uses of animals, and thus feminists could relate more readily with the enslavement of the animal for man's purposes such women equated their loss of dignity and the effacement of their civil rights with how animals were treated in research. For example, suffragettes were among the early animal rights protestors, as exemplified by the Brown Dog matter (Lansbury 1985; Powell 1988).

It may be more than coincidence that in the 1960s and 1970s, and into the 1980s, the Canadian seal hunt gained international notoriety. The image, projected each March on television and in the news media, of a sealer with a club or a hakapick standing over a white, wide-eyed seal pup, became repugnant to the majority of people, both in Canada and elsewhere. It benefited little to state that all evidence suggested that the hakapick rendered the animals unconscious immediately, and thus insensitive to pain, and that the method fulfilled the requirements for humane slaughter.

The 'protest' industry flourished during this period, initially through the efforts of Brian Davies, who first established in Canada a 'Save the Seals' campaign. Later, when it became obvious that this attracted the attention and interest of the public who were willing to donate their money for a single animal welfare issue, the International Fund for Animal Welfare (IFAW) was established. Other groups, which included Greenpeace and the US-based Fund for Animals, were also involved. The RSPCA also sent its veterinarian, who countered the reports of representatives from the International Society for Protection of Animals (ISPA).

The protests against the seal hunt resulted, in 1983, in a ban on importation of seal pelts in Europe and the eventual death of the industry. A subsequent protest against trapping of furbearers has resulted in the virtual death of that industry as well. Some 500 000 Canadian jobs (one-tenth of which were aboriginal) were linked to the fur industry (Harvey 1990, Moloney 1991).

Thus, the protest industry became rich and there were created numerous groups which became animal welfare profiteers (Rowsell 1984), preparing more printed matter with mass distribution, in order to increase their revenue. It became obvious that the animal protest movement had become an industry in itself.

During the past 15 years, animal groups have discovered that direct mail funding is almost as good as minting money, realizing that, for every dollar spent, the return is likely to be three or four times that amount (Rowan 1991).

A questionable practice is where fundraising materials are claimed to be 'educational' or 'stimulating activism'. IFAW which, as noted, began its fundraising activities during the Canadian seal hunt, continues to use direct mail campaigns, employing horrific photographs, for example, dogs being bound and cooked in South Korea (Cumming 1986). Specific accounting is rarely given for funds received for a particular purpose. The funds raised do little to educate, and the accuracy of the portrayal of the actual situation in the field is questionable.

The animal rights movement

Although for the purposes of this chapter our prime interest is in the animal welfare societies who have worked for an improvement in livestock animal welfare, this review would be incomplete without referring to another group of animal welfarists whose reason for participation in animal welfare issues had little to do with livestock, but with opposition to vivisection. It is important to note their existence because, as will be pointed out later, their influence in today's society has created a more intense interest in all animal issues, not the least of which is the welfare of livestock.

In Victorian England, antivivisectionists were vociferous (French 1975). Their influence culminated with the passage of the Cruelty to Animals Act 1876. It is believed that many women who later became suffragettes deplored the treatment of women by physicians, particularly those women who were reduced to being subjects for the teaching of medical students; women were shabbily treated by the doctors of the day, and working-class women were stereotyped as 'raucous vocal animals' (Lansbury 1985).

From these beginnings, the British Union for the Abolition of Vivisection (BUAV) became the voice for the antivivisection movement opposed to the use of animals in research. As the SPCAs, the roots of this British organization extended into other countries with the formation of antivivisection societies.

In the USA, the National Anti-Vivisection Society (NAVS) was followed by the American Antivivisection Society (AAV) and the New England Anti-Vivisection Society (NEAVS). These last three societies, along with BUAV, continue to maintain a high profile. Today, such organizations have proliferated and include the World League Against Vivisection, the Society for the Protection of Animals Liable to Vivisection, the Friends Animal Welfare and Anti-vivisection Society, the Society for the Protection of Animals in North Africa, and the Society for United Prayer for the Prevention of Cruelty to Animals Especially with Regard to the Practice of Vivisection (Henshaw 1989). Such societies engage in dialogue with those opposed to factory farming and the fur trade.

The animal rights/liberation movements had their beginnings in the 18th and 19th centuries, albeit without the use of the present terminology. For instance, the theologian, Humphrey Priment, wrote in 1776 of 'the duty of mercy and the sin of cruelty to brute animals'. Additionally, the theme of animal rights can be identified in the writing of poets such as Pope, Goldsmith, Burns, Blake, Coleridge, Wordsworth, Byron and Shelley, the last being a vegetarian. Perhaps the most familiar and oft-cited quotation was that of the philosopher, Jeremy Bentham, who wrote: 'The Question is not, Can they reason, nor Can they talk, but, Can they suffer' (quoted in Wood 1990). Undoubtedly, these pioneers laid the foundation on which today's animal rights movement has been built; however, writings for the most part dealt with beasts of burden, livestock and free-living species.

The individual most often described as the 'Father' of the animal rights movement is Richard Ryder who, in the late 1960s and early 1970s, formed the Oxford Group, which began the struggle for animal rights. It included not only Ryder, but also Andrew Linzey and Stephen Clark, along with three young Oxford Philosophers, Roslind and Stanley Godlovitch and John Harris (Regan 1991). Ryder, while a member of this Oxford Group, coined the term 'speciesism' in 1970, equating it with racism.

In 1973, Peter Singer published his review *Animals, Men and Morals* (Singer 1973). This was followed by Ryder's publication in 1975 of *Victims of Science: The Use of Animals in Science* (Ryder 1975). During that same year, Singer, who was influenced by Ryder and the Oxford Group, published his now world-famous and widely read publication, *Animal Liberation* (Singer 1975). This book became known as the 'Bible' of the animal rights/liberation movements.

It was during this period that Ryder became a Board member of the RSPCA and later its Chairman. The RSPCA during this period has changed its attitudes significantly, but has remained steadfast in its objective of preventing avoidable suffering, thus maintaining the concept of its name.

It was also during this period that Richard Ryder became involved with the Canadian seal hunt, although in no way could he be described as one of the 'animal welfare profiteers'. He, along with theologian Andrew Linzey, helped organize the 1977 Cambridge Conference on Animal Rights at Cambridge University, the proceedings of which were later published as *Animal's Rights: A Symposium* (Paterson and Ryder 1979). Ryder himself drafted a 'Declaration Against Speciesism' that was signed by 150 of the delegates (Ryder 1989). This declaration stated:

> Inasmuch as we believe that there is ample evidence that many other species are capable of feeling, we condemn totally the infliction of suffering upon our brother and sister animals, and the curtailment of their enjoyment, unless it be necessary for their own individual benefit.

> We do not accept that a difference in species alone (any more than a difference in race) can justify a wanton exploitation or oppression in the name of science or sport, or for food, commercial profit or other human gain.

> We believe in the evolutionary and moral kinship of all animals and we declare our belief that all sentient creatures have rights to life, liberty and the quest for happiness.

> We call for the protection of these rights.

These publications opened the floodgates to an ever-increasing number of individuals, some of whom were looking for a cause and others who had been active in various protest movements, for example in the 1960s against the Vietnam War. Coupled to this activism was a trend toward urbanization; few people clung to the traditions of rural life or had any understanding of the animals they sought to 'liberate' (Loew, quoted in Malcolm 1991).

Vegetarianism had been the practice of many, not because of concern for animal welfare, but because of religious and familial beliefs. However, many of the pioneers in the animal rights/liberation movements were not vegetarians. Richard Ryder himself, as late as 1976, continued to eat fish. Others continued to be meat eaters. With the advent of the 1980s, health also became an important factor for many people; a substantial number turned away from meat and joined the vegetarians and the ever-increasing number of vegans who spurn any animal product. Many of the disciples of vegetarianism today claim that it is because of their belief in animal rights that they spurn the flesh of animals.

The animal rights movement flourished in England during the 1970s, notably with Animal Welfare Year (1976/77). In 1978/79, supported by the conventional animal welfare societies, animal rights activists developed a political campaign to 'Put Animals into Politics' (Hollands 1980).

Precisely how the animal rights movement has improved animal welfare as opposed to the contributions of traditional animal welfare societies, is difficult to document. However, there is no doubt that they have helped foster an increased awareness of the animal issues on the part of the general public as well as the politicians. One has only to observe the tremendous increase over the past 15 years of various Bills introduced in the US Congress and Senate to recognize the response of politicians to the vociferous and emotional arguments generated by a still relatively small proportion of the population.

However, while their influence is considerable in suggesting the targets for legislation, it is the veterinarians in various departments of Agriculture who have the most input in the final drafts; nonetheless, such individuals must reflect the will of the politicians who have introduced the legislation.

Animal rights groups are worldwide in distribution. However, some of those that are now listed amongst the 'animal rights' groups are still traditionally the basic animal welfare societies whose objective is the prevention of cruelty. Their inclusion is the result of what has happened to the term 'animal rights', which has no genuinely clear definition, but often relates to establishing a balance between human rights and animal rights. Lists of such organizations are included in various reports (Dickinson 1989; Magel 1989; Anon 1991a). These sources will not provide the names of all of the various groups involved in the animal rights/liberation/animal welfare movements, but will suffice to indicate that the movement is well established as a worldwide entity.

The spectrum of viewpoints among all of the voices who claim they are speaking on behalf of the animals of the world, is wide. At one extreme are those who would end all uses of animals for any purpose that would benefit humankind, including the possession of pets or companion animals. Their philosophy is stripped of all of the accompanying verbiage of, for example, those who would like to see animals returned to natural surroundings (the aim of the environment and ecological groups). To abolitionists, farm animal welfare is a misnomer for, they ask, how can improving the animal's lot be considered welfare, when the animal is going to be used and even slaughtered for profit or for human benefit?

'Welfarist' societies on the other hand accept that animals are going to be used for some purpose by humankind. Thus, they are willing to work within the system in order to effect improvements in the welfare and well-being of the animals themselves. There are many examples of this worldwide.

Probably the most important in the UK is the RSPCA (see above). A group which often strays to the left of the middle ground is Compassion in World Farming (20 Lavant St., Petersfield, Hampshire, England GU32 3EW), which publishes the magazine *AgScene*. Finally mention must be made of the Farm

Animal Welfare Council (FAWC), an independent council which serves an advisory function to the UK's Ministry of Agriculture, Fisheries and Food (MAFF). One of its recent reports dealt with the enforcement of farm animal welfare legislation (Farm Animal Welfare Council 1990). It is this group's responsibility to ensure legislation is written and capable of application and enforcement.

Codes of Practice for Livestock Animal Welfare have also been published in the United Kingdom and form the basis for any cruelty charges which may be laid against livestock owners. From 1992 stockpersons and all those involved in caring for livestock are required to have knowledge of these Codes of Practice and to have undertaken training programmes to ensure their knowledge and capabilities (Robert Darrock, personal communication).

Another organization which has more recently appeared on the scene, and which is providing information and leadership in farm animal welfare, is the Cambridge Centre for Animal Health and Welfare (CCAHW: Department of Clinical Veterinary Medicine, Madingley Road, Cambridge, England CB3 0ES). The organization's primary objective is to 'bridge the gap between wide divisions of opinions' about farm animals. It recently produced its first publication, a survey of opinions on what may, or should be their consequences on the way animals are treated (Hill and Sainsbury, 1990).

Two organizations which promote responsible animal welfare are the Universities Federation for Animal Welfare (UFAW) and the Humane Slaughter Association (HSA: 8 Hamilton Close, South Mimms, Potters Bar, Herts, England AN6 EQD). These highly respected bodies have produced many excellent publications on livestock well-being (e.g. Universities Federation for Animal Welfare 1980, 1981, 1982) and, indeed, produced a document on humane slaughter two decades ago (HSA 1971).

In 1989, the World Association for Transport Animal Welfare and Studies (TAWS) was founded in the UK (G J R Hovell, c/o Department of Physiology, Parks Road, Oxford, England OX1 3PT). Its role is to encourage research and bring veterinarians, scientists and lay people together to work for draft animals, of which there are some 400 million in the world (Singleton 1989).

In Canada, under the auspices of Agriculture Canada, Codes of Practice have been developed for all of the domestic species (Agriculture Canada, Communications Branch, Ottawa, Ontario, Canada K1A 0C7) (Agriculture Canada 1986, 1988, 1989a, 1989b, 1989c, 1990). The first, published in 1980, was entitled *Recommended Code of Practice for Handling Chickens from Hatchery to Slaughterhouse*; the latest revision to this was published in 1989 (Agriculture Canada 1989c). The most recent Code is the *Beef Code of Practice*; slated for publication in January 1992, a tentative version was published in the July, August and September 1991 issues of *Cattlemen Magazine*.

The Canadian Federation of Humane Societies (CFHS) has participated on the committee which developed these Codes, as have representatives of the

Canadian Veterinary Medical Association (CVMA), the Canadian Association for Laboratory Animal Science (CALAS), the Canadian Cattlemen's Association (CCA), and the Canadian Council on Animal Care (CCAC).

While the enforcement of these Codes of Practice has not taken the same strides as those made in the UK, an effort is being made by Agriculture Canada to ensure that the codes are practised.

In Canada a new Act, with a short title of the Health of Animals Act or Bill C-66, has been passed. It relates to 'disease and toxic substances that may affect animals or that may be transmitted by animals to persons and respecting the protection of animals', and was given royal assent on 19 June 1990 (available from Canadian Government Printing Centre, Supply and Services Canada, Ottawa, Ontario, Canada K1A 0S9). This Act replaced the old Animal Disease and Protection Act 1974. (Although the latter Act was formulated in consultation with representatives of the CFHS, the Federation played no part in development of the new Health of Animals Act.) Under the Health of Animals Act, Agriculture Canada veterinarians will have the ability to ensure that Codes of Practice are being followed in various regions across Canada.

A lack of similar guidelines for agricultural animals in the USA was felt most acutely by the agricultural research community. Therefore, in the spring of 1986, there began an effort to develop guidelines for the care and use of agricultural animals in agriculture research and teaching. This reached fruition in 1988, when a *Guide for the Care and Use of Agricultural Animals* was published by a consortium of scientific and professional organizations, industrial groups and government agencies (Curtis 1989) (available from Association headquarters, 309 West Clark Street, Champagne, IL 61820, USA).

Although many animal welfare organizations in the USA have expressed opinions on Livestock Intensive Management Practices (LIMP), only two will be mentioned. The Washington-based Animal Welfare Institute (AWI: PO Box 3650, Washington, DC 20007, USA), which produces the Animal Welfare Institute Quarterly newsletter, recently published *Factory Farming—The Experiment that Failed* (AWI 1988). In 1955, the AWI spawned the Society for Animal Protective Legislation (SAPL), whose contacts with numerous members of the US Congress and Senate are employed to promote legislation affecting livestock animal welfare.

A second organization is Animal Rights International: Coalition to Abolish the LD$_{50}$ and Draize Tests, Coalition for Non-Violent Food (Box 214, Planetarium Station, New York, NY 10024, USA) headed by Henry Spira. As noted, Spira first became recognized for his efforts to ban the Draize (eye irritancy) test and LD$_{50}$ toxicity test, but he has since taken on the livestock industry, contending that 95% of animal suffering is in factory farming (Spira 1986). He states that, because there are five billion farm animals 'suffering from birth to slaughter each year' every one per cent reduction in their suffering can accomplish more than all other animal campaigns put together (Clifton

1990). Spira is considered 'one of the leading moderate figures in the national [animal rights] movement' (Venant and Treadwell 1990).

The dark side of the animal rights movement

It would be improper if readers were left with the impression that animal rights organizations merely differ in viewpoint from the more traditional animal welfarist groups. Many of the former believe that the only way to effect change is to take positive action against individuals involved in the specific industries or institutions associated with the use of animals. The farm community in the UK, for example, has not gone untouched. The terrorist Animal Liberation Front (ALF) had its beginnings with the Hunt Saboteur's Association in the 1960s (Henshaw 1989). ALF founder, Ronnie Lee, was first a member of the (Luton) HSA, which is thought to be 'genuinely opposed to violence'. Former members of the HSA subsequently formed the Hunt Retribution Squad (HRS) which desecrated the cross on the grave of the Duke of Beaufort, a Master of the Hunt at Badminton parish church in Gloucestershire. Its press release said the HRS had planned to 'remove the corpse from the grave and scatter him around Worcester Lodge. We also planned to remove his head and despatch it to Princess Anne, a fellow blood junkie'. It is estimated that damage to farms and laboratories in the UK totals at least 6 million per year (Henshaw 1989). Not only were specific farms vandalized, but some farmers had their barns and dwellings burnt, slaughterhouses were ransacked, and 'Meat is Murder' was scrawled on the windows of butcher's shops.

In the USA, Wannall (1991) noted that, although animal activists claim compassion for creatures, they are 'soft on violence'. Animal rights activities prompted an editorial in *Live Animal Trade and Transport Magazine* entitled 'Terrorism on the Farm'. Noting the 'significant economic issues at stake', it suggested that an anti-terrorism department be established in each school of agriculture, and a similar staff function in each private enterprise (Anderson 1989). The animal rights organization Physicians Committee for Responsible Medicine (PCRM) has recently developed its own four food groups, including legumes and grains, but excluding meat and milk (Drexler 1991). The well-known, fast-growing animal rights organization, People for the Ethical Treatment of Animals (PETA), while it claims to have no connection with the Animal Liberation Front in the USA, becomes the depository of information stolen during ALF raids and distributes it to the media. PETA implies that it is merely the fortunate recipient of the information and that it believes that the public should be made aware of how strongly the ALF feels about the issues and take action with their own hands.

ALF spokesperson, Margo Tannenbaum, recently stated that her group's goal is 'elimination of the livestock industry'. Increasingly, remote farms are being attacked (Hillinger and Stein 1989).

More recently, PETA has used personalities such as a well-known Canadian country singer to publicly proclaim that 'Meat Stinks'.

One PETA action which was abhorrent to most people was to place an advertisement in the Des Moines Register which equated the slaughter of food animals with the ghastly serial murders perpetrated by Jeffrey Dahmer, who killed and dismembered a dozen men in his Milwaukee apartment. The advertisement stated:

> Milwaukee . . . July 1991 . . . They were drugged and dragged across the room . . . Their legs and feet were bound together . . . Their struggles and cries were unanswered . . . Then they were slaughtered and their heads sawn off . . . The body parts were refrigerated to be eaten later . . . Their bones were discarded with the trash. It's Still Going On . . . If this leaves a bad taste in your mouth, become a vegetarian.

Even the founder/publisher of the *Vegetarian Times* commented that PETA had 'seemed to exceed the boundaries of good taste' (Anon 1991c).

In Canada, the Animal Liberation Front claims to have burnt barns in the Toronto area, according to boasts in its own newsletter (Anon. 1986).

While livestock producers have been (rightly) disturbed by these actions, they themselves have taken positive steps to inform the general public and educate city dwellers about modern agricultural practices and their concern for the welfare of the animals they raise. If the ALF has done anything, it has galvanized farmer's opinions against those promoting animal rights, and has effectively removed any middle ground for discussion that may have been present amongst members of the farming community and the animal welfare communities.

Conclusions

Although animal welfare societies have played a role, both nationally and internationally, in the prevention of avoidable suffering among farm animals, the zeal and activities of the terrorist Animal Liberation Front and the philosophies of many in the animal rights movement have dulled some of the sensitivities (and indeed, alienated) many in the agricultural industry and legislature who might have pressed for the development of effective, realistic and enforceable legislation.

The urbanization of modern society, Franklin Loew's 'urban prism', through which we see animals (Malcolm 1991) has removed most of us from daily contact with livestock. Those responsible for enforcement of legislation, including Departments of Agriculture, must exercise their responsibilities in an environment of mutual trust and respect. By so doing, the animal will become the beneficiary.

Neither the legislators nor those in the animal welfare movement should forget the importance of trust, for the development of bureaucratic and burdensome legislation may represent good politics (which no doubt also fosters re-election of representatives), but does little to protect and improve the welfare and well-being of livestock.

The key to animal welfare lies primarily with the farmer or the stockperson caring for the animals on a daily basis (Anon. 1991f). These individuals should be encouraged to be attentive and well-trained in the conduct of their responsibilities. Additionally, as each farmer and stockperson knows, animals that are stressed, either by improper care, poor environments or disease, are less productive. Animal welfare societies interested in preventing unnecessary suffering should make greater efforts to encourage appropriate training and selection of individuals who are going to be caring for the animals, rather than striving only for legislative means to improve animal welfare. This applies not only to the animal on the farm, but the animal in transportation, at auction yards, and at the time of slaughter.

10 THE IMPACT OF BIOTECHNOLOGY ON ANIMAL HEALTH AND WELFARE
W Sybesma

Biotechnology
Historical development
New biotechnology (NBT)
Future prospects and consequences
The future of animal health, welfare, biotechnology and ethics in Europe
General discussion and conclusions

Biotechnology is capable of introducing mouse genes into tobacco plants so that those plants can produce animal proteins. This example, from the work of Hiatt et al. (1989), clearly demonstrates the impact of this new technology, which has probably unlimited potential but is at the same time of great concern for several groups in our society. The challenge is enormous, not only for scientific research but also for animal and veterinary science. It is important to try to specify the consequences for animal health and welfare, the environment and the final product because the whole world and the human species itself will be profoundly affected by this new technology.

In this chapter we deal with these scientific aspects and with the prospects and perspectives for the health and welfare of livestock.

Biotechnology

Definition

Biotechnology is just another word for a group of technologies which have existed for a long time. It is very important to specify a particular technique in order to discuss its impact and its significance in given areas. The European Community defines biotechnology as follows: 'all techniques which exploit or cause induced organic changes in biological material, micro-organisms, plants and animals or techniques which use biological methods to induce changes in an organic material.' The Organization for Economic Co-operation and

Development (1988) gives the following definition: 'Biotechnology is the application of scientific and engineering principles to the processing of materials by biological agents to provide goods and services.' Biological agents in this sense are microorganisms, viruses, bacteria, cells or parts of cells of any kind including algae, insects, mammals and plants.

Brewing, bread baking and tofu preparation are examples of production techniques which go back thousands of years. They belong to the field of classical biotechnology (CBT). By the use of the most up-to-date technology man can build a fully computerized brewery, so CBT becomes part of modern biotechnology (MBT).

New biotechnology is a term used for another part of modern biotechnology and consists of special technologies such as gene manipulation, hybridoma technology, gene mapping and gene transfer by micro-injection in embryos, for instance. These technologies are now common in many scientific fields, including animal production and veterinary science. For the sake of clarity the OECD definition is preferred.

As indicated previously it is important when dealing with biotechnology to distinguish between:

- hybridoma technology
- genetic engineering or rDNA technology
- micromanipulation of embryos, including gene transfer

Historical development

Science from the Historical point of view

The concern of the general public about these new developments has a lot to do with their perceptions of the role of science. How can this be explained?

Scientific research has always had its place in human history. In Greek civilization, myth was the prevailing element in society's thinking. The forces of the natural environment determined this. Later in history the ontological phase can be distinguished, ontology being the branch of metaphysics which deals with the nature of being. In this phase the investigator distances himself from the object of study. He is at that moment not part of the natural environment but has become a watcher. Ontology was followed by the functional phase: this articulates the functional element of thinking. Here participation and distance determine the approach to the reality around us.

For many centuries agriculture and veterinary science had the characteristics of the mythical phase. Only in the second half of the 19th century—later in fact than in other areas—was there a change towards the ontological and functional phases.

Secularization was one of the reasons that the functional differentiation between science and non-science (i.e. morals, ethics) took place. This is nicely demonstrated by the history of the Royal Society, which was founded in 1662. Robert Hooke drafted the articles in which he described the tasks as follows:

> to improve the knowledge of natural things and all the useful arts, manufactures, mechanick practices, engynes and inventions by experiments (not meddling with Divinity, Metaphysics, Moralls, Politicks, Grammar, Rhetoric and Logick).

King Charles II officially approved the Charter and its privileges, which were as follows:

> We have given. . .that they. . .enjoy mutual intelligence and knowledge with. . .strangers and foreigners. . .without any molestation and corruption. . .provided [this be] in matters or things philosophical, mathematical and mechanical.

This meant that ethical and political considerations were exempted. The responsibility of the researchers was officially limited, which was accepted at that time. By so doing the distinction between morals and science was clear for everyone to see. Science got its own domain. Within this framework science had a completely free hand in this so-called period of 'Enlightenment'.

However, nowadays, this 'freedom' is being questioned. Developments like the nuclear explosion at Chernobyl, not to mention other technological disasters, upset the public, creating public fear of unrestricted scientific developments and its applications. This apprehension operates at two levels in our society:

(i) The level of the concern of the general public about scientific development.
(ii) The level of individual choice with regard to the acceptance of certain scientific applications (Medawar 1984; Laeyendecker 1989)

With regard to the first level, the Royal Society point of view, namely that science is neutral both politically and morally is still valid. However, selection of research topics and the application of research results are definitely not neutral. Funtowicz and Ravets (1990) put it this way:

> Science has become increasingly capital-intensive and rather intimately connected with technology and political power. Therefore it has lost its ideological function as the unique bearer of the true. So-called 'normal' science based on 'puzzle-solving' within an unquestioned 'paradigm' or

accepted picture of the world [cited definition of Thomas Kuhn] is not able to give answers on the challenges of global environmental and other complex and technical issues. Therefore a new scientific method neither value free nor ethically neutral has to be developed. This method is called 'post-normal' science. Normal and post-normal science can in a dialogue safeguard the quality of the health and safety of the world. The question of the impact of [the release of] genetically engineered organisms is part of these challenges. They warn us against pseudo-science creating pseudo-myths through computer modelling which can be called GIGO (Garbage in Garbage out).

This is in short how science and research face new challenges which are by no means all attributable to new biotechnology.

Animal Production and Veterinary Science

What can we say in respect of the development of animal production and veterinary science. Hoffmann (1987), in an article on the effects of beta-agonists on growth and carcass quality, notes that Justus von Liebig (1803–1873) was the pioneer of the change from myth to functional research. Up to that time no goal-oriented measures of plant growth existed. Liebig made it clear that:

a. mineral nutrient requirements are different for different plant species, and
b. one nutrient cannot substitute for another.

This insight led to the 'law of minimum', which recognized 'that the nutrient which is present in the smallest amount relative to the amount required, determines the yield'; this was quite revolutionary. By application of this insight through scientific research, new sources of productivity in agriculture have been tapped.

Furthermore Hoffmann points to the fact that next to animal nutrition, animal breeding and genetic selection have exerted the greatest impact on the productivity of animal production. For instance, fertility and meatiness in pigs have shown much progress. Another landmark worth mentioning in this respect is the recognition of the importance of animal hygiene and its application, which includes maintenance of a proper environment together with disease control and eradication regimes. The hygienic approach arose from the work of great pioneers like Pasteur and Koch in the last part of the 19th century.

Veterinary schools had already been established in the 18th century. In January 1762 we see in Lyon 'une école pour le traitement des bestiaux' followed by comparable institutions in Paris (1765), Copenhagen (1773),

Vienna (1777), Hanover (1784) and London (1791). First of all these institutions were initiated by the equestrian interests of royal households and other aristocratic establishments. Around 1750 Europe had been particularly harassed by rinderpest, although anthrax and sheep pox also took their toll (Offringa 1971). Scientific discoveries made by Koch on the aetiology of tuberculosis, rinderpest, typhus, Texas fever, etc. and by Pasteur on the theory of the existence of microorganisms and work with rabies, made treatment, prevention and pretreatment through immunization feasible. We have now progressed to a state where the limitation of animal production due to infectious diseases belongs more or less to the past, especially with the introduction of antibiotics and coccidiostats, etc. in our century.

Hoffmann (1987) signals a new natural limit to this scientific approach, but at the same time makes it clear that the pharmacological approach still offers new perspectives. However, public concern with this pharmacological approach has halted some very fruitful scientific development. As he states, despite numerous meetings involving the EC, WHO and FAO, in which the application of anabolic sex hormones was found not only to be safe but also very efficient, the EC commission considered the use of these compounds unacceptable. Hence, this is not a biological limit but an administrative one based on public fear. How did the public fear come about?

In Politiek and Bakker (1982) a neat survey is given of different areas where progress has been made in the 20th century, culminating in intensive farming. This relates to economic and structural developments, animal health and welfare of all livestock species. The overall impression is of very great progress.

However, there is no progress without setbacks. Intensive farming has been termed by some a 'bio-industry', which suggests that more industrial methods have replaced traditional farming practices. Ruth Harrison (1964) speaks about 'animal machines' and the 'new factory farming industry'. In the case for intensive farming of food animals Curtis (1987) stresses the positive role which intensive farming has on food prices, i.e. food supply, and believes that animals' basic needs are being met in most intensive production systems. However Mickley and Fox (1987) state that this revolution in American agriculture has led to the demise of American farming. They are of the opinion that animal husbandry has been changed into animal technology where the health and well-being of the animals are sacrificed in the name of efficiency and productivity. They point to examples such as the battery cage for laying hens and the tethering of sows. Furthermore they mention occupational and consumer health hazards.

Frankenhuis et al. (1989) give the following details on the development of intensive farming. In 1946, 12 weeks were required to rear a broiler of 1200 g. Today, half the time and less food are used to rear a bird of 2000 g. Laying hens now produce 290 eggs/year compared with 143 eggs/year in 1920, an increment of 2.5/year. The Veterinary care of the laying hen up to 20 weeks of age comprises 18 different vaccine combinations administered in 10 vaccinating sessions. Nevertheless one still speaks about threatening cumulus clouds of Newcastle disease and infectious bronchitis which might endanger the poultry flock. All this started in 1940 with just one vaccination against fowl pox.

A similar kind of evolution has taken place with pigs. Genetic selection for growth considerably improved the meat:fat ratio. But new problems of stress susceptibility and meat quality occurred, and the phenomena of transport death, pale, soft, exudative (PSE) meat and dark, firm, dry (DFD) meat came to prominence in animal production research.

In cattle, the breeding of double-muscled animals especially in Western Europe, has been blamed for problems with mobility and calving (King and Menissier 1980).

Greater stocking densities in poultry and pig housing increase infection pressure and infection rate, and the use of vaccines and massive use of antibiotics to keep fast-growing stock healthy does not prevent an often labile physiological equilibrium from being disturbed.

Not only are health and welfare involved but also environmental problems and the quality of food products are at the heart of concerns expressed by our society over the intensive farming revolution.

Environmental issues

The link between animal production and pollution is nowadays well known, although many other industries are equally culpable. In the Netherlands alone the pig industry produces approximately 15 million tonnes of manure every year; such vast quantities, if mishandled, can threaten ground water and hence, potentially, the drinking water supply. Another livestock pollutant is ammonia, discharge of which is contributing to acid rain, which has caused devastation of the forests. Draconian measures will have to be taken, not only in the Netherlands, if the problem of manure disposal is to be eliminated. The Dutch government wants to resolve these problems within one generation. What is presently happening in the Netherlands is just an indication of what is happening and will happen elsewhere in Europe.

Food quality

Intensive farming systems are able to produce very efficiently large quantities of food. In the dairy industry quality control has always been of prime concern. In the meat industry we see a different picture. Although meat inspection could, generally speaking in the past, cope with negative quality aspects, current concerns over residues and microorganisms like *Salmonella* and *Campylobacter* make traditional meat inspection practices out of date or inadequate. In meat, for instance, one can make the distinction between negative and positive quality aspects. Negative aspects comprise residues and bacterial contamination, whereas positive aspects cover good colour, consistency, taste, tenderness and conformation of the carcass.

Wholesomeness is the ultimate goal (Hoffmann 1987). Many consumers no longer trust the safety of the food chain, and meat inspection systems have great difficulty in guaranteeing wholesomeness. This is partly due to the publicity over such issues as listeria, salmonella in chickens and eggs and botulism in yogurt. Publicity concerning bovine spongiform encephalopathy (BSE) the so-called 'mad cow disease', and contaminated mineral water have contributed to this atmosphere of mistrust. On the other hand the habits of the consumer have also changed considerably. Although they insist on eating healthily, they do not want a return to the days before convenience food with the hours of preparation entailed.

Furthermore a section of consumers desire good housing conditions for farm animals, resulting in, for example, free-range systems for laying hens and fattening pigs. Here so-called emotional quality aspects are involved, bringing ethical issues to the fore.

Conclusion

We may conclude that highly successful animal production systems, born of scientific progress, now face rising criticism, with pollution, animal welfare and food quality the main issues. New limits are now being set for the further development of animal production. What role will new biotechnology (NBT) play in this context? Can it solve the existing technical problems and can it also help to resolve the issues arising in this climate of increasing restriction. Will it even intensify negative feelings about animal production? Scientists cannot ignore the increasing concern about morals and ethics; researchers are no longer exempted from responsibility for the ultimate consequences of their work. Structures have to be provided in which an exchange of views and information can help to clarify the real intentions and real goals of research in order to reach a mutual understanding.

New biotechnology (NBT)

Hybridoma technology—monoclonal antibodies

In 1975 Köhler and Milstein developed the hybridoma technique. This technique is based on the fusion of two types of cells, mouse B-lymphocytes from the spleen and tumour cells from bone marrow, the so-called myeloma cells. This hybridoma has the genetic information for producing antibodies on one side (from the lymphocyte) and an unlimited growth potential on the other side (from the myeloma cell). A revolutionary biological entity is created which is able to produce *in vitro* specific antibodies, *the monoclonal antibodies* (MCA), in contrast to the conventional polyclonal antibodies. These specific antibodies can be evoked against all kinds of antigens, and offer new and exciting perspectives for therapeutic and diagnostic use.

An important aspect is the possibility of freezing the cell cultures. Antibody-producing clones may be stored in liquid nitrogen and retrieved at any given time. Furthermore the MCAs can be produced in unlimited quantities, barring financial constraints. This availability of large quantities of monoclonals with identical characteristics makes therapeutic use feasible and has made them very important for standardizing immunological assays (Booman 1988). Raybould (1989) stresses that passive immunization by MCA application, in growth promotion for instance, sometimes has advantages over administration of the hormone preparation itself. It evokes endogenous growth hormone secretion, which does not have the side-effects of genetically engineered hormones like pST (porcine somatotrophin). pST has to be administered daily, posing a practical problem (De Meyer et al. 1988). Booman (1989) prefers this kind of immuno-neutralization over active immunization, which is not very reproducible. Raybould (1989) distinguishes the following applications for MCAs:

a. MCA based immunoassays for monitoring ovulation and detecting pregnancies in cattle.
b. MCA based rapid immunodiagnostics for early identification of disease outbreaks.
c. MCAs against specific infectious agents.
d. MCAs used as therapeutic modifiers of specific physiological functions, for instance promoting superovulation or promoting growth.
e. MCAs against immunoglobulins and specific cell surface markers for immunodiagnosis and for immunotherapy in several diseases and certain types of tumour.

Veterinary applications of MCAs

The first MCAs were of murine origin. However, homologous MCAs are preferred from the immunological viewpoint, but it is not easy to construct hybridomas from other species. Booman et al. (1989) produced bovine/murine cell lines by fusing bovine lymphoid cells with a mouse myeloma cell line. The

361

ratio between numbers of bovine and murine chromosomes, bovine and mouse cell-surface Ig (immunoglobulin) and secretion of bovine Ig were assessed. In one case fusion resulted in 32 growing hybrid colonies after 6–8 weeks of culture. The hybrid cells contained variable numbers of chromosomes, ranging between 53 and 112 with a mean of 67.6 ± 12.6. The percentage of bovine chromosomes ranged between 0 and 29 with a mean of 14.8 ± 8.4. Only two colonies were positive for bovine cell-surface Ig and were secreting bovine IgM.

In experiments (with PMSG neutralizing efforts) murine MCA (mMCA) elicited an anti-mouse immune response whereas bovine MCA (bMCA) did not. The conclusion was that for repeated passive immunization in cattle homologous antibodies are to be preferred over heterologous antibodies. This example is cited to show that prospects do not always turn into real opportunities.

In polyclonal antisera where antibodies are derived from multiple distinct B-lymphocyte clones, cross-reactivity is a major problem. The discriminating abilities of MCAs are potentially very great. However, because of the selection for a single antigenic determinant, their affinity is far below conventional antisera. Mixing MCAs is often a solution (Booman 1988). The use of MCAs has improved the quality of several diagnostic systems, and MCAs can be raised against all kinds of antigens. In combination with the ELISA technique, MCAs are extensively used in diagnostic tests which are easy to use in the barn or in the field. In the case of pregnancy and oestrus determination these tests have been found to be very helpful. MCA-containing immunoassays have been brought onto the market for parasites, neonatal diarrhoea, respiratory diseases, brucellosis and other infectious diseases (Raybould 1989).

Reproductive applications of MCAs

In the assessment of oestrus and pregnancy in cattle a milk progesterone test is very effective. The bovine oestrous cycle is characterized by an abrupt fall in peripheral plasma progesterone levels between the third and second day before oestrus. Since this fall is not seen in pregnant animals early pregnancy diagnosis is feasible at 3 weeks after insemination by the determination of progesterone levels in milk, which accurately reflect those in plasma (Booman et al. 1984). This test is also applicable to buffaloes (Nasir Hussain Shah et al. 1988).

MCAs also have a possible use in sex determination. H-Y antigen is a histocompatibility antigen which is only present on the surface of male cells. Therefore early detection in embryonic development seems feasible (Kroo and Goldberg 1976). Booman et al. tried to produce specific, high-affinity, monoclonals against H-Y antigen of the mouse. With the help of an enzyme immunoassay, bovine embryos of 6–7 days were tested. The rate of fluorescence is the determining criterion, with fluorescing embryos positive and hence male. Table 10.1 lists the results.

Discussion and Conclusions

This part of NBT is biologically revolutionary because cells with completely different functions are fused to act as one entity. Furthermore these new cell systems are capable of producing antibodies against all kinds of antigens; not only proteins, steroids and toxins will also form antibodies.

The use of MCAs in human and veterinary medicine and also animal production has opened new approaches to therapy and diagnosis. For example in 1991 the FDA approved the first monoclonal antibody conjugate, called Orthozyme-CD-5+ which is used for the treatment of acute graft versus host disease (GvHD). It is made of a mouse MCA specific for the CD-5 binding site on mature T-lymphocytes and a toxin called the ricin A chain. The MCA homes in on the T-lymphocyte and the toxin kills the cell responsible for the disease (Eisner 1991). In veterinary medicine one of the first applications of MCA's was to protect neonatal calves against diarrhoea caused by enterotoxigenic *E. Coli* through oral administration (Sherman and co-workers 1987, cited by Raybould 1989).

The greatest impact of MCAs on animal health and welfare, now and in the future, is through better and quicker diagnostic techniques for disease and pregnancy. These offer the farmer direct information on the spot, and enable him to take therapeutic action early in an infection. The use of MCAs for diagnosis is thus a management tool for both the veterinarian and the farmer, increasing the profitability of the farm by enabling more efficient use of livestock but without any harmful effects.

rDNA Technology

The discovery of the structure of DNA by Crick and Watson in 1953 opened the way to what is now called genetic engineering or genetic manipulation. DNA is a component of the genetic material of all living creatures which means that all possible combinations are feasible. The basic DNA unit is made up of deoxyribose sugar, phosphate and one of four bases—adenine, guanine, cytosine and thymine. DNA (deoxyribonucleic acid) codes for the amino acid components that make up proteins in the body. The code is determined by the sequence of the four bases. The total genetic information in a cell is called the genome, which consists of several chromosomes. Every chromosome comprises many genes, which are linked by intervening stretches of non-coding DNA. The code is transcribed by RNA polymerase and duplicated as mes-

Table 10.1 Numbers of embryos and accuracy of sex determination in each category of fluorescent and non-fluorescent bovine embryos sexed under improved conditions (from Booman et al. 1989).

	No. of embryos observed		No. of readable karyotypes	No. of embryos sexed correctly		
	Fluorescent	Non-fluorescent		Fluorescent	Non-fluorescent	Total
H-Y-positive embryos	35 (36%)	–	5	5/5 (100%)	–	5/5 (100%)
H-Y-negative embryos	–	45 (47%)	14	–	9/14 (64%)	9/14 (64%)
Intermediate embryos	5 (5%)	8 (8%)	3	1/1 (100%)	1/2 (50%)	2/3 (67%)
Total	40 (42%)	53 (55%)	22 (23%)	6/6 (100%)	10/16 (63%)	16/22 (73%)

senger RNA, which penetrates into the cell's cytoplasm where the process of translation transforms the code into the specific protein. By recombination of the genetic material a new genotype can be constructed.

Through analysis and mapping of an organism's genotype, it is possible to construct a new genotype or to repair a damaged chromosome (gene therapy). Because the DNA code is universal it is possible to use recombinant DNA techniques to introduce eukaryotic genes, for example from vertebrates, into simple prokaryotes such as bacteria. The production of hormones or hormone-like substances by microorganisms is such an example. In contrast, transgenic animals are the result of the insertion by way of micro-injection of foreign genetic material into one of the two pronuclei of the zygote. Here the germ line is directly involved. Another possibility is to introduce foreign DNA into embryonic stem cells.

The expression of the novel genes (heterologous DNA) in the host organism is the most essential part of this technique. Integration in the host DNA molecule of both the foreign DNA and a suitable promoter sequence is required. With GH genes a zinc-regulatable mettalothionein (MT) is often used (Pursel et al. 1989). The transgenic animal is a new entity made by human hand. Bacteria (prokaryotes) as well as vertebrates (eukaryotes), human included, may be the subject of this manipulation.

Veterinary application

Genetic engineering has made available a host of new techniques, especially in the field of diagnosis and immunization.

Vaccines

One area of genetic engineering that has benefited vaccine manufacture is the production of *synthetic peptides*. The new techniques have overcome the technical problems found with former chemical methods of synthesis, meaning that peptides can now be produced whatever their size and structure. Genetically engineered synthetic peptides are used for viral vaccine production, e.g. foot-and-mouth disease vaccine. Similarly, the new techniques can be used to assemble *subunit vaccines* consisting of non-viable (non-replicative) and non-infectious portions of the pathogenic agent that are still capable of eliciting a protective immune response. This means that from the pathogenic point of view the vaccines are safe.

Expression of target antigens in prokaryotic hosts for instance *E. coli*. *E. coli* offers a useful expression host for the production of unmodified prokaryotic proteins or viral gene products. Polio virus, rabies virus and influenza virus are used for that purpose. The use of *Live attenuated recombinant viruses* is an alternative approach based on genetic engineering compared to the production of protein subunits. It is possible to insert a gene for a protective antigen from one virus into a different virus that is attenuated. Usually antigens from vaccinia virus and adenovirus are the attenuated factor. *Live attenuated adenoviruses* have been used as antigen-generating vehicles to trigger immune responses. Adenovirus vectors may be directed to express viral antigens at a specific site where the local immune response is crucial to provide protection against the disease. Therefore this approach is used in rotavirus vaccines (Yong Kang 1989).

Recombinant cytokines

Lawman et al. (1989) reviewed the impact on recombinant DNA technology on the prospect of the use of cytokines in veterinary medicine. Cytokines are soluble, non-antibody factors secreted by lymphocytes, monocytes and macrophages. They play an important role in the activation of the immune system as so-called immunomodulators. The group of interleukins and all kind of growth stimulating factors for granulocytes, macrophages, B-cell maturation, interferon production and erythropoietin production have to be mentioned in this respect. The new biotechnology techniques make large quantities of purified immunomodulators available for researchers in this field. These compounds have to be seen as a viable adjunct to the non-conventional approaches to vaccine development.

Diagnostics

The technique of using DNA probes as a diagnostic tool has led to very sensitive tests for detecting microorganisms. The sensitivity of these tests has been greatly increased by use of the polymerase chain reaction (PCR), which is theoretically capable of finding a few microorganisms per sample. Indeed, DNA polymerase was hailed as molecule of the year in 1989 (Levy Guyer and Koshland 1989).

DNA and RNA hybridization techniques, using nucleic acid probes, have already proved to be of great value in detecting the following diseases: Bovine herpes virus, dengue virus, papillomavirus and enterotoxigenic *E. coli*. The technique of DNA fingerprinting is now used for genotypic analysis (Beaty and Carlson 1989). Genetically engineered antigen-constructed vaccines induce antibody patterns that are totally different from those induced by the 'natural' virus. This makes possible discrimination between vaccination titres and titres derived from natural infection, which will mean improved control measures.

The utilization and control of these biotechnological procedures in veterinary science are described by Blancou (1990).

Disease Resistance

Analysis of the genome can lead to the discovery of gene defects. Although this area is of more importance in human medicine it could be of some importance in veterinary science (Schwenger 1990). For example, genetic selection for disease resistance based on the major histocompatibility complex (MHC) might help to boost natural resistance against certain diseases, for instance Marek's disease in chickens and *Theileria annulata* and *T. parva* in cattle (Zijpp et al. 1989; Gogolin-Ewens et al 1990). These techniques are at present being extensively studied in animal breeding.

Animal Production Aspects

Transgenic animals

rDNA techniques are capable of introducing new characteristics into an animal. Ward et al. (1990) report their results with the transfer of foreign DNA into domestic animals, especially sheep. They distinguish the following areas of physiology amenable to genetic manipulation:

1. Hormonal status
2. Metabolic pathways
3. Structural proteins
4. Disease resistance
5. Behavioural characteristics

Simons et al. (1987) were able to produce sheep beta-lactoglobulin transgenic mice. Ebert (1989) reported the successful injection of rat growth hormone gene (rGH) into fertilized pig zygotes. The enhanced growth rate was sustained during the growing period compared to littermates without this rGH. Pursel et al. (1989) used bovine growth hormone transgenic pigs (bGH) and showed that their metabolic and physiological equilibrium more or less collapsed. Two successive generations of pigs expressing the bGH gene showed significant improvements in both daily weight gain and feed efficiency and a marked reduction in subcutaneous fat. However, the long-term elevation of bGH was generally detrimental to health, with such problems as arthritis, gastric ulcers, dermatitis and cardiomegaly. Furthermore the success rate of the production of transgenic pigs was very low. Depending on the method of calculation only 0.98% of the injected eggs were transformed into transgenic offspring. Ward et al. (1990) noticed the same phenomenon of elevated growth hormone levels in their transgenic sheep which led to greatly reduced fat content and higher basal metabolic rate and heat production. All animals died before 12 months of age. The main hurdle to success is the transcriptional control of the inserted genes. Additionally, the low efficiency of the technique poses a big problem. Wagner (1988) suggests a method of transgenic animal formation in which the negative effects of growth hormone expression in transgenic pigs may be overcome by restricting the duration of expression of the foreign genes to only a portion of the life of the pig.

Expression of the growth hormone gene affects the organism's entire physiology, with profound consequences. In contrast, by confining transgenic expression to an organ system, like the mammary gland, less problems arise. In the Netherlands research is underway in which a cow's genetic make-up is altered so that it will produce milk containing substances with biomedical applications or allow the milk as a whole to be used as food additives for children to prevent diarrhoea. Furthermore it might be possible to produce anti-mastitis proteins, like lactoferrin: Van Brunt (1988) labels this approach as molecular farming. Hence, it is the way in which the expression of the implanted gene is regulated that chiefly determines how the animal's behaviour, and consequently welfare, will be affected.

Products of prokaryotic organisms

Genetic engineering extensively uses microorganisms for the production of foreign proteins. A gene for a particular protein is integrated in the DNA of the microbe, located in so-called plasmids. After insertion and integration of the desired gene the protein is produced. The colonies of such treated bacteria serve as factories, manufacturing large quantities of proteins suitable for vaccines, diagnostic reagents and hormone-like substances, for example. Bovine (bST) and porcine somatotrophin (pST) are such biochemical products which have already been used extensively for research purposes.

Bovine Somatotrophin

Dave Baumann from Cornell University showed in the early 1980s the potency and the potential of recombinant somatotrophin preparations for boosting milk yield. Since then an enormous amount of work has been devoted to this milk yield-stimulating compound. A recent review has been published with regard to food safety (Juskevich and Guyer 1990).

A series of experiments covering three lactations has been reported by Oldenbroek et al. (1989). The main results can be summarized as follows:

1. In all three lactations the somatotrophin treatment (once every 28 days, subcutaneously) significantly increased milk yield (7%).
2. The response was better on a diet of concentrates than on mainly roughage.
3. Somatic cell counts in milk tended to increase.
4. No adverse effects on fertility and health, including culling rate, were found.

In the USA the Food and Drugs Administration (FDA) has released safety data showing that milk from treated cows presents no increased health risk to consumers (Juskevich and Guyer 1990). However, there still remains considerable controversy between some pressure groups and scientists as to whether this produce of the New Biotechnology should be introduced onto the market. Until now only the former USSR, Romania, Czechoslovakia, Argentina and South Africa have accepted the scientific evidence which shows that the product is safe. One important element in the discussion is that because of the socioeconomic consequences for the farmer it should not be allowed to be used freely.

Porcine Somatotrophin

Porcine somatotrophin is in a quite different position since the desired effect is not restricted to one organ, as is the case with bGH in cattle. In the experiments so far subcutaneous doses have to be administered daily, which is quite a disadvantage.

In a symposium in 1988 in the Netherlands (V.d. Wal et al. 1988) various aspects of the economics, health, food safety and consumer acceptability were considered. In a dose response study with pigs injected daily the animals were found to grow 20% faster, consumed 19% less feed and had a food conversion ratio of 36% greater than controls (McLaren et al. 1990). Verstegen et al. (1990) found a 19% improvement in rate of weight gain. Daily protein gain increased 31% till 39% more with decreasing fat gain. The daily heat production rose 12%. The effect on the meat quality has been assessed by De Meyer et al. (1988). The results are listed in Table 10.2. It seems from these data that

Table 10.2 Effect of daily injections of recombinant pST on carcass characteristics (fresh-killed) (from Demeyer et al. 1989)

Daily pST dose (mg)	0	1.5	3	6
Backfat thickness (mm)	24.4	22.7	21.9	17.6
Length (cm)	79.9	78.3	79.9	80.3
Meat (%)	59.5	61.9	61.5	64.8
pH 30 min. p.m. (long. dorsi)	5.9	5.9	5.9	5.8
Temp. (°C) 30 min. p.m. (long. dorsi)	40.7	41.1	40.8	41.3

the meat quality in a meatier carcass is hardly affected. Without doubt pST is a very powerful instrument in improving the efficiency of pig production. However, as said before, practical difficulties such as the need for daily injections prevent its commercial use at the present time.

Regulatory Aspects of bST and pST

Norcross et al. (1989) report that somatotrophins will be approved and regulated in the USA in a manner similar to endogenous hormones like oestradiol, progesterone and testosterone.

The somatotrophins are being produced by bacteria; a particular variety (K12) of *Escherichia coli* is used for the production of bST. The FDA in the USA feels that this genetically engineered strain poses no greater threat to the environment than unmodified organisms.

Other Compounds

Apart from the somatotrophins, very potent so-called repartitioning agents exist which have similar effects on carcass growth and composition (Hanrahan 1987). Beta-agonists like cimaterol and clenbuterol increase feed efficiency by approximately 10% and can improve carcass characteristics, giving a better lean/fat ratio. These compounds can be given with the daily feed. The effects have been observed in bovines (Allen et al. 1987; Boucque et al. 1987), sheep (Duquette et al. 1987; Hanrahan et al. 1987), pigs (Bekaert et al. 1987; Cole et al. 1987; Van Weerden 1987; Wallace et al. 1987) and poultry (Dalrymple et al. 1987; Scholtyssek 1987). It seems that they offer good alternatives to somatotrophins in improving meat production efficiency.

Animal Breeding Aspects

The elucidation of the structure of DNA in 1953 by Watson and Crick has ultimately enabled the mapping and characterization of specific genes. Since 1988 James Watson has headed the Human Genome Project, a three billion dollar project of the US National Institutes of Health (NIH) that aims to map and interpret important regions of the human genome, and eventually the entire genetic message.

One of the aims is to track down the genes that cause the 4000 or so hereditary diseases. The same idea is attractive for use in animal husbandry, albeit targeting genotypes for quality traits. Deciphering genetic instructions for superior livestock could revolutionize animal breeding.

Genetic Markers

Genetic markers are DNA sequences which correlate with certain genes and hence with certain production characteristics. These markers can be identified using DNA probes. The DNA of the organism under scrutiny is digested with restriction enzymes, which cleave the DNA at specific sites along its length. The resulting DNA fragments are separated by an electrophoretic technique known as Southern blotting, and identified using gene probes. The restriction sites can be used as markers to map genes. They also show variation between individuals, a phenomenon called restriction fragment length polymorphism (RFLP). Certain RFLP patterns have been employed as DNA fingerprinting.

RFLP is useful in different ways:

- determination of parentship (DNA fingerprinting)
- detection and mapping of genetic defects
- detection and mapping of genetic markers for production traits
- mapping genes for transfection or transgenesis

The fact that a particular marker is found to be associated with quantitative genetic characteristics for growth and milk production can be used in selection of these traits. In this respect the major histocompatibility complex (MHC) has to be mentioned. The MHC is a gene cluster that encodes various components of the immune system. It is thus related to blood group composition and functions as a genetic disease resistance indicator (Zijpp et al. 1989).

Micromanipulation of the embryo

Although it is a very substantial part of the new biotechnology, micromanipulation itself is just another mechanical technique. We have already mentioned the crucial role micro-injection plays in the transfection of genes. After fertilization the pre-embryo develops from eight cells into a morula with 16–32 cells. Then the blastocyst is formed, comprising a hollow sphere of cells (trophoblast) surrounding a fluid-filled cavity (blastocoel), within which lies the inner cell mass (ICM). Everything is wrapped in the zona pellucida. Stem cells from the ICM can be extracted, treated and inserted into the blastocoel of another animal. A chimaera is then the possible result.

By using nuclear transplantation clones can be formed. This involves using enucleated mature oocytes to receive cells originating from blastomeres. Genetically identical individuals can thus be produced. Splitting embryos is used for producing identical twins or quadruplets (Picard and Betteridge 1989). In the area of gene therapy a so-called 'biolistic' approach has been developed. Tungsten pellets coated with genes are shot at very high velocities into animal cells (Watts 1990).

All these techniques lean heavily on the availability of *in vitro* conservation of embryonic tissues. *In vitro* fertilization is one aspect of this 'externalization' of the fertilization processes, as are AI, embryo transfer and embryo freezing. It also makes possible research using embryonic microsurgery. The PCR technique makes it possible to determine at the single-cell stage desired sequences in the DNA molecules of the chromosomes, including X or Y sequences (sex) or special markers for certain traits.

Future prospects and consequences

Prospects and constraints

The new biotechnology provides novel and exciting areas for research and applications in veterinary medicine as well as in animal production. We have already concluded that in intensive farming all kind of constraints appear due to, for instance, problems with quality assurance, pollution and welfare. Does NBT offer help to overcome these problems or will it add to the objections against any further development of intensive farming?

Advantages of the new technology might include the following:

1. The growing pressure of infectious diseases might be alleviated by the rDNA techniques, e.g. through development of new vaccines.
2. Discrimination between natural infection sources is easier because of the differences in antibody characteristics between the vaccine antigen and the natural virus antigen.
3. rDNA techniques greatly improve the scope of diagnostic assessment of all kinds of diseases.
4. MCAs offer a wide variety of applications whether of therapeutic or diagnostic nature.
5. Transgenic animals have the potential for enhanced or novel forms of production.
6. The production of clones offers the way for an accelerated multiplication of superior animals.

However, at the same time several objections can be raised. To name a few:

1. If actual constraints which now exist in intensive farming are lifted, this might create in the system even more serious problems with regard to health and welfare.
2. Effective rDNA products like somatotrophin alarm certain consumers and are seen by some as a threat to the socio-economic structure of farming in Europe and the USA.
3. The proliferation of genetic clones will diminish genetic variety to such an extent that genetic disease resistance will be diminished.
4. Transgenic animal production may lead to monopolies of big companies, especially if these animals are patentable.

It should be noted that the products of the hybridoma technique, the MCAs, may cause problems because of their heterologous nature (Booman 1988). In addition the rDNA technique and the creation of transgenic animals and transgenic products may cause health and welfare problems. Pursel et al. (1989) noted various physical and physiological aberrations in transgenic bGH pigs. But Oldenbroek et al. (1989) were unable to detect health problems in cattle after a three-lactation treatment with bovine somatotrophin. Microinjection in embryos has hitherto raised little criticism with regard to animal health and welfare. However, the success rate for transgenic embryos is very low (about 6%). This means that large proportions of donors have to be superovulated and ovary punctured. This practice might be regarded as welfare-unfriendly.

Improvement of existing practices by way of NBT, whether it is in the field of diagnosis or immunization will in general not meet much resistance. Genetic engineering and *in vitro* fertilization give the most concern. Fox (1988) compares the discovery of genetic engineering with the splitting of the atom in physics. This technique is able to release forces which might go beyond the control of society. It is a potential Pandora's box. He claims that if genetic manipulation means the enhancing of productivity and efficiency it is unlikely to contribute to the animal's health and welfare. Fox states that, because of prohibitive cost limitations, it presents a potentially serious animal welfare concern. In other words, further genetic engineering to improve animals' welfare will not be cost-effective, since the primary goals of livestock and poultry genetic engineering will be production—and profit-oriented. Full provision for animals' welfare (and for their basic freedoms essential for the development, expression and experiencing of their intrinsic nature) is frustrated, truncated and deformed. The question is valid. Who will decide what kind of research is undertaken and applications implemented? Several professional and non-professional categories are involved in the decision-making process (Mepham 1988).

The role of the different professional and non-professional categories in future decisions

Mepham (1988) divides those involved in future decision-making into five categories (see below). He formulated recommendations or criteria for decision-making on proposed biotechnological innovations and stressed the need for evaluations according to these criteria. Not only physiological but special procedural criteria have to be used. Every category has its own responsibility in this revolution.

The scientific community

At the beginning of this chapter we concluded that in principle science may still be regarded as neutral both morally and politically. But, as we also added, the selection of research projects and the implementation of the results are not. Governments and the European Community set priorities for research and therefore continuous interaction exists between these two bodies and the scientists. Guidelines and regulations have to incorporate not only health and welfare aspects but also moral issues.

The livestock farming community

Within the farming community the veterinarian plays an especially important role. The task of the veterinarian has already shifted from curative to preventive medicine. The modern farm manager sees the veterinarian as a specialist of animal health problems which interfere in the economics of the daily farming process. Intensive farming requires a high educational level. The new tools, like diagnostic kits, help the farmer to improve even further the level of his operation. The veterinarian may profit from these innovations because better management decisions can be made on the spot on the basis of immediate information on disease or reproduction data. Ethical considerations also play an important part in these categories; the health and welfare of the animals has to be assured. How far ethics can be used as a guideline is still debatable. This is not only true for the farmer, but for the veterinarian as well. In view of these rapid developments a new professional ethical code for veterinarians is needed (Rutgers 1990).

The lay public—attentive and inattentive

Mepham (1988) made a distinction between two categories of the lay public: the biotechnologically attentive and the biotechnologically inattentive. As there is already concern about food safety and the way food is produced, the new biotechnology brings even more doubt. Animal rights activists claim that domestic animals and wild animals have rights independent of the value human beings place on them. A still-growing group in society supports the notion that animals have a so-called intrinsic value, which give them certain rights to be treated humanely. In this category, to which in fact we all belong, the hazards of modified organisms, i.e. viruses, plants and animals, give concern. Risk assessment is something which has to be paramount before implementation or even research is considered.

Less developed countries

In the industrialized countries high input-high output agriculture is the norm and can feed the population. In the non-industrialized countries more than 400 million people still do not have adequate nourishment. Furthermore agricultural productivity per capital is falling (Dargie 1989). The new biotechnology may help to overcome a lot of the constraints. rDNA technology allows for better control of disease; trypanosomiasis is an example which might be successfully attacked using these modern techniques. However, one may not expect Western pharmaceutical companies to develop vaccines or therapeuticals for tropical diseases which exist only in certain poor areas of the world. Even existing diagnostic tools are too costly. A sad example can be found in human medicine where blood for transfusion purposes cannot be screened for the AIDS virus in some poor countries because it is too costly. The expectation is that NBT will enlarge the existing gap between the developed and the developing countries unless governments world-wide express their willingness to make these technologies widely available through international organizations like the FAO, the International Atomic Energy Agency (IAEA), and international institutes such as the International Livestock Centre of Africa (ILCA) in Addis Ababa.

Of course growth promotors, embryo transfer techniques and transgenic animals have little future if animal feed supplies are not adequate. Furthermore, a satisfactory veterinary infrastructure is required if the small farmer is to benefit (Dargie 1989).

The future of animal health, welfare, biotechnology and ethics in Europe

Introduction

The European Community is designing a programme for the future health and welfare of livestock. For some of the draft regulations fixed terms and years are already targeted. Although in this special programme no specific role has been devoted to biotechnology as such it will go without saying that beneficial spin-offs will undoubtedly be used for the practical implementation of future plans.

This programme has the following elements. The crucial issue for the future of livestock health in Europe is the guarantee of free trade in healthy animals and animal products. The European Community aims at the abolition of veterinary controls at borders of all member states, hence it is necessary to develop a policy of further improvement in the harmonization of the EC internal market. Inspections by the competent veterinary authorities of the sending country and the import inspection at the border will be replaced by random inspection at the final destination. The introduction of such a liberal system is hampered by the existing large differences in the animal health status of member states. Furthermore, harmonization of the import conditions for imports from third countries is still to be achieved. The central and essential part of this policy is, of course, efficient disease control.

Disease control

An approach taking into account the nature of specific diseases and their risks for the Community is envisaged. It is necessary to differentiate between:

1. Compulsory notifiable epizootic diseases which pose a serious threat to the economy. This group contains classical swine fever, African swine fever and foot-and-mouth disease;
2. Contagious diseases which are notifiable on a herd basis and which have a significant effect on farming or on individual animals, e.g. tuberculosis, brucellosis;
3. Diseases which may be made declarable and can be eradicated from individual herds on a voluntary 'health scheme' basis, e.g. IBR, leptospirosis;
4. Zoonotic diseases for which special Community action is justified in support of local operations to eliminate pockets of infection, e.g. rabies;
5. Fish diseases for which special Community action is justified.

In order to achieve these aims several actions are required by the EC as well as by the individual member states. National Health schemes must be in accordance with these EC strategies.

In this respect it is important to note that regulations need to cover regional instead of national boundaries. This system has already been put into practice in the eradication of classical swine fever (CSF) and African swine fever (ASF) in various countries. A directive for bovine leukosis control within the Community already lays down rules on determining herds, regions and member states which can be deemed to be leukosis free. The differences in health status between member states will require extra effort on the part of the EC to achieve effective control and/or eradication. One of the consequences of the new policy is restriction of vaccination against certain diseases, like foot-and-mouth disease and CSF.

National health schemes

National health schemes have to be complementary to EC policy. Registration of herds or flocks is the keystone of such disease control. In general the following requirements must be met:

a. registration of all operations;
b. minimum requirements for the keeping of particular species;
c. availability of reliable information systems which are capable of providing rapid information about outbreaks of disease;
d. clear instructions on the tasks and division of responsibility of the different authorities involved.

There should be no question of the competence of the local as well as national and international authorities, including general veterinary practitioners, animal health centres, national veterinary services, meat inspection services and last but not least the European Community Veterinary Inspectorate. The latter will become increasingly important, especially with regard to ensuring compliance with Community legislation by:

a. inspecting livestock in third countries prior to import into the Community;
b. public health inspections;
c. coordination of action taken in member states;
d. inspections of installations in member states.

In this respect the training and exchange of veterinary personnel and the strengthening of reference laboratories for both public and animal health needs attention. Of utmost importance is the implementation of a reliable system for animal identification. New technologies such as transponders may make it possible in the near future to link individual animal registration to a national computer database (Lambooy 1991).

Animal welfare

Coordinated agricultural and veterinary research has been stimulated by the Commission of the European Community. Over 20 seminars were held in the 1980s, proceedings of which were published in 52 volumes in the series *Current topics in veterinary medicine and animal science*. The basic idea behind these efforts was to formulate common opinions and provide objective data for policy decisions. Part of the programme has been devoted to farm animal welfare, published as an evaluation report for 1979–1983, *Farm Animal Welfare Programme* (Tarrant 1984).

What has been stated before with regard to the EC animal disease situation holds true also for the animal welfare situation. Large differences exist between member states both with respect to legislation on and public opinion. Scientific research in this field has been strongly supported by the Community.

The European Parliament has for some time been seeking to implement new directives with regard to such issues as:

1. The intensive rearing of veal calves;
2. The keeping of laying hens;
3. The intensive rearing of pigs;
4. The transport of farm animals.

Separate legislation will be required for each of these sectors and will seek to cover the following:

Veal calves: individual crates should be abolished in favour of a system of group housing. The diet should contain roughage and adequate amounts of iron for the normal development of a calf. The production of white veal is to be regarded as unethical and such a rearing system is to be prohibited.

Laying hens: the battery cage system is to be phased out taking into account the Council directive of 1986 which contains minimum standards.

Intensive rearing of pigs: the minimum age of weaning of piglets is to be three weeks, and afterwards a non-slatted or non-perforated surface as a lying/rest area must be provided. Castration of male pigs is not necessary if slaughtered before sexual maturity. The close confinement of sows in cell stalls or tethering of sows is to be discontinued.

Transport of farm animals: existing directives on transport are to be applied more rigorously by competent authorities. Directives are needed to further specify conditions for the transport of live animals of particular farm species, and too little is known of these subjects because of inadequate research. More attention to the design and construction of vehicles used to transport farm livestock is a prerequisite of good welfare legislation.

Despite the existing differences of opinion in member states on these proposed measures common rules have to be applied equally throughout the whole community.

Legislation on welfare is at present being undertaken in several European countries. In the Netherlands the so-called Law on Health and Welfare for Animals is now being issued and accepted by the parliament. It is the third in a trio which covers the whole range of veterinary activities. Already in force is the law on veterinary drugs and preparations and one laying down official rules veterinarians have to follow in fulfilling their professional responsibilities.

Zootechnics

Community zootechnical rules must be established by 1992 for all breeding animals, their semen, ova and embryos. An appropriate breeding association must give proof of registration if sold. Veterinary guarantees regarding diseases including tuberculosis, brucellosis, leukosis, foot-and-mouth disease, campylobacteriosis, and infectious bovine rhinotracheitis are required. In this area biotechnology of all kinds, such as embryo transfer, embryo splitting and cloning, is used and not only welfare but also ethics are involved.

Biotechnology

NBT will undoubtedly have a huge impact on the future development of agriculture in Europe. Hence the need to find new goals and to adjust and direct the Commission's policy. Cantley, head of CUBE (Concertation Unit for Biotechnology in Europe), at a symposium in 1988 (Cantley 1988), formulated future strategy with regard to the special role of biotechnology as follows:

1. The overall continuing, long-term goal:
*   The beneficial application of biotechnology to the maintenance and improvement of health and well-being, local environments and the global ecosystem.

2. Major policies with specific implications for biotechnology:
*   Competitiveness and innovation in the bio-industries, with particular reference to the formation and growth of small and medium-sized enterprises.
*   Harmonized internal market (regulations, patents, standards).
*   Research (basic, pre-competitive and infrastructure), development and training.
*   International collaboration (scientific, technological and industrial).

3. Other current priority actions in support of the above goals and policies:

- European biotechnology information policy (for infrastructure and competitiveness).
- Communication: public, consumers, political leaders and legislators.

In 1984 the Commission established a Biotechnology Steering Committee. Action has been undertaken through planning the programmes known as BRIDGE (Biotechnology for Innovation, Development and Growth in Europe) for 1990–1994, and ECLAIR (European Collaborative Linkage of Agriculture and Industry) for 1988–1993, which is also based on biotechnological research and development. Furthermore, action on regulations, intellectual properties and demonstration projects are all in the remit of this Steering Committee.

One of the ultimate goals is to use biotechnology for the benefit of humankind in such a way that the human population, which will rise from the current 4 billion to a likely 10 billion, can be sustained. With respect to veterinary science, animal health, feedstuffs and the regulation of veterinary medicines derived from biotechnology, Cantley outlined the very complicated approaches which will be necessary in order to benefit from these new developments (Cantley 1990). This effort has to consider not only the environment and the use of animal surpluses, but also the economic structures and the acceptability to consumers and politicians of the use of the biotechnology.

Legislation

Cantley (1990) dealt very extensively with the complicated process of regulating biotechnological applications, especially in veterinary medicine. In a review of the International Office of Epizootics, Glosser and Goham (1990) describe the regulation of biotechnology in the USA and Canada, while Millis (1990) reviews them in Asia and Oceania (1990).

In Europe several countries are trying to produce workable regulations for scientists which are also acceptable to the lay public. The German government has a proposed law for 'Protection against the dangers of modern genetic manipulation' which is still under debate. In France as yet no special regulations for biotechnology research have been issued.

In the UK the Advisory Committee on Genetic Manipulation (ACGM) of the Health and Safety Executive has drafted guidelines in the 'Transgenic Animals Guidance Note'. ACGM requires advance notification of any plans to use viral vectors or to release transgenic animals, and warns that it will be tough on both (Newmark 1989). For large animals a well-fenced field is sufficient and the welfare of such animals is adequately dealt with by existing legislation. However, the consumption of transgenic animals or their products by humans or animals would be subject to consideration by the Advisory Committee on Novel Foods and Processes.

In the Netherlands biotechnology research is subjected to the 'Environmental Dangerous Substances' law of the Department of Housing, Urban and Rural Planning and Environmental Control. This law covers genetic material, microorganisms and viruses and genetically modified organisms. A special DNA Advisory Committee advises the government on research plans regarding this matter. The Department of Agriculture proposes in the new 'Health and Welfare of Agricultural Animals' law a prescreening system for biotechnology research projects in the field of genetic engineering and cloning with large animals.

In Denmark an Environment and Gene Technology Act, issued in 1986 by the Department for the Environment, forbids the deliberate release of genetically engineered organisms and cells. In certain cases, however, the Minister may give exemption to this prohibition.

Throughout Europe safety and ethics both play an important role in the conflict between public anxiety and industrial profits (Hodgson 1990). In Germany, Denmark and the Netherlands several clashes have been reported between pressure groups, industry and government about research and research applications, predominantly with genetically engineered plants. The European Commission's directive on genetically engineered organisms (1988) allows their release into the environment under certain conditions. The introduction of genetically modified organisms (GMO) and products which consist partly of GMOs is possible. GMOs are organisms which might be obtained by techniques like rDNA, micro-infection, micro-encapsulation, nuclear transplantation, organelle transplantation, cell fusion and genetic manipulation of viruses. This therefore applies to transgenic animals and to preparations like somatotrophins and to modified vaccines.

The Directive should promote free trade between the EC countries but it is in conflict with the Danish legislation on this matter. The Commission requires notification in advance with adequate information about the identification and characteristics of the GMO, the information required for risk analysis, the geography of the introduction site, the conditions of the deliberate introduction and the control and emergency measures. Notwithstanding this Directive the use of bovine somatotrophin was prohibited after December 1990 (according to the Committee on Agriculture, Rural Development and Fisheries) because in the authorization process of such a product the social and economic consequences for agriculture should be included (draft report CARDF, December 1989). If these limitations are adopted great problems will arise for the veterinary pharmaceutical industry in Europe.

A Senior Advisory Group on Biotechnology (SAGB) was set up in 1989 by nine of Europe's largest chemical companies (including ICI, Hoffmann-La Roche and Ciba Geigy) in order to combat what they saw as the EC muddled policies towards industry. The group has consistently argued that existing product-safety legislation should be sufficient. The advisory group hopes that the EC will treat genetically engineered products according to their inherent characteristics, not to their method of manufacture (Aldhous 1992).

Concluding remarks

International co-operation and concerted action will certainly boost the development of biotechnological research, applications and products. On the European level programmes like BRIDGE and ECLAIR together with national research programmes will guarantee this. More than ever before the involvement of the general public and the consumer has to be part of the decision-making process because ethics, the potential effects on the environment, and the implications for human genetic manipulation make such involvement at an early stage very necessary.

It will not be easy to find practical systems, for instance pre-screening of research projects and/or implementation, with appropriate criteria that will allay public concerns. This will only happen if these research efforts solve most of the problems for which intensive farming is now blamed. The new biotechnology thus offers fresh challenges for better animal health and welfare in the future.

It is not easy to be exact about welfare requirements. However, directives and draft directives have already benefited from concerted activities and research. Hence legislation concerning animal husbandry methods in Western Europe has been stimulated. One example is the recommendation for minimum space in the cages of the battery system for laying hens, which has been transferred into national laws with the ultimate goal of abandoning the system in 1995.

Ethics

With regard to the application of and research in biotechnological products, ethical aspects figure prominently. Whether it is rDNA research with transgenic animals or embryo research, the immediate health and welfare of the animal is only part of the wider debate. The main issues in this respect are:

1. A feeling of incalculability—caused by the perception of biotechnology as amorphous and impenetrable. More precise identification of the various techniques—hybridomas, rDNA technology, micro-infection, cloning and enzyme technology—would help in this respect. A Dutch consumer organization, called SWOKA, questioned 1729 persons of 16 years and above and showed that 43% had never heard of biotechnology, and of the other 57% two-thirds had wrong ideas about it.

2. The creation of new forms of life. The modification of the genetic structure of an organism is regarded as an interference in the principles of nature. Furthermore the 'new' animal is prone to patenting. Where do we draw the line?

3. The animal is an object worthy of moral consideration. The use of animals for experimentation and for producing food is often questioned. In Western Europe animals are, generally speaking, receiving increasing respect, and the norms of the human-animal relationship are shifting. The animal's so-called intrinsic value demands extra care from its keepers.

4. The consequences for the quality of human life and the environment. New organisms introduced into our environment may bring new hazards: diseases, new materials, and diminishing genetic variation. The process may also lower the threshold for genome manipulation generally which might increase the pressure for human genome manipulation.

5. Socio-economic consequences. If biotechnological products are monopolized in one way or another (e.g. patents, market control) national and international competition will be endangered. Multinationals could be able to dictate the market. Large farming operations might profit more than small farms due to the extra investment requirements.

6. Fear about controllability. This originates from the conviction that research is autonomous and most of the time is invisible and secret. Examples of negative effects on the ecology due to research applications strengthen this fear. Democratic control has failed too often in the past.

A Dutch governmental Advisory Commission on Ethics and Biotechnology (1990) concluded that more information is urgently needed about the techniques themselves and their impacts. This will also help to define more precisely the limits of acceptance of certain forms of transgenic organisms. Growing awareness about the so-called intrinsic value of animals demands the formulation of handy criteria, while risk assessment of the likely impact on human life and the environment is also essential. Investigations of the socio-economic consequences are strongly recommended, as is the institution of proper democratic controls on the development of biotechnological methods. Therefore a prescreening system for approval of research projects and their applications should be framed in law.

General discussion and conclusions

In Europe in the future NBT offers animal health and welfare many possibilities. Technical breakthroughs have already materialized in vaccine production and diagnostics. These developments as fruits of NBT can only be regarded as very useful. Transgenic animals expressing foreign genes can be reliably produced, albeit still at a low efficiency. More research is necessary to understand how selected physiological processes relate to isolated genes, before the effect of a certain gene transfer may be predicted. Gene mapping is of crucial importance (Ward et al. 1990).

Genetic engineering in animals and microorganisms in order to obtain hormonal compounds has met a lot of resistance. Although the evidence is not always there, animal health and welfare are thought to be unfavourably affected. Furthermore, ethical questions arise when, for instance, species barriers are no longer respected. There is also the fear that genetic engineering in animals facilitates genetic manipulation and eugenics in humans.

These ethical objections can be brought into focus by the provision of full information at every stage of research or application. The scientific community has, in this respect, a heavy responsibility. This relates also to aspects of environmental pollution in every sense. The need is for the development of new procedures and new systems which are able to cope with the psychological as well as the technical spin-offs. In the food industry, for instance, quality assurance systems and integrated control systems have to be developed in order to guarantee food safety (Snijders et al. 1989).

Neutral scientific research no longer exists. In several countries guidelines, regulations and laws on biotechnologies have already been made. This revolutionary scientific evolution requires all groups concerned to reassess their own values and attitudes. Setting up new professional ethical codes is part of this process. In this context the ideas of 'post-normal' science, in which both insiders and outsiders play an equal role in reaching the right decisions, need further attention (Funtowicz and Ravetz 1990). A solely utilitarian application leads to aggravation of the present problems in intensive farming systems.

If applied in accordance with the views of all interested parties the acceptable part of the new biotechnology will undoubtedly be very useful for everyone. The EC, together with its member states, is already integrating these new developments within their future plans and programmes, especially in the field of animal health and welfare.

REFERENCES

Abbitt B, Ball L, Kitlo G P (1978) Effect of three methods of palpation for pregnancy diagnosis per rectum on embryonic and foetal attrition in cows. *Journal of the American Veterinary Medical Association* **272**: 973–78.

Adler H C (1974a) Retsmedicin i moderne vetinaermedicin Medlemsbl. *Den danske Dyrlaegeforening* **57**: 949–50.

Adler H C (1974b) In: Folsh D W (ed) *The ethology and ethics of farm animal production.* EAAP Publication No. 24, p 14.

Advisory Commission on Ethics and Biotechnology (1990) *Ethics and biotechnology in animal research* (Dutch) National Agricultural Research Council, Wagenigen, pp 1–18.

Agnes F, Sartorelli P, Abdi B H, Locatelli A (1990) Effect of transport, loading or noise on blood biochemical variables in calves. *American Journal of Veterinary Research* **51**: 1679–81.

Agnew J E, Sutton P P, Pavia D, Clarke S J (1986) Radio aerosol assessment of mucociliary clearance: towards definition of a normal range. *British Journal of Radiology* **59**: 147–51.

Agricultural Research Council (1980) *The nutrient requirements of farm livestock. No. 2, ruminants.* 2nd edn. Commonwealth Agricultural Bureau, Farnham Royal.

Agricultural Research Council (1982) *The nutrient requirements of farm livestock. No. 3, pigs.* 2nd edn. Commonwealth Agricultural Bureau, Farnham Royal.

Agriculture Canada (1986) *Recommended code of practice for care and handling of pigs.* Publication 1771/E.

Agriculture Canada (1988) *Recommended code of practice for the care and handling of mink.* Publication 1819/E.

Agriculture Canada (1989a) *Recommended code of practice for the care and handling of special fed veal calves.* Publication 1821/E.

Agriculture Canada (1989b) *Recommended code of practice for the care and handling of ranched fox.* Publication 1831/E.

Agriculture Canada (1989c) *Recommended code of practice for the care and handling of poultry from hatchery to processing plant.* Publication 1757/E.

Agriculture Canada (1990) *Recommended code of practice for the care and handling of dairy cattle.* Publication 1853/E.

AHMS 1 (1984) *Health management information pack, fertility packages.*

British Veterinary Association, London.

AHMS 2 (1985) *Health management information pack, the young ones.* British Veterinary Association, London.

Aldhous P (1972) Biotech lobby pressures EC. Nature **355**: 289.

Algers B (1982a) Animal health in flatdeck rearing of weaned piglets. *Zentralblatt für Veterinärmedizin* **31**: 1–13.

Algers B (1982b) Early weaning and cage rearing of piglets: Influence on behaviour. *Zentralblatt für Veterinärmedizin* **31**: 14–24.

Algers B (1984) Short communication. A note on behavioural responses of farm animals to ultrasound. *Applied Animal Behaviour Science* **12**: 387–91.

Algers B, Viske D (1990) Segerstad-projektet. Värphöns i framtidens miljö. *Svensk Veterinär Tidning* **42**: 307–8.

Algers B, Linder A, Oden K, Svedberg J (1984) *Health and behaviour in laying hens in different cages.* Swedish University of Agricultural Science Department of Animal Hygiene, Report 10. Skara, Sweden, 61 pp.

Allen M (1991) Getting the best from the laboratory—sampling and despatch. *In Practice* **13**(2): 58–9, 68.

Allen P, Quirke J F, Tarrant P V (1987) Effects of cunaterol on the growth, food efficiency and carcass quality of Friesian cattle. In Hanrahan J P (ed) *Beta-agonists and their effects on animal growth and carcass quality.* Elsevier, London/New York, pp 83–93.

Anderson D (1989) Terrorism on the farm, an editorial. *Live Animal Trade and Transport Magazine* **1**(3): 2–3.

Anil M H, Fordham D P, Rodway R G (1990) Plasma β-endorphin increase following electrical stunning in sheep. *British Veterinary Journal* **146**: 476–7.

Animal Welfare Institute (1988) *Factory farming: the experiment that failed.* Animal Welfare Institute, Washington.

Anon (1969) Seek international law for protection of animal rights. *Halifax Chronicle Herald*, October 9.

Avon (1980) *Report of the United Kingdom House of Commons Agriculture Committe for the session 1979–80.*

Anon (1986a) Action reports. *Animal Liberation Front Canada Front Line News.* 8.

Anon (1986b) *The works and benefits of the Pig Health Control Association.* Pig Health Control Association, Cambridge.

Anon (1990a) Farm animal welfare in Europe. *Animals International* **10**(32): 7.

Anon (1990b) RSPCA: 100 years. *Canadian Council on Animal Care Resource* **15**(1): 4.

Anon (1991a) Top 200 Animal Rights groups. *Animal Rights Reporter* **3**(8): 5–6.

Anon (1991b) World Veterinary Association policy statement on animal welfare, well-being and ethology. *World Veterinary Association Bulletin* **7**(2): 38–9.

Anon (1991c) The bacon made him do it. *The Washington Times*, August 9, F2.

Anon (1991d) Deafening stridency: Revulsion and PETA. Let the reader decide (editorial). *Des Moines Register*, August 9, 12A.

Anon (1991e) U.S. news. *Canadians for Health Research Diary* **5**(3): 8–10.

Anon (1991f) Stockmanship paramount in promoting welfare. *Veterinary Record* **129**(2): 22.

Anon (1991g) The CVMA Humane Practices/Animal Welfare Committee: A review and steps forward. *Canadian Veterinary Journal* **32**:273–6.

Anon (1992) Ontario Veterinary College establishes new chair in animal welfare. *At Guelph* **36**(9): 1.

Appleby M C, Lawrence A B (1987) Food restriction as a cause of stereotypic behaviour in tethered gilts. *Animal Production* **45**: 103–10.

Art T, Desmecht D, Amory H, Delogne O, Buchet M, Leroy P, et al. (1990) A field study of post-exercise values of blood biochemical constituents in jumping horses: Relationship with score, individual and event. *Journal of Veterinary Medicine A* **37**: 231–9.

Artursson K, Wallgren P, Alm G V (1989) Appearance of interferon-a in serum and signs of reduced immune function in pigs after transport and installation in a fattening farm. *Veterinary Immunology and Immunopathology* **23**: 345–53.

Bäckström L (1973) Environment and animal health in piglet production. A field study of incidences and correlations. Thesis. *Acta Veterinaria Scandinavica* **41**(Suppl): 240 pp.

Bakken G (1981) An epidemiological study of bovine mastitis. *Thesis*. Oslo, 91 pp.

Baldwin B A (1983) Operant conditioning in farm animals and its relevance to welfare. In Schmidt D (ed) *Indicators relevant to farm animal welfare*. Martinus Nijhoff, The Hague, pp 117–20.

Balsbaugh R K, Curtis S E (1979) Pigs know best—turn on the heat when they need it. *Research Minnesota University Agricultural Experiment Station* **21**: 8–9.

Barnett J L, Cronin G M, Winfield C G (1981) The effects of individual and group penning of pigs on total and free plasma corticosteroids and the maximum corticosteroid binding capacity. *General and Comparative Endocrinology* **44**: 219–25.

Barnett J L, Hemsworth P H, Newman E A, McCallum T H, Winfield C G (1989) The effect of design of tether and stall housing on some behavioural and physiological responses related to the welfare of pregnant pigs. *Applied Animal Behaviour Science* **24**: 1–12.

Barnouin J (1980) Continuous eco-pathological surveillance of monitored herds of ruminants, I. Objectives and strategy; II. Coding system and data verification. *Ann. Rech. Vet.* **11**: 341–66.

Bassett J M, Hinks N T (1969) Microdetermination of corticosteroids in ovine peripheral plasma: effects of venepuncture, corticotrophin, insulin and glucose. *Journal of Endocrinology* **44**: 387–403.

Baxter M R (1989) Intensive housing: the last straw for pigs. *Journal of Animal Science* **67**: 2433–40.

Baxter M R, Schwaller C (1983) Space requirements for sows in confinement. In Baxter S H, Baxter M R, McCormack J A C (eds) *Farm animal housing and welfare*. Martinus Nijhoff, The Hague. pp 181–95.

Baxter S H (1984) *Intensive pig production: environmental management and design*. Granada Publishers, London.

Beaty B J, Carlson J O (1989) Nucleic acid hybridization: application to diagnosis of microbial infections and to genotype analysis. In Babink L A, Phillips J P, Moo-Young M (eds) *Animal biotechnology*. Pergamon Press, Oxford, pp 108–35.

Bee D (1986) Observations on lameness in a Hampshire, U.K. practice. In Weaver A D (ed) *Proceedings 5th International Symposium on Disorders of the Ruminant Digit*. University of Missouri-Columbia, Columbia, MO, 65211 USA.

Bendixen P H, Vilson B, Ekesbo I, Åstrand D B (1986a) Disease frequencies of tied zero-grazing dairy cows and of dairy cows on pasture during summer and tied during winter. *Preventive Veterinary Medicine* **4**: 291–306.

Bendixen P H, Vilson B, Ekesbo I, Åstrand D B (1986b) Disease frequencies in Swedish dairy cows. I. Dystokia. *Preventive Veterinary Medicine* **4**: 307–16.

Bendixen P H, Vilson B, Ekesbo I, Åstrand D B (1988a) Disease frequencies in dairy cows in Sweden. III. Parturient paresis. *Preventive Veterinary Medicine* **5**: 87–97.

Bendixen P H, Vilson B, Ekesbo I, Åstrand D B (1988b) Disease frequencies in dairy cows in Sweden. V. Mastitis. *Preventive Veterinary Medicine* **5**: 263–74.

Bengtsson G, Ekesbo I, Jacobsson S O (1967) Ett presumtivt fall av gödselgasförgiftning. *Svensk Veterinär Tidning* **17**: 248–54.

Bennett C (1991) BVA Animal Welfare Foundation. The profession's own charity. *Veterinary Record* **128**(17): 394.

Berkenbosch F, van Oers J, del Rey A,

Tilders F, Besedovsky H (1987) Corticotrophin releasing factor-producing neurons in the rat activated by interleukin-1. *Science* **238**: 524–6.

Besedovsky H, del Rey A, Sorkin E, Dinarello C A (1986) Immunoregulatory feedback between interleukin-1 and glucocorticoid hormones. *Science* **233**: 652–4.

Beuving G (1983) Corticosteroids in welfare. Research of laying hens. In Smidt D (ed) *Indicators relevant of farm animal welfare*. Martinus Nijhoff, Boston, pp 47–53.

Blackshaw J K (1981) Some behavioural deviations in weaned domestic pigs: persistent inguinal nose thrusting and tail and ear biting. *Animal Production* **33**: 325–32.

Blancou J (1990) Utilisation and control of biotechnological procedures in veterinary science. *Rev. sci, tech. Off. int. Epiz.*, **9**(3): 641–59.

Blaxter K L (1979) The limits to animal production. *Veterinary Record* **105**: 5–9.

Blood D C, Radostits O M (1989) *Veterinay medicine*, 7th edn. Baillière Tindall, London.

Blood D C, Studdert V P (1988) *Ballière's Comprehensive Veterinary Dictionary*. Ballière Tindall, London, p 265.

Blood D C, Morris R S, Williamson N B, Cannon C M, Cannon R M (1978) A health programme for dairy herds 1. objectives and methods. *Australian Veterinary Journal* **54**: 207–15.

Blowey R W (1975) A practical application of metabolic profiles. *Veterinary Record* **97**: 324–7.

Blowey R W (1985) *A veterinary book for dairy farmers*. Farming Press, Ipswich.

Blowey R W, Sharp M W (1989) Digital dermatitis in dairy cattle. *Veterinary Record* **122**: 505–8.

Boissy A, Bouissou M F (1988) Effect of early handling on heifer's subsequent reactivity to humans and to unfamiliar situations. *Applied Animal Behaviour Science* **20**: 259–73.

Booman P (1988) Application of monoclonal antibodies in animal production: A review. *Livestock Production Science* **18**: 199–215.

Booman P, Tieman M, Wiel D F M van de, Schakenraad J M, Koops W (1984) Production and characterisation of anti-progesterone monoclonal antibodies for pregnancy diagnosis in cattle. In Houwink E M, Meer R R van der (eds) *Innovations in biotechnology*. Elsevier, Amsterdam, pp 259–66.

Booman P, Tieman M, Zaane D van, Bosma A A, Boer G F de (1990) Construction of a bovine murine heteromyeloma cell line; production of bovine monoclonal antibodies against rotavirus and pregnant mare serum gonadotrophine. *Veterinary Immunopathology* **24**: 211–26.

Booman P, Kruijt L, Veerhuis R, Hengst A M, Tieman M, Ruch F E (1989) Sexing bovine embryos with monoclonal antibodies against the H-Y antigen. *Livestock Production Science* **23**: 1–16.

Booth J M (1988) Progress in controlling mastitis in England and Wales. *Veterinary Record* **122**: 299–302

Boucquè Ch V, Fiens L O, Sommer M, Cottyn B G, Buysse F X (1987) Effects of the beta agonist cimaterol on growth, feed efficiency and carcass quality of finishing Belgian white-blue beefbulls. In Hanrahan J P (ed) *Beta agonists and their effect on animal growth and carcass quality*. Elsevier Applied Science Publishers, pp 93–106.

Boxberger J (1983) Wichtige verhaltensparameter von kuehen als grundlagen zur verbesserung der stalleinrichtung habilitation. *Technische Universität München-Weihenstephan*.

Boyce J R (1990) Animal Welfare Committee looks at animal rights. *Journal of the American Veterinary Medical Association* **196**(1): 17–18.

Boyne R, Arthur J R (1979) Alterations of neutrophil fraction in selenium deficient cattle. *Journal of Comparative Pathology* **89**: 151–8.

Brambell F W R (1965) *Report of the technical committee to enquire into the welfare of animals kept under intensive livestock husbandry systems*. (Cmd.

2836). H.M. Stationery Office, London.

Brantas G C (1980) The pre-laying behaviour of laying hens in cages with or without laying nests. In Moss R (ed) *The laying hen and its environment*. Martinus Nijhoff, The Hague, pp 227–34.

Breazile J E (1988) The physiology of stress and its relationship to mechanisms of disease and therapeutics. *Veterinary Clinics of North America: Food Animal Practice* 4: 441–80.

Bremel R D, Gangwer M I (1978) Effect of adrenocorticotrophin injection and stress on milk cortisol content. *Journal of Dairy Science* 61: 1103–8.

Boddie G F (1946) *Veterinary diagnosis*, 2nd edn., Oliver & Boyd.

Broom D M (1983) Stereotypies as animal welfare indicators. In Schmidt D (ed) *Indicators relevant to farm animal welfare*. Martinus Nijhoff, The Hague, pp 81–7.

Broom D M (1986) Indicators of poor welfare. *British Veterinary Journal* 142: 524.

Broom D M (1988) The scientific assessment of animal welfare. *Applied Animal Behaviour Science* 20: 5–19.

Brown F, Bomford R H (1989) Synthetic peptides in animal health. In Babiuk L J, Phillips J P, Moo-Young M (eds) *Animal Biotechnology*. Pergamon, Oxford, pp 1–19.

Bruce J M (1979) Heat loss from animals to floors. *Farm Buildings Progress* 55: 1–4.

Buré R G (1987) New concepts in the rearing of piglets after conventional suckling periods. In Marx D, Grauvolg A, Schmidt D (eds) *Welfare aspects of pig rearing* European Communities Publications 10776, Luxembourg, pp 34–42.

Bush I E (1957) The physio-chemical state of cortisol in blood. *CIBA Foundation Colloquia on Endocrinology* 11: 263–85.

Bush I E, Ferguson K A (1953) The secretion of the adrenal cortex in the sheep. *Journal of Endocrinology* 10: 1–8.

Campbell I L, Davey A W F, McDowall F H, Wilson G F, Munford R E (1964) The effect of adrenocorticotrophic hormone on the yield, composition and butterfat properties of cow's milk. *Journal of Dairy Research* 31: 71–9.

Canadian Federation of Humane Societies (1988) *Surface livestock transportation in Canada: A survey*. CFHS, Suite 102-30 Concourse Gate, Nepean, Ontario, Canada K2E 7V7.

Cannon W B (1935) Stresses and strain of homeostasis. *American Journal of Medical Science* 189: 1–14.

Cantley M F (1988) Biotechnology, competitiveness and acceptability: the challenge to Europe. In Wal P van der, Nieuwland S J, Politiek R D (eds) *Biotechnology for control of growth and product quality in swine. Implications and acceptability*. Pudoc, Wageningen, pp 5–11.

Cantley M F (1990) Regulatory aspects of biotechnology in Europe, with particular reference to veterinary science. In Blancou J (ed) *Rev. sci. tech. Off. int. Epiz.*. 9(3): 695–713.

Cariolet R, Dantzer R (1984) Motor activity of tethered sows during pregnancy. *Annales Recherches Vétérinaires* 15: 257–60.

Carpenter E (1980) *Animals and ethics*. Watkins, London.

Carter P D, Johnston N E, Corner L A, Jarrett R G (1983) Observations on the effect of electroimmobilisation on the dehorning of cattle. *Australian Veterinary Journal* 60: 17–19.

Cermak J P (1987) *Proceedings of the BCVA meeting held in London* pp 173–82.

Clarkson, Faull (1990) *Handbook for the sheep clinician*. Liverpool University Press.

Clason A, Everitt B (1986) Ekonomiska förluster vid mastit. *SHS-material Juverinflammationer och deras bekämpande, Eskilstuna*.

Clemens E T, Schultz B O, Brumm M C, Jesse G W, Mayes H F (1986) Influence of market stress and protein level on feeder pig hematologic and blood chemical values. *American Journal of Veterinary Research* **47**: 359–62.

Clifton M (1990) Out of the cage. The movement in transition. *The Animals' Agenda* **10**(1): 26–30.

Codes of Recommendations for the Welfare of Livestock (1968) Miscellaneous Revisions Act 1 Part 1, Ministry of Agriculture, Fisheries and Food, Surbiton, Surrey. (updated between 1983–87).

Colam-Ainsworth P, Lunn G A, Thomas R C, Eddy R G (1989) Behaviour of cows in cubicles and its possible relationship with laminitis in replacement dairy heifers. *Veterinary Record* **125**: 573–5.

Collick D W, Ward W R, Dobson H (1989) Associations between types of lameness and fertility in dairy cows. *Veterinary Record* **125**: 103–6.

Collins M, Algers B (1984) *The effects of stable dust on farm animals*. Swedish University of Agricultural Science Department of Animal Hygiene, Report 12. Skara, Sweden, 21 pp.

Council of Europe (1976) *No. 87: European Convention for the Protection of Animals kept for farming purposes*, Strasbourg.

Cowley G, Hager M, Drew L, Namuth T, Wright L, Murr A, et al. (1988) Of pain and progress. *Newsweek*, 26 December, pp 50–9.

Crestani F (1990) Effets comportementaux de l'endotoxine et de l'interleukine-1 chez le rat et la souris—Bases cellulaires. *Doctoral Neurosciences*, Université de Bordeaux II.

Cronin G M (1985) The development and significance of abnormal stereotyped behaviors of tethered sows. PhD Thesis, University of Wageningen, The Netherlands.

Cronin G M, Wiepkema P R (1984) An analysis of stereotyped behaviours in tethered sows. *Annales Recherches Vétérinaires* **15**: 263–71.

Cronin G M, Tartwijk J M F, van der Hel W, Verstegen M W (1985) The influence of degree of adaptation to tether-housing by sows in relation to

behaviour and energy metabolism. *Animal Production* **42**: 257–68.

Cumming B G (1986) Human and animal rights. *Policy Options Politiques*, September, pp 19–23.

Curtis S E (1983) *Environmental management in animal agriculture*. Iowa State University Press, Iowa.

Curtis S E (1987) A case for intensive farming of food animals. In Fox M W, Mickley L D (eds) *Advances in animal welfare 1986/1987*. Martinus Nijhoff, Boston/Dordrecht/Lancaster, pp 245–56.

Curtis S E (1989) Guidelines for agricultural animals in science and animals. Addressing contemporary issues. In Guttman H E, Mench J A, Simmons R C (eds) *Proceedings of a Scientists Center for Animal Welfare symposium, June 22–25, 1988, Washington, DC*. Scientists Center for Animal Welfare, 4805 St. Elmo Avenue, Bethesda, MD 20814.

Curtis S E, Hurst R J, Gonyou H W, Jensen A H, Muehling A J (1989) The physical space requirement of the sow. *Journal of Animal Science* **67**: 1242–9.

CVMA Human Practices/Animal Welfare Committee (1991) A review and steps forward. *Canadian Veterinary Journal* **32**: 273–6.

Dantzer R (1986) Behavioral, physiological and functional aspects of stereotyped behavior: a review and a re-interpretation. *Journal of Animal Science* **62**: 1776–86.

Dantzer R, Kelley K W (1989) Stress and immunity: an integrated view of relationships between the brain and the immune system. *Life Sciences* **44**: 1995–2008.

Dantzer R, Mormède P (1983a) De-arousal properties of stereotyped behaviour: evidence from pituitary-adrenal correlates in pigs. *Applied Animal Ethology* **10**: 233–44.

Dantzer R, Mormède P (1983b) Stress in farm animals: a need for reevaluation. *Journal of Animal Science* **57**: 6–18.

Dantzer R, Mormède P (1985) Stress in domestic animals: A psychoneuroendocrine approach. In Moberg G P (ed) *Animal Stress*. American Physiological Society, Bethesda, pp 81–95.

Dantzer R, Arnone M, Mormède P (1984) Effects of frustration on behaviour and plasma corticosteroid levels in pigs. *Physiology and Behaviour* 24: 1–4.

Dantzer R, Bluthé R M, Tazi A (1986) Stress-induced analgesia in pigs. *Annales Recherches Vétérinaires* 17: 147–51.

Dantzer R, Mormède P, Bluthe R M, Soissons J (1983a) The effect of different housing conditions on behavioural and adrenocortical reactions in veal calves. *Reproduction and Nutrition Development* 23: 501–10.

Dantzer R, Mormède P, Henry J P (1983b) Significance of physiological criteria in assessing animal welfare. In Schmidt D, (ed) *Indicators relevant to farm animal welfare*, Martinus Nijhoff, Boston pp 29–37.

Dantzer R, Mormède P, Henry J P (1983c) Physiological assessment of adaptation in farm animals. In Baxter S H, Baxter M R, MacCormack J A C (eds) *Farm animal housing and welfare*. Martinus Nijhoff, The Hague, pp 8–20.

Dargie J D (1989) Helping small farmers to improve their livestock. *IAEA Yearbook 1989*, IAEA, Vienna, pp B 35–B 55.

Davies C P (1991) Deposition and clearance of inhaled particles of different size in calves of two ages. *Journal of Aerosol Science* (in press).

Dawkins M S (1980) *Animal suffering. The science of animal welfare*. Chapman and Hall, London.

Dawkins M S (1983a) *Animal Behaviour* 11: 1199–205.

Dawkins M S (1983b) Battery hens name their price: consumer demand theory and the measurement of animal needs. *Animal Behaviour* 31: 1195–205.

Dawkins M S (1990) From an animal's point of view: consumer demand theory and animal welfare. *Behavioural Brain Science* (in press).

De Koning R (1984) Injuries in confined sows—incidence and relation with behaviour. *Annales Recherches Vétérinaires* 15: 205–14.

Demeyer D, Verbeke R, Voorde G van de, Fabry J, Roover E de, Dalrymple R H (1989) In Wal P van der, Nieuwland G J, Politiek R D (eds) *Biotechnology for control of growth and product quality in swine. Implications and acceptability*. Pudoc, Wageningen, pp 191–201.

De Silva M, Kiehm D J, Kaltenbach C C, Dunn T G (1986) Comparison of serum cortisol and prolactin in sheep sampled by two methods. *Domestic Animal Endocrinology* 3: 11–16.

Deviche P (1985) Behavioral response to apomorphine and its interaction with opiates in domestic pigeons. *Pharmacology Biochemistry and Behaviour* 22: 209–14.

De Wilt J (1985) Behaviour and welfare of veal calves in relation to husbandry system. PhD thesis, University of Wagneningen, The Netherlands.

Dickinson L (1989) *Victims of vanity*. Summerhill Press, Toronto.

Diesch S (1988) Development and application of animal health information systems. In Ekesbo I (ed) *Environment and Health. Proceedings of the 6th International Congress on Animal Hygiene, 14–17 June 1988, Skara, Sweden*, pp 185–9.

Dobson H (1983) *A radio-immunoassay laboratory handbook*. Liverpool University Press, Liverpool.

Dohoo I R, Martin S W (1984) Disease, production and culling in Holstein-Friesian cows. *Preventive Veterinary Medicine* 2: 655–90.

Donaldson A I (1978) Factors influencing the dispersal, survival and deposition of airborne pathogens of farm animals. *Veterinary Bulletin* 48: 83–94.

Done-Currie J R, Hecker J F, Wodzicka-Tomaszewka M (1984) Behaviour of sheep transferred from pasture to an animal house. *Applied Animal Behaviour Science* 20: 121–30.

Drew B (1980) The effect of progesterone treatment on the fertility of dairy cows. Paper presented to the European

Association of Animal Production, 1–4 September 1980.

Drexler M (1991) Let them eat grain. *Boston Globe Sunday Magazine*, July 14.

Droke E A, Loerch S C (1989) Effects of parenteral selenium and vitamin E on performance, health and humoral immune response of steers new to the feedlot environment. *Journal of Animal Science* **67**: 1350–9.

Dryden A L, Seabrook M F (1986) An investigation into some components of the behaviour of the pigstockman and their influence on pig performance and behaviour. *Journal of Agricultural Manpower Society* **1**: 44–52.

Ducrot Ch, Arnould B, Berthelon Ch, Calavas D (1988) Obviousness of the factors of risk of the lambs perinatal mortality from a survey made on 92 ovine farms in the south east of France. In Ekesbo I (ed) *Environment and Health. Proceedings of the 6th International Congress on Animal Hygiene, 14–17 June 1988, Skara, Sweden*, pp 147–51.

Duff S R I (1988) Abnormalities in the axial skeleton of the broiler breeding fowl. *Avian Pathology* **17**: 239–58.

Duncan I J H (1975) *Deutsche Geflugal wirkschaft und Schweine Production* **33**: 815.

Duncan I J H (1978a) The interpretation of preference tests in animal behaviour. *Applied Animal Ethology* **4**: 197–200.

Duncan I J H (1978b) *First Danish Seminar on Poultry Welfare in Egg Laying Cages*. The National Committee for Poultry and Eggs, pp 81–8.

Duncan I J H, Dawkins M S (1983) The problem of assessing 'well-being' and 'suffering' in farm animals. In Smidt D (ed) *Indicators relevant to farm animal welfare*, Marinus Nyholt, 14.

Duncan I J H, Filshie J H (1979) The use of radio telemetry devices to measure temperature and heart rate in domestic fowl. In Amlaner C J, Macdonald D W (eds) *A Handbook of Biotelemetry and Radio Tracking*. Pergamon Press, Oxford, pp 579–88.

Duncan I J H, Wood-Gush D G M (1972) Thwarting of feeding behaviour in the domestic fowl. *Animal Behaviour* **20**: 444–51.

Duquette P F, Rickes E L, Dison G, Hedrick A B, Capozzi F P, Convey E M (1987) L 644,696 improves growth and carcass composition of lambs. In Hanrahan J P (ed) *Beta-agonists and their effects on animal growth and carcass quality*. Elsevier, London/New York, pp 119–27.

Dvorak M (1968) The effect of traumatic stress on the leukocyte blood picture in the course of the postnatal development of piglets. *Acta University Agriculture Brno* **37**: 537–44.

Ebert K M (1989) Gene transfer through embryo micro infection. In Babiuk L A, Phillips J P, Moo-Young M (eds) *Animal biotechnology*. Pergamon, Oxford, pp 233–51.

Eddy R G (1978) Use of the prostaglandin analogue cloprostenol for oestrus synchronization in dairy herds with seasonal calving patterns. *Proceedings of XII World Congress of Buiatrics, Mexico City, 1978*.

Eddy R G (1980) Analysing dairy herd fertility. *In Practice* **2**: 25–7.

Eddy R G (1981) The application and some economic implications of a fertility control programme in dairy herds. Thesis for FRCVS.

Eddy R G (1982a) Marketing of a herd recording scheme to farmer clients. *Proceedings of XII World Congress on Cattle Diseases, Amsterdam*, pp 633–6.

Eddy R G (1982b) Dealing with errors in computerized dairy herd recording. *Proceedings of the XII World Congress on Cattle Diseases, Amsterdam*.

Eddy R G, Clark P J (1987) Oestrus prediction in dairy cows using an ELISA progesterone test. *Veterinary Record* **120**: 31–4.

Eddy R G, Esslemont R J (1973) A computer based recording scheme for health in dairy cows. In Grunsell, Wright (eds) *The Veterinary Annual No. 14*. Wright, Bristol, pp 32–7.

Edmondson P W (1989) An economic

justification of 'Blitz' therapy to eradicate *Streptococcus agalactia* from a dairy herd. *Veterinary Record* **125**: 591–3.

Edwards S A, Riley J E (1986) The application of the electronic identification and computerized feed dispensing system in dry sow housing. *Pigs News and Information* **7**: 295–8.

Eilers C (1983) What sort of person reads Agenda? Responses to our reader survey. *The Animals' Agenda*, May/June, pp 26–7, 38.

Eisner R (1991) Technological breakthrough form the basis of biotech's new ware. *The Scientist* **5**(19): 4–9.

Ekesbo I (1966) Disease incidence in tied and loose housed dairy cattle and causes of this incidence variation with particular reference to the cowshed type. Thesis. Acta Ag. Scand. Suppl. 15, 74 pp.

Ekesbo I (1973) Animal health, behaviour and disease prevention in different environments in modern Swedish animal husbandry. *Veterinary Record* **93**: 36–40.

Ekesbo I (1983) Ethical problems in keeping and breeding farm animals. In Berg K, Trangøyke K E (ed) *Research Ethics*. New York, A R Liss, pp 167–83.

Ekesbo I (1984) Methoden der Beurteilung von Umwelteinflussen auf Nutztiere unter besonderer Berucksichtigung der Tiergesundheit und des Tierschutzes. *Wiener Tierärztliche Monatsschrift* **71**: 186–90.

Ekesbo I (1988) Health and welfare of farm animals and their impact on the livestock industry. In (ed) *Proceedings VI World Conference on Animal Production, July 1988, Helsinki*, pp 102–11.

Ekesbo I, Nilsson J, Oltenacu P A (1991) A disease recording programme for dairy herds. *Proceedings 7th International Congress on Animal Hygiene, August 1991, Leipzig*, pp 14–19.

Ellersieck M R, Veum T L, Durham T L, McVickers W R, McWilliams S N, Lasley J F (1979) Response of stress susceptible and stress resistant Hampshire pigs to electrical stress. II.

Effects on blood levels and blood minerals. *Journal of Animal Science* **48**: 453–8.

Emmans G C, Charles D R (1977) Climatic environment and poultry feeding in practice. In Haresign W, Swan H (eds) *Nutrition and the climatic environment*. Butterworths, London, pp 31–50.

Eskew M L, Scholz R W, Reddy C C, Todhunter D A, Zarkower A (1985) Effects of vitamin E and selenium deficiencies on rat immune function. *Immunology* **54**: 173–80.

Esslemont R J (1973) *A study of the economic and husbandry aspects of the manifestation and detection of oestrus in large dairy herds*. PhD Thesis, University of Reading.

Esslemont R J, Eddy R G, Ellis P R (1977) Planned breeding in autumn calving dairy herds. *Veterinary Record* **100**: 426–7.

Eurogroup for Animal Welfare (1988) *Analysis of major areas of concern for animal welfare in Europe* Eurogroup for Animal Welfare, Brussels.

European Commission (1985) *Abnormal Behaviour in Farm Animals*

FAO *Animal Health Yearbook (FAO-WHO-OIE)*. UN Food and Agriculture Organization, Rome.

Farm Animal Welfare Advisory Committee (1970) *Report on effect of welfare codes of practice*. Ministry of Agriculture, Fisheries and Food, Surbiton, Surrey.

Farm Animal Welfare Council *Welfare Codes of Practice*. Ministry of Agriculture, Fisheries and Food, Surbiton, Surrey.

Farm Animal Welfare Council (1990) *Report of the enforcement working group*. Ministry of Agriculture, Fisheries and Food, Publ. no. PB0124. Surbiton, Surrey, England KT6 7NF.

Farmer R W, Pierce C E (1974) Plasma cortisol determination: radioimmunoassay and competitive protein binding compared. *Clinical Chemistry* **20**: 411–14.

Faye B, Fayet J C, Barnouin J, Bro-

chart M (1988) Pathological associations in dairy farms. Individual and herd data. In Ekesbo I (ed) *Environment and Health. Proceedings of the 6th International Congress on Animal Hygiene, 14–17 June 1988, Skara, Sweden*, pp 35–45.

Fell L R, Shutt D A, Bentley C J (1985) Development of a salivary cortisol method for detecting changes in plasma 'free' cortisol arising from acute stress in sheep. *Australian Veterinary Journal* 62: 403–6.

Forbes J M (1986) *The voluntary food intake of farm animals.* Butterworths, London.

Ford E J H, Robinson I P, Evans J (1990) An enzyme-linked immunoassay for the measurement of the concentration of cortisol in sheep plasma. *Research in Veterinary Science* 48: 262–3.

Fox L, Butler W R, Everett R W, Natzke R P (1981) Effect of adrenocorticotrophin on milk and plasma cortisol and prolactin concentrations. *Journal of Dairy Science* 64: 1794–800.

Fox M (1988) Genetic engineering biotechnology: animal welfare and environmental concerns. *Applied Animal Behaviour Science* 20: 83–94.

Frankena K, Noordhuizen J P, Villeberg P, van Voorthuysen P F, Goelema J O (1990) Episcope: computer programs in veterinary epidemiology. *Veterinary Record* 126: 573–6.

Frankenhuis M T, Nabuurs M J A, Bool P H (1989) Veterinary care and worries and intensive animal husbandry (Dutch). *Tijdschrift voor Diergeneeskund* 114(24): 1237–48.

Fraser A F (1989) Welfare and well-being (letter). *Veterinary Record* 125(12): 332.

Fraser A F, Broom D M (1990) *Farm animal behaviour and welfare*, 3rd edn. Baillière Tindall, London.

Fraser D (1975) The effect of straw on the behaviour of sows in tether stalls. *Animal Production* 21: 59–68.

Fraser D (1978) Observations on the behavioural development of suckling and early weaned piglets during the first six weeks after birth. *Animal Behaviour* 26: 22–30.

Fraser D (1987a) Attraction to blood as a factor in tail-biting by pigs. *Applied Animal Behaviour Science* 17: 61–8.

Fraser D (1987b) Mineral-deficient diets and the pig's attraction to blood: implications for tail-biting. *Canadian Journal of Animal Science* 67: 909–18.

Fraser D, Phillips P A, Thompson B K (1986) A test of a free access two-level for fattening pigs. *Animal Production* 42: 269–74.

French R D (1975) *Antivivisection and medical science in Victorian society.* Princeton University Press, Princeton, NJ.

Friend T H, Gwazdauskas F C, Polan C E (1978) Change in adrenal response from free stall competition. *Journal of Dairy Science* 62: 768–71.

Fry J P, Sharman D P, Stephens D B (1981) Cerebral dopamine apomorphine and oral activity in the neonatal pig. *Journal of Veterinary Pharmacology Therapy* 4: 193–207.

Fuller M F (1987) Methods of protein evaluation for non-ruminants. In Ørskov E R (ed) *Feed science.* Elsevier, Amsterdam, pp 81–101.

Funtowicz S, Ravetz J (1990). Postnormal science: A new science for new times. *Scientific European* October, pp 20–3.

Garry R C, Passmore R, Warnock G M, Durnin J (1955) *Studies on expenditure of energy and consumption of food by miners and clerks, Fife, Scotland (1952).* Medical Research Council Special Report No. 289. MRC, London.

Gibbs D M (1984) Dissociation of oxytocin, vasopressin and corticotrophin secretion during different types of stress. *Life Sciences* 35: 489–91.

Gilmour M I, Taylor F G R, Wathes C M (1989) Pulmonary clearance of *Pasteurella haemolytica* and immune responses in mice following exposure to titanium dioxide. *Environmental Research* 50: 184–94.

Glosser J W, Gorham J R (1990) Regulation of biotechnology in the United

States and Canada. In Blancou J (ed). *Rev. Sci, tech. Off. int. Epiz.*, **9**(3): 681–94.

Gloster J, Sellars R F, Donaldson A I (1982) Long distance transport of foot and mouth disease virus over the sea. *Veterinary Record* **110:** 47–52.

Gogolin-Ewens K J, Meensen E N T, Scott P C, Adams T E, Brandon M R (1990) Genetic selection for disease resistance and traits of economic importance in animal production. In Blancou J (ed). *Rev. sci. tech. Off. int. Epiz.*, **9**(3): 865–96.

Gonyou H W, Hemsworth P H, Barnett J L (1986) Effects of frequent interactions with humans on growing pigs. *Applied Animal Behaviour Science* **16:** 269–78.

Goodger W J, Ruppanner R (1982) Why the dairy industry does not make greater use of veterinarians. *Journal of the American Veterinary Association* **181:** 706–10.

Gorewit R C (1981) Pituitary, thyroid and adrenal responses to clonidine in dairy cattle. *Journal of Endocrinological Investigation* **4:** 135–9.

Grandin T, Curtis S E, Tayor I A (1987) Toys, mingling and driving reduce excitability in pigs. *Journal of Animal Science* **65:** 230 (Abstract).

Greanville P, Moss D (1985) The emerging face of the movement. *The Animals' Agenda*, March/April, 10–11, 36.

Griffin D R (1976) *The question of animal awareness.* Rockefeller University Press, New York.

Grommers F J (1967) Dairy cattle housing health. *Thesis, Utrecht*, 124 pp.

Gross W B, Siegel H A (1983) Evaluation of the heterophil: lymphocyte ratio as a measure of stress in chickens. *Avian Disease* **27:** 972–9.

Grunsell C S G, Penny R H C, Wragg S R, Allcock J (1969) The practicability and economics of veterinary preventive medicine. *Veterinary Record* **84:** 26–41.

Hager M, Cowley G, Drew L, Namuth T, Wright L, Murr A, et al. (1988) Of pain and progress. *Newsweek*, December 26, pp 50–9.

Hanrahan J P (1987) *Beta-agonists and their effects on animal growth and carcass quality.* Elsevier, London/New York.

Hanrahan J P, Fitzsimons J M, McEwan J C, Allen P, Quirke J F (1987) Effects of the beta agonist cimaterol on growth, food efficiency and carcass quality in sheep. In Hanrahan J P (ed) *Beta-agonists and their effects on animal growth and carcass quality.* Elsevier, London/New York, pp 106–19.

Hargreaves A L, Hutson G D (1990) Some effects of repeated handling on stress responses in sheep. *Applied Animal Behaviour Science* **26:** 253–65.

Harrison R (1964) *Animal machines. The new factory farming industry.* Vincent Stuart, London.

Hart B L (1988) Biological basis of the behavior of sick animals. *Neuroscience and Biobehavioral Reviews* **12:** 123–37.

Harvey I (1990) Fur trade fights back. *Saturday Sun*, March 24, pp 28–9.

Hattingh J, Ganhao M, Kay G (1989) Blood constituent responses of cattle to herding. *Journal of the South African Veterinary Association* **60:** 219–20.

Hemsworth P H, Barnett J L (1987) The human-animal relationship and its importance in pig production. *Pig News and Information* **8:** 133–6.

Hemsworth P H, Brand A, Willems P (1981a) The behavioural response of sows to the presence of human beings and its relation to productivity. *Livestock Production Science* **8:** 67–74.

Hemsworth P H, Barnett J L, Hansen C (1981b) The influence of handling by humans on the behaviour, growth and corticosteroids in the juvenile female pig. *Hormones and Behavior* **15:** 396–403.

Hemsworth P H, Gonyou H W, Dziuk P J (1986a) Human communication with pigs: the behavioural response of pigs to specific human signals. *Applied Animal Behaviour Science* **15:** 45–54.

Hemsworth P H, Barnett J L, Hansen C, Gonyou H W (1986b) The influence of early contact with humans on subsequent behavioural response of pigs to humans. *Applied Animal Behaviour Science* 15: 55–63.

Hemsworth P H, Barnett J L, Hansen C (1986c) The influence of handling by humans on the behaviour, reproduction and corticosteroids of male and female pigs. *Applied Animal Behaviour Science* 15: 303–14.

Hemsworth P H, Barnett J L, Hansen C (1987) The influence of inconsistent handling by humans on the behaviour, growth and corticosteroids of young pigs. *Applied Animal Behaviour Science* 17: 245–52.

Hemsworth P H, Barnett J L, Coleman G J, Hansen C (1989) A study of the relationships between the attitudinal and behavioural profiles of stockpersons and the level of fear of humans and reproductive performance of commercial pigs. *Applied Animal Behaviour Science* 23: 301–14.

Hennichs K, Plym-Forshell K (1984) *Feeding barriers for tied dairy cows. An animal health evaluation*. Swedish University of Agricultural Science Department Hygiene, Report 11, Skara, Sweden, 56 pp.

Henshaw D (1989) *Animal warfare* Fontana-Collins, London.

Herd K M (1989) Serum cortisol and 'stress' in cattle. *Australian Veterinary Journal* 66: 341.

Hiatt H, Cafferkey R, Bowdish K (1989) Production of antibodies in transgenic plants. *Nature* 342: 76–8.

Hill J R, Sainsbury D W B (eds) (1990) *Farm animal welfare. Who cares? How?* Cambridge Centre for Animal Health and Welfare, Cambridge, UK.

Hillinger C, Stein M A (1989) Militant vegetarians tied to attacks on livestock industry. *The Boston Globe*, November 23.

Hindson J (1982) Sheep health schemes. *In Practice* 4: 53–8.

Hindson J (1989) Examination of the sheep flock before tupping. *In Practice* 11: 149–55.

Hodgson J (1990) When ethics and biotechnology collide. *Scientific European* (Supplement to *Scientific American*), April, pp 24–7.

Hoffmann B (1987) Introductory remarks in relation to beta-agonists and their effects on growth and carcass quality in farm animals. In Hanrahan J P (ed) *Beta-agonists and their effect on animal growth and carcass quality*. Elsevier, London/New York, pp 1–12.

Hofmann K (1987) The meat quality issue (Der Begriff Fleischqualitat. *Fleischwirtschaft* 67(1): 44–9.

Högsved O, Holtenius P (1968) *Proceedings V International Meeting Cattle Diseases*, Opatija, pp 1081–7.

Hollands C (1980) *Compassion is the bugler. The struggle for animal rights*. MacDonald, Edinburgh.

Hopwood D, Christie J (1986) *Marketing in agricultural practices*. University of Lancaster Press.

House of Commons Agricultural Committee Session 1979–80 Minutes of evidence, UK Agricultural Departments, Annex A p 80.

Howard C J, Stott E J, Thomas L H, Gourlay R N, Tayler G (1987) Protection against respiratory disease in calves induced by vaccines containing respiratory syncytial virus, parainfluenza 3 virus, *Mycoplasma bovis* and *M. dispar*. *Veterinary Record* 121: 372–6.

Hubbert W T, McCulloch W F, Schnurrenberger P R (eds) (1975) *Diseases transmitted from animals to man*, 6th edn. Charles C. Thomas, Springfield, IL.

Hughes B O (1982) Feather pecking and cannibalism in domestic fowls. In Bessei W (ed) *Disturbed behaviour in farm animals*. Verlag Eugen Ulmer, Stuttgart, pp 138–46.

Hunter E J, Broom D M, Edwards S A, Sibly R M (1988) Social hierarchy and feeder access in a group of 20 sows using a computer controlled feeder. *Animal Production* 47: 139–48.

Hurst L (1991) Humane society in another dogfight. *The Toronto Star*, July 14.

International Air Transport Association (1991) *IATA live animals regulations*, 18th edn. IATA, Montreal.

Jensen P (1980) An ethogram of social interactions patterns in group-housed dry sows. *Applied Animal Ethology* **6**: 341–50.

Jensen P (1982) An analysis of agonistic interactions patterns in group-housed dry sows, aggression regulation through an 'avoidance' order. *Applied Animal Ethology* **9**: 47–61.

Jensen P, Algers B, Ekesbo I (1986) Methods of sampling and analysis of data in farm animal ethology. *Tierhaltung, Band 17*. Birkhäuser Verlag, Basel, 86 pp.

Johnson S K, Johnson A R, Keefer C L, Silcox R W (1990) Blood constituents during the estrous cycle and early pregnancy in dairy cows. *Theriogenology* **34**: 701–7.

Jointex (1976) Preventive medicine in practice. *Veterinary Record* **98**: 349–50, 371.

Juskevich J C, Guyer C G (1990) Bovine growth hormone: human food safety evaluation. *Science* 249–4971, 875–84.

Kelly J M (1990) Why are cows culled? *Proceedings of the British Cattle Veterinary Association*. Glasgow.

Kelly J M, Whitaker D A, Smith E J (1988) A dairy herd health and productivity service. *British Veterinary Journal* **144**: 470–80.

Kelley R W (1980) Stress and immune function: A bibliographic review. *Annales Recherches Vétérinaires* **11**: 445–78.

Kempson S A, Currie R J W, Johnston A M (1989) Influence of biotin on pig claw horn: a scanning electron microscope study. *Veterinary Record* **124**: 37–40.

Kendrick K M, Keverne E B, Baldwin B A (1987) Intracerebroventricular oxytocin stimulates maternal behavior in sheep. *Neuroendocrinology* **46**: 56–61.

Kerr M G (1989) *Veterinary laboratory medicine: clinical biochemistry and maematology*. Blackwell Scientific Publications, Oxford, 270pp.

Kiley-Worthington M (1977) *Behavioural problems of farm animals*. Oriel Press, Stockfield.

King J W B, Menissier F (eds) (1980) *Muscle hypertrophy of genetic origin and its use to improve beef production*. CEC seminar. Martinus Nijhoff, The Hague.

Kirkwood J K, Webster A J F (1984) Energy budget strategies for growth in mammals and birds. *Animal Production* **38**: 147.

Kleiber M (1961) *The fire of life*. Wiley, New York.

Kluger M J (1979) *Fever—Its biology, evolution and function*. Princeton University Press, Princeton.

Kroo C J, Goldberg E H (1976) Detection of H-Y (male) antigen on 8-cell mouse embryos. *Science* **193**: 1134–5.

Krueger J M, Walter J, Dinarello C A, Wolff S M, Chedid L (1984) Sleep promoting effects of endogenous pyrogen (interleukin-1). *American Journal of Physiology* **246**: R994–R999.

Kyle R (1990) The downward spiral of cattle veterinary practice. *Veterinary Record* **127**: 465–7.

Ladewig J (1984) The effect of behavioural stress on the episodic release and circadian variation of cortisol in bulls. In Unshelm J, Van Putten G, Zeeb K (eds) *Proceedings of the International Congress of Applied Ethology in Farm Animals*. KTBL, Germany, pp 339–42.

Ladewig J, Ellendorff F (1983) The sleep-waking pattern and behaviour of pigs kept in different husbandry systems. In Smidt D (ed) *Indicators relevant to farm animal welfare*. Martinus Nijhoff, Boston, pp 55–65.

Laeyendecker L (1989) The pillars of Hercules passed by (Dutch): Sense problems in modern culture. In Adriaansens H F M (Dutch), Culemborg, Lemma, pp 55–83.

Lambooy E (ed) (1991) Automatic electronic identification systems for farm animals. *Report EUR 13198*, EN, Brussels, Luxembourg.

Lansbury C (1985) *The old brown dog. Women, workers and vivisection in Edwardian England*. University of Wisconsin Press, Madison.

Lawman M J P, Campos M, Bielfeldt Ohmann H, Griebel P, Babiuk L A (1989) Recombinant cytokines and their therapeutic value in veterinary medicine. In Babuik L J, Phillips J P, Moo-Young M (eds). *Animal Biotechnology*. Pergamon, Oxford, pp 63–106.

Lawrence A B, Appleby M C, Mac-Leod H A (1988) Measuring hunger in the pig using operant conditioning: the effect of food restriction. *Animal Production* 47: 131–8.

Leech F B, Vessey M P, Macrae W D, Lawson J R, Mackinnon D J, Morgan W J B (1964) *Brucellosis in the British dairy herd (1960/61)*. HMSO, London.

Leshner A I (1978) *An introduction to behavioural endocrinology*. Oxford University Press, Oxford.

Levy F, Poindron P (1987) The importance of amniotic fluids for the establishment of maternal behaviour in experienced and inexperienced ewes. *Animal Behaviour* 35: 1188–92.

Levy Guyer R, Koshland D E (1989) The molecule of the year. *Science* 246: 1543–4.

Lindqvist J-O (1974) Animal health environment in the production of fattening pigs. A study of disease incidence in relation to certain environmental factors, daily weight gain and carcass classification. *Acta Veterinary Scandinavica* (Suppl.) 51: 1–78.

Loew F M (1990) Animal welfare. A voice of one's own. *Veterinary Economics*, May, p 104.

Looker D (1991) Animal rights ad irks meat producers. *Des Moines Register*, August 9, p 1A.

Lyon M, Robbins T (1975) The action of central nervous system stimulant drugs: a general theory concerning amphetamine effects. In Essman W, Valzell L (eds) *Current developments in psychopharmacology*. Spectrum, New York, pp 81–163.

McCarthy D O, Kluger M J, Vander A J (1985) Suppression of food intake during infection: is interleukin-1 involved? *American Journal of Clinical Nutrition* 42: 1179–82.

McCarthy D O, Kluger M J, Vander A J (1986) Effect of centrally administrated interleukin-1 and endotoxin on food intake of fasted rats. *Physiology and Behavior* 36: 745–9.

McDonald P, Edwards R A, Greenhalgh J F D (1988) *Animal Nutrition*, 4th edn. Oliver & Boyd, Edinburgh.

McFarlane J M, Curtis S E (1989) Multiple concurrent stresses in chicks. 3. Effects on plasma corticosterone and the heterophil:lymphocyte ratio. *Poultry Science* 68: 522–7.

McFarlane J M, Boe K E, Curtis S E (1988) Turning and walking by mated gilts in modified gestation crates. *Journal of Animal Science* 66: 326–33.

McGlone J J (1985a) Aerolized androstenone reduces pig aggressive and submissive behavior. *Texas Technic University Swine Report*.

McGlone J J (1985b) Olfactory cues and pig agonistic behavior: evidence for a submissive pheromone. *Physiology and Behavior* 34: 195–8.

McGlone J J (1986) Influence of resources on pig aggression and dominance. *Behavioural Processes* 12: 135–45.

McGlone J J, Curtis S E (1985) Behavior and performance of weanling pigs in pens equipped with hide areas. *Journal of Animal Science* 60: 20–4.

McLaren D G, Bechtel P J, Grebner G L, Novakofski J, McKeith F K, Jones R W, et al. (1990) Dose response in growth in pigs infected daily with porcine somatotrophin from 57 to 103 kilograms. *Journal of Animal Science* 68(3): 640–50.

Machlin L J, Horins M, Hertelendy F, Kipnis D M (1968) Plasma growth hormone and insulin levels in the pig. *Endocrinology* 82: 369–76.

MAFF (1978) Condition scoring of dairy cows. Leaflet G12. HMSO, London.

MAFF (1979) Pig health and production recording. Booklet no. 2075, HMSO, London.

MAFF (1982) Rearing autumn born Friesian dairy heifers. Booklet no. 2379, HMSO, London.

MAFF (1983) Brucellosis—a history of the disease and its eradication from cattle in Great Britain. HMSO, London.

MAFF (1984) Dairy herd fertility and reproductive terms and definitions. Booklet no. 2476, HMSO, London.

Magel C R (1989) *Keyguide to information sources in animal rights.* Mansell, London; McFarland, Jefferson, North Carolina.

Malcolm C (1991) Animal research: Views are changing. *Santa Barbara News-Press*, January 29.

Mardsen D, Wood-Gush D G M (1986) A note on the behaviour of individually-penned sheep regarding their use for research purposes. *Animal Production* **42**: 157–9.

Martin S W, Meek A H, Davis D G, Johnson J A, Curtis R A (1981) Factors associated with morbidity and mortality in feedlot calves. The Bruce County Beef Project, Year Two. *Canadian Journal of Comparative Medicine* **45**: 103–12.

Marx D, Schuster H (1980) Ethologische wahlversuche mit früabgesetzten ferkeln wärend der flatdeckhaltung. I—Mitteilung: Ergebnisse des ersten abschnitts der untersuchungen zur tiergerechten fussbodengeshaltung. *Deutsche Tierärtzliche Wochenschrift* **87**: 369–75.

Marx D, Schuster H (1982) Ethologische wahlversuche mit frühabgesetzten ferkeln während der flatdeckhaltung. II—Mitteilung: Ergebnisse des zweiten abschnitts der untersuchungen zur tiergerechten fussbodengeshaltung. *Deutsche Tierärtztliche Wochenschrift* **89**: 313–18.

Mathison G W (1984) *B-vitamins and related compounds in ruminant nutrition.* Hoffman La Roche, Basle, Switzerland.

Matter F (1989) Die Enstreuproblematik in der Legehennenhaltung aus hygienischer Sicht *Schlussbericht zum Forschungsprojekt 014.86.4 Sept. 1989 Schweizerische Geflügelschule.*

Mayer H K, Lefcourt A M (1987) Failure of cortisol injected prior to milking to inhibit milk ejection in dairy cattle. *Journal of Dairy Research* **54**: 173–7.

Maylin G A, Rubin D S, Lon D H (1980) Selenium and vitamin E in horses. *Cornell Veterinarian* **70**: 272–89.

Maynard L A, Loosli J K (1979) *Animal Nutrition*, 7th edn. McGraw-Hill, New York.

Medawar P (1984) *The limits of science.* Oxford University Press.

Menissier F, Foulley J L (1979) *Current Topics in Veterinary Medicine* **4**: 30–87.

Mepham T B (1988) Criteria for the public acceptability of biotechnological innovations in animal production. In Heap R B, Prosser C G, Lamming G A (eds) *Biotechnology in growth regulation. Symposium, September 18–20, Institute of Animal Physiology, Babraham, U.K.*

Metz J H M (1987) The response of farm animals to humans. In Seabrooks F M (ed) *The role of the stockman in livestock production and management.* European Communities Publications 10982, Luxembourg, pp 23–39.

Meunier-Salaün M C, Vantrimponte M N, Raab A, Dantzer R (1987) Effect of floor area restriction upon performance, behaviour and physiology of growing finishing pigs. *Journal of Animal Science* **64**: 1371–7.

Mickley L D, Fox M W (1987) The case against intensive farming of food animals. In Fox M W, Mickley L D (eds) *Advances in animal welfare 1986/1987.* Martinus Nijhoff, Boston/Dordrecht/Lancaster, pp 257–72.

Miller W M, Harkness J W, Richard M S, Pritchard D G (1980) *Research in Veterinary Science* **28**: 267–74.

Millis N F (1990) Biotechnology in veterinary science: regulations in Asia and Oceania. In Blancou J (ed). *Rev. sci. tech. Off. int. Eniz.*, 9(3): 715–32.

Mitchell G, Hattingh J, Ganhao M F (1988) Stress in cattle assessed after handling, after transport and after slaughter. *Veterinary Record* **123**: 201–5.

Moloney P (1991) Hudson's Bay ending

321 years of fur sales. *The Toronto Star*, January 31, p A2.

Monteith J, Mount L E (1974) *Heat loss from animals and man*. Butterworths, London.

Mormède P, Dantzer R (1978) Pituitary-adrenal influences on avoidance behaviour of pigs. *Hormones and Behavior* 10: 285–97.

Mormède P, Bluthé R M, Dantzer R (1983) Neuroendocrine strategies for assessing welfare: application to calf management systems. In Schmidt D (ed) *Indicators relevant to farm animal welfare*. Martinus Nijhoff, The Hague, pp 39–46.

Mormède P, Dantzer R, Bluthé R M, Caritez J C (1984) Differences in adaptive abilities of three breeds of Chinese pigs. Behavioural and neuroendocrine reactions. *Genetic Selection and Evaluation* 16: 85–102.

Morris R S, Williamson N B, Blood D C, Cannon R M, Cannon C M (1978) A health programme for dairy herds. 3. Changes in reproductive performance. *Australian Veterinary Journal* 54: 231–46.

Morris R S, Blood D C, Williamson N B, Cannon C M, Cannon R M (1978) A health programme for dairy herds. 4. Changes in mastitis prevalence. *Australian Veterinary Journal* 54: 247–51.

Morrison W D, MacMillan I, Bate L A, Otten L (1986) Behavioural observations and operant procedures using microwaves as a heat source for young chicks. *Poultry Science* 65: 1516–21.

Morrow D A (1966) Fertility control programs *Veterinary Medicine* 61: 474.

Muirhead M R (1976) Veterinary problems in intensive pig husbandry. *Veterinary Record* 99: 288–92.

Muirhead M R (1978) Constraints on productivity in the pig herd. *Veterinary Record* 102: 228–31.

Muirhead M R (1980) The pig advisory visit in preventive medicine. *Veterinary Record* 106: 170–3.

Muirhead M R (1983) The role of the veterinarian as a swine management consultant. *International Swine Update* 2: 1–2.

Nagy K A (1987) Field metabolic rate and food requirement scaling in mammals and birds. *Econological Monographs* 57: 111–28.

Napier J (1974) Introductory address. In: Stress in farm animals. Proceedings of joint symposium of the Society for Veterinary Ethology/Royal Society for the Prevention of Cruelty to Animals, London, May 25–26. *British Veterinary Journal* 130: 85–6.

Nasir Hussain Shah S, Koops W, Samad H A, Wiel D F M van de (1988) A simple enzyme immunoassay of milk progesterone for monitoring fertility in dairy buffaloes. *Theriogeneology* 30(2): 211–15.

National Research Council (1988) *Nutrient requirements of dairy cattle, swine, etc*. National Academy Press, Washington D.C.

Nehring A (1981) One answer to the confinement pig problem. *International Journal of Study Probability* 2: 256–9.

Newby T J, Miller B, Stokes C R, Hampson D, Bourne F J (1985) Local hypersensitivity reactions to dietary antigens in early weaned pigs. In Cole D J A, Haresign W (eds) *Recent advances in pig nutrition*. Butterworths, London, pp 211–20.

Newmark P (1989) Guidelines produced for the use of transgenic animals in research. *Nature* 337: 295.

Norcross M A, Carnevale R A, Brown E A, Post A R (1989) Biotechnology and the control of growth and product quality in swine: safety of edible products. In Wal P van der, Nieuwland G J, Politiek R D (eds) *Biotechnology for control of growth and product quality in swine. Implications and acceptability*. Pudoc, Wageningen, pp 169–79.

Nygaard A, Oybwad I R (1969) How wide should the manager be? Institute for Bysningsteknikk, Norges Landbrukshogskole, Saertrykk, 121.

Oester H, Fröhlich E (1989) Alternative systems in Switzerland. In Kuit A R, Ehlhardt D A, Blokhuis H J (eds) *Agriculture. Alternative improved housing systems for poultry. Proceedings of a seminar, 17–18 May 1988, in the Community programme for the coordination of agricultural research, Spenderholt, Centre, Beekbergen, The Netherlands.*

Offringa C (1971) From the early history of veterinary science in The Netherlands (Dutch). In Numans S R, Mathijsen A H hM, Dunk H W van der, Poel J M G van der (eds) *From Gildestein to the Uithof* (Dutch). Veterinary Faculty of Utrecht, pp 7–31.

Ojo-Amaize E A, Solimonu L S, Williams A I O, Akinwolere O A O, Shabo R, Alm G V (1981) Positive correlation between degree of parasitaemia, interferon titres and natural killer cell activity in *Plasmodium falciparum*-infected children. *Journal of Immunology* **127**: 2296.

Oldenbroek J K, Garssen G J, Napel J ten, Verplanke J C, Brown A C G, Jonker L G (1989) The effect of treatment of dairy cows of different breeds with recombinantly derived bovine somatotrophin in a sustained delivery vehicle in three successive lactations. Contribution to the 40th Annual Meeting of the EAAP, August 27–31, Dublin, Ireland.

Oliverio A (1987) Endocrine aspects of stress: central and peripheral mechanisms. In Wiepkema P R, van Adrichem P W M (eds) *Biology of stress in farm animals: an integrative approach.* Martinus Nijhoff, Dordrecht, pp 3–12.

Oltenacu P A, Bendixen P H, Vilson B, Ekesbo I (1988) Evaluation of the tramped teats-clinical mastitis disease complex. Risk factors and interrelationships with other diseases. In Ekesbo I (ed) *Environment and Health. Proceedings of the 6th International Congress on Animal Hygiene, 14–17 June 1988, Skara, Sweden,* pp 46–50.

Organization for Economic Co-operation and Development (1988) *Long term economic impacts of biotechnology. An international survey.* Definitions-5. Committee for Scientific and Technological Policy. OECD.

Orr C L, Hutcheson D P, Grainger R B, Cummins J M, Mock R E (1990) Serum copper, zinc, calcium and phosphorus concentrations of calves stressed by bovine respiratory disease and infectious bovine rhinotracheitis. *Journal of Animal Science* **68**: 2893–900.

Otterness I G, Seymour P A, Golden H W, Reynolds J A, Daumy G O (1988) The effect of continuous administration of murine interleukin-1 in the rat. *Physiology and Behavior* **43**: 797–804.

Palmer S E (1981) Use of the portable infra-red thermometer as a measure of increasing limb surface temperature in the horse. *American Journal of Veterinary Research* **42**: 105–8.

Palya W L, Zacny J P (1980) Stereotyped adjunctive pecking by caged pigeons. *Animal Learning Behaviour* **8**: 293–300.

Parrott R F, Misson B H, Baldwin B A (1989) Salivary cortisol in pigs following adrenocorticotrophic hormone stimulation: comparison with plasma levels. *British Veterinary Journal* **145**: 362–6.

Paterson D, Ryder R D (eds) (1979) *Animal rights: a symposium.* Centaur Press, London.

Paterson J H, Linzell J L (1974) Cortisol secretion rate, glucose entry rate and the mammary uptake of cortisol and glucose during pregnancy and lactation in dairy cows. *Journal of Endocrinology* **62**: 371–83.

Payne J M et al. (1970) *Veterinary Record* **87**: 150.

Payne J M, Payne S (1987) *The metabolic profile test.* Oxford University Press, Oxford.

Pearce G P, Paterson A M, Pearce A N (1989) The influence of pleasant and unpleasant handling and the provision of toys on the growth and behaviour of male pigs. *Applied Animal Behaviour Science* **23**: 27–37.

Peplowski M A, Mahan D C, Murray F A, Moxon A L, Cantor A H, Ekstrom K E (1980) Effect of dietary and injectable vitamin E and selenium in weanling swine antigenically challenged with sheep red blood cells. *Journal of Animal Science* **51**: 344–51.

Perry G C, Patterson R L S, McFic H J H (1980) Pig courtship behaviour: pheromonal properties of androstene steroids in male submaxillary secretions. *Animal Production* **31**: 191–5.

Petherick J C, Baxter S H (1981) Modelling the static spatial requirement of livestock. In McCormack J A D (ed) *Modelling, design and evaluation of agricultural buildings*. Aberdeen, August 1981, Seminar CIGR, pp 75–82.

PHCA (1986) *The works and benefits of the Pig Health Control Association*. PHCA, Hadingley, Cambridge, UK.

Phillips P A, Fraser D, Thompson B K (1987) A farrowing crate design to promote sow movement. *American Society Agricultural Engineering Report*.

Phillips W A, Juniewicz P E, Zavy M T, Von Tungeln D L (1989) The effect of the stress of weaning and transport on white blood cell patterns and fibrinogen concentrations of beef calves of different genotypes. *Canadian Journal of Animal Science* **69**: 333–40.

Picard L, Betteridge K J (1989) The micro manipulation of farm animal embryos. In Babiuk L J, Phillips J P, Moo-Young M (eds) *Animal Biotechnology*. Pergamon, Oxford, pp 141–79.

Plym-Forshell K (1986) *Studies on health and behaviour in fatteners in three different feeding systems*. Swedish University of Agricultural Science Department of Animal Hygiene, Report 16, Skara, Sweden, 66 pp.

Politiek R D, Bakker J J (eds) (1982) *Livestock production in Europe. Perspectives and prospects*. Elsevier, Amsterdam.

Poulos P, Reiland S, Olsson S, Elwinger K (1978) *Acta Radiologica* (Suppl.) **358**: 277–98.

Powell A (1988) The story of the brown dog. *Liberator*, November/December, pp 24–5.

Prathaban S, Gnanaprakasam (1990) Study of plasma fibrinogen level of Indian crossbred cows in health and disease. *Indian Veterinary Journal* **67**: 453–6.

Prathaban S, Nagarajan V U (1984) Study on plasma fibrinogen levels in health and disease of Indian buffaloes. *Cheiron* **13**: 232–5.

Price E O (1984) Behavioural aspects of animal domestication. *Quarterly Review of Biology* **59**: 1–31.

Pritchard D G (1989) Analysis of risk factors for infection of cattle herds with *Leptospira hardjo*. *Proceedings of the Society for Veterinary Epidemiology and Preventive Medicine, Exeter*. pp 130–8.

Pursel V G, Hammer R E, Bolt D J, Palmiter R D, Brinster R L (1990) Integration, expression and germ-line transmission of growth-related genes in pigs. In Hansel W, Weir B J (eds) Genetic engineering of animals. *Journal of Reproduction and Fertility* Supplement **41**: 77–87.

Pursel V G, Pinkert C A, Miller K F, Bolt D J, Campbell R G, Palmiter R D, et al. (1989) Genetic engineering of livestock. *Science* **244**: 1281–8.

Raybould T J G (1989) Applications of monoclonal antibodies in animal health and production. In Babiuk L J, Phillips J P, Moo-Young M (eds) *Animal biotechnology*. Pergamon, Oxford, pp 21–39.

Reiland S (1975) Osteochondrosis in the pig. A morphologic and experimental investigation with special reference to the leg weakness syndrome. *Thesis, Stockholm*, 118 pp.

Regan T (1991) The more things change. *Between the Species*. Spring, pp 110–16.

Ricker J P, Shoog L A, Hirsch J (1987) Domestication and the behaviour genetic analysis of captive population. *Applied Animal Behaviour Science* **18**: 91–103.

Robert S, De Passille A-M B, St Pierre N, Dubreuil P, Pelletier G, Petitclerc D, et al. (1989) Effect of the stress of injections on the serum concentration of cortisol, prolactin and growth hormone in gilts and lactation sows. *Canadian Journal of Animal Science* **69**: 663–72.

Rose R J, Ilkiw J E, Arnold K S, Backhouse J W, Sampson D (1980) Plasma biochemistry in the horse during 3-day event competition. *Equine Veterinary Journal* 12: 132–6.

Ross C C, Daley W D R (1988) Sensor performance in monitoring and control systems for animal housing. *Proceedings of the Third International Livestock Environment Symposium*. American Society of Agricultural Engineering, St Joseph, MI.

Rowan A N (1991) Money and mail (letter). *The Animals' Agenda*, September, pp 6–7.

Rowsell H C (1984) Public concern and the animal welfare profiteer. Presented at Canadian Association for Laboratory Animal Science 23rd Annual Symposium, Quebec, Quebec, June 24. *CALAS Newsletter* 16(6): 106, 111–15.

Rowsell H C (1991a) Transportation of animals. A global animal issue. In *Proceedings on Animal Welfare, 24th World Veterinary Congress, Rio de Janeiro, Brazil, August 19–24* (in press).

Rowsell H C (1991b) The Canadian Council on Animal Care—Its guidelines and policy directives: The veterinarian's responsibility. *Canadian Journal of Veterinary Research* 55: 205.

Rushen J P (1984) Stereotyped behaviour adjunctive drinking and the feeding period of tethered sows. *Animal Behaviour* 32: 1059–68.

Rushen J P (1985) Stereotypies, aggression and the feeding schedules of tethered sows. *Applied Animal Behaviour Science* 14: 137–47.

Rutgers L J E (1990) Looking for a specifically professional code in a justifiable animal husbandry (Dutch). In Politiek R D (ed) *Prominent Developments*. Pudoc, Wageningen, pp 202–13.

Ryder R (1975) *Victims of science. The use of animals in science*. Davis-Poynter, London.

Ryder R (1989) *Animal revolution: Changing attitudes towards speciesism*. Basil Blackwell, Oxford, England; Cambridge, Massachusetts.

Sainsbury D W B, Sainsbury P (1988) *Livestock health and housing*, 3rd edn. Baillière Tindall, London.

Saloniemi H (1980) Udder diseases in dairy cows—field observations on incidence, somatic and environmental factors, and control. *Journal of the Scientific Agricultural Society of Finland* 52: 85–184.

Sambraus H H (1985) Stereotypies. In Fraser A F (ed) *Ethology of farm animals*. Elsevier, Amsterdam, pp 431–41.

Sanhouri A A, Jones R S, Dobson H (1991) Pentobarbitone inhibits the stress response to transport in male goats. *British Veterinary Journal* 147: 42–8.

Sapolsky R, Rivier C, Yamamoto G, Plotsky P, Vale W (1987) Interleukin-1 stimulates the secretion of hypothalamic corticotrophin-releasing factor. *Science* 238: 522–4.

Sayers G (1950) The adrenal cortex and homeostasis. *Physiological Reviews* 30: 241–320.

Schalm O W, Jain N G, Carroll E J (1975) *Veterinary Hematology*, 3rd edn. Lea & Febiger, Philadelphia.

Schlichting M C, Andreae U, Thielscher H-H, Smidt D (1983) Application of an integrated system of indicators in animal welfare research. In Smidt D (ed) *Indicators relevant to farm animal welfare*. Martinus Nijhoff, Boston, pp 215–21.

Schutt D A, Fell L F (1985) Comparison of total and free cortisol in bovine serum and milk or colostrum. *Journal of Dairy Science* 68: 1832–4.

Schwenger B (1990) Control of genetic defects. In Blancou J (ed) *Rev. sci. tech. Off. int. Epiz.* 9(3): 897–910.

Schwlam J W, Tucker H A (1978) Glucocorticoids in mammary secretions and blood serum during reproduction and lactation and distributions of glucocorticoids, progesterone and oestrogens in fractions of milk. *Journal of Dairy Science* 61: 550–60.

Seabrook M F (1984) The psychological interaction between the stockman and his animals and its influence on performance of pigs and dairy cows. *Veterinary Record* **28**: 84–7.

Seabrook M F (1987) *The role of the stockman in livestock productivity and management*. European Communities Publications 10982, Luxembourg.

Seabrook M F (1990) Reaction of dairy cattle and pigs to humans. In Zayan R, Dantzer R (eds) *Social stress in domestic animals*. Kluwer, Dordrecht, pp 110–20.

Seawright G L (1976) Remote temperature monitoring in animal health management. *United States Animal Health Association's 80th Annual Meeting, Florida*, pp 214–30.

Seligsohn U, Rapaport S C, Kuefler P R (1973) Extra-adrenal effect of ACTH on fibrinogen synthesis. *American Journal of Physiology* **224**: 1172–9.

Selye H (1936) A syndrome produced by diverse nocuous agents. *Nature* **138**: 32–3.

Selye H (1946) The general adaptation syndrome and the disease of adaptation. *Journal of Clinical Endocrinology and Metabolism* **6**: 117–23.

Selye H (1950) *The physiology and pathology of stress. A treatise based on the concepts of the general adaptation syndrome and the diseases of adaptation*. Acta Inc., Montreal, Canada, 822 pp.

Selye H (1973) The evaluation of the stress concept. *American Scientist* **61**: 692–9.

Serjsen K, Vestergaard M, Neimann-Sørenson A (1989) *Use of somatotrophin in livestock production*. Elsevier, London.

Sharman D F, Stephens D B (1974) The effect of apomorphin on the behaviour of farm animals. *Journal of Physiology* **242**: 25–7.

Simons J P, McClenaghan, Clark J A (1987) Alteration of the quality of milk by expression of sheep betalactoglobulin in transgenic mice. *Nature* **328**: 530–2.

Simonsen H B (1977) Velfaerdsuiveau i husdryproducktionen. *Danske Vet. Tiddski* **60**(6): 272–4.

Singer P (1973) Animals, men and morals. *New York Review of Books,*

Singer P (1975) Animal liberation. *New York Review of Books,*

Singer P (1990) The significance of animal suffering. *Behavioural Brain Science* (in press).

Singleton W B (1989) Summary. In Cockrill W R (ed) *Proceedings of symposium: Working Animals International. December 12, Oxford, UK*, pp 71–3.

Sloet van Oldruitenbourgh-Oosterbaan M M, Wensing Th, Bareneveld A, Breukink H J (1991) Heart rate, blood biochemistry and performance of horses competing in a 100 km endurance ride. *Veterinary Record* **128**: 175–9.

Smedegaard H H (1982) Pododermatitis circumscripta. *Dansk Veterinär Tidskrift* **65**: 558–69.

Smith F B (1983) Meteorological factors influencing the dispersion of airborne diseases. *Philosophical Transactions of the Royal Society, London* **B302**: 439–50.

Smith K L, Conrad H R, Amiet B A, Schoenberger P S, Todhunter D A (1985) Effect of vitamin E and selenium dietary supplementation in mastitis in first lactation dairy cows. *Journal of Dairy Science* **68**(Suppl. 1): 190–1 (Abstract).

Snijders J M A, Smeets J F M, Harbers A H M, Logtestijn J G van (1989) The evolution of meat inspection of slaughter pigs. *Fleischwirtschaft* **69**(2): 1422–4.

Spallholz J E, Martin J L, Gerlach M L, Heinzerling R H (1975) Injectable selenium: Effect on the primary immune response of mice. *Proceedings of the Society of Experimental Biology and Medicine* **148**: 37–40.

Spira H (1986) Here's what you can do to make a difference. Factory farming. *Animal Rights Coalitions Coordinators Report '86* September, p 4.

Spira H (1991) Alternatives and future challenges. The *Johns Hopkins Center for Alternatives to Animal Testing— Special 10th Anniversary Edition* **9**(1): 8.

Stephens A J, Esslemont R J, Ellis P R (1982) DAISY in veterinary practice.

Planned animal health and production services and small computers. In Gunsell, Hill (eds) *Veterinary Annual No. 22.* Wright, Bristol, pp 6–17.

Stephens D B (1980) Stress and its measurement in domestic animals. A review of behavioural and physiological studies under field and laboratory situations. *Advances in Veterinary Science and Comparative Medicine* 24: 179–210.

Stolba A, Wood-Gush D G M (1984) The identification of behavioural key features and their incorporation into a housing design for pigs. *Annales Recherches Vétérinaires* 15: 287–98.

Stolba A, Baker N, Wood-Gush D G M (1983) The characterisation of stereotyped behaviour in stalled sows by informational redundancy. *Behaviour* 87: 157–82.

Svedberg J (1976) Studies of connections between environment and health in poultry herds. Information of an on-going investigation. *2. Congress of the International Society for Animal Hygiene, Zagreb, Collected Reports*, pp 282–6.

Svedberg J (1980) Some environmentally evoked changes and lesions in laying hens. In Willinger H (ed) *Proceedings of the 3rd International Congress on Animal Hygiene, Vienna, 1980*, pp 198–9.

Svedberg J (1988a) The connection between environment and foot conditions in laying hens. In Ekesbo I (ed) *Environment and Animal Health. Proceedings of International Congress on Animal Hygiene*, Vol. I, Report 20. Department of Animal Hygiene, Skara, pp 125–30.

Svedberg J (1988b) Feed pelleting process and salmonella infection in broilers. In Ekesbo I (ed) *Environment and Animal Health. Proceedings of International Congress on Animal Hygiene*, Vol. II, Report 21. Department of Animal Hygiene, Skara, pp 826–30.

Swedish Ministry of Agriculture (1988) *Swedish Code of Statutes* SFS, 1988:539. Animal Protection Ordinance.

Tarrant P V (ed) (1984) *Farm animal welfare programme. Evaluation report 1979–1983.* CEC, Brussels/Luxembourg.

Tazi A, Dantzer R, Crestani F, Le Moal M (1988) Interleukin-1 induces conditioned taste aversion in rats: a possible explanation for its pituitary-adrenal stimulating activity. *Brain Research* 473: 369–71.

Teige J E, Tollersrud S, Lund P, Larsen H J (1982) Swine dysentery. The influence of dietary vitamin E and selenium on the clinical and pathological effects of *Treponema hyodysenteriae* infection in pigs. *Research in Veterinary Science* 32: 95–100.

Tennessen T (1989) Coping with confinement—features of the environment that influence animals' ability to adapt. *Applied Animal Behaviour Science* 22: 139–49.

Tennessen T, Price M A, Berg R T (1984) Comparative responses of bulls and steers to transportation. *Canadian Journal of Animal Science* 64: 333.

Thomas L H (1978) Disease incidence and epidemiology—the situation in the UK. In Martin W B (ed) *Respiratory diseases in cattle.* Martinus Nijhoff, The Hague, pp 57–65.

Thurley D C (1977) Some factors predisposing to perinatal lamb mortality. *Proceedings of the 2nd Seminar of the New Zealand Veterinary Assocation Sheep Society.* Massey University, New Zealand, pp 95–103.

Tielen M J M (1974) Incidence and the prevention by animal care of lung and liver affections of fattening pigs. Thesis, Med. Landb. Hogeschool, 141 pp.

Traystman R J (1990) The goal of animal welfare, animal 'rights' and anti-vivisectionist groups in the United States. *Journal of Neurosurgical Anaesthesiology* 2(3): 153–8.

Turner M J B, Gurney P, Crowther J S W, Sharp J R (1984) An automatic weighing system for poultry. *Journal of Agricultural Engineering Research* 29: 17–26.

Underwood E J (1980) *Mineral nutrition of livestock.* Commonwealth Agricultural Bureau, Slough.

Udomprasert P, Williamson N B (1990) The DAIRY champ program. A computerised recording system for dairy herds. *Veterinary Record* **127**: 256–62.

Universities Federation for Animal Welfare (1971) *Humane killing and slaughterhouse techniques.* UFAW, South Mimms, UK.

Universities Federation for Animal Welfare (1980) *Self-awareness in domesticated animals.* UFAW, South Mimms, UK.

Universities Federation for Animal Welfare (1981) *Alternatives to intensive husbandry systems.* UFAW, South Mimms, UK.

Universities Federation for Animal Welfare (1982) *Stockmanship on the farm.* UFAW, South Mimms, UK.

Unshelm J (1983) Applicability of indicators in animal welfare research. In Smidt D (ed) *Indicators relevant to farm animal welfare.* Martinus Nijhoff, Boston, pp 225–32.

Valpy M (1991) Humane Society's rules under the gun. *Toronto Globe and Mail*, June 25, p A6.

Van Brunt J (1988) Molecular farming: transgenic animals as bioreactors. *Biotechnology* **6**(10): 1145–54.

Van der Kolk J H (1990a) The bovine pituitary adrenocortical axis and adaptive abilities of three breeds of Chinese pigs. Behavioural and neuroendocrine reactions. *Genetic Selection and Evaluation* **16**: 85–102.

Van der Kolk J H (1990b) The bovine pituitary adrenocortical axis and milk yield. *Veterinary Quarterly* **12**: 114–20.

Van der Mei J (1987) Health aspects of welfare research in veal calves. In Schlichting M C, Smidt D (eds) *Welfare aspects of housing systems for veal calves and fattening bulls.* CEC, EUR 19717 EN.

Van Putten G (1979) *Proceedings 1st Conference on the Protection of Farm Animals.* RSPCA, London.

Van Putten G (1982) Handling of slaughter pigs prior to loading and during loading in a lorry. In Moss R (ed) *Transport of animals intended for breeding, production and slaughter.* Martinus Nijhoff, The Hague, pp 15–25.

Van Putten G, Elshof W J (1982) Inharmonious behaviour in veal-calves. In Bessei W (ed) *Disturbed behaviours in farm animals.* Verlag Eugen Ulmer, Stuttgart, pp 61–71.

Venant E, Treadwell D (1990) biting back. *Los Angeles Times*, April 12, p E1.

Verstegen M W A, Hel W van der, Henken A M, Huisman J, Kanis E, Wal P van der, et al. (1990) Effect of exogenous porcine somatotrophin administration on nitrogen and energy metabolism in three genotypes of pigs. *Journal of Animal Science* **68**(4): 1008–16.

Vilson B (1973) Environment and health in 1000 dairy herds. *Proceedings 1st International Congress for Animal Hygiene, October 1973, Budapest*, 41 pp.

Vilson B (1976) Dairy cattle health in different environments. Preliminary results from a four-year Swedish study. In Ivos J (ed) *Proceedings 2nd International Congress for Animal Hygiene, September 1976, Zagreb*, pp 135–40.

Visek W J (1978) The mode of growth promotion by antibiotics. *Journal of Animal Science* **46**: 1447–69.

Wagner Th E (1988) Direct modification of the livestock genome. In Wal P Vd, Nieuwhof G J, Politiek R D (eds) *Biotechnology for control of growth and product quality in swine. Implications and acceptability.* Pudoc, Wageningen, pp 77–87.

Waltner-Toews D, Martin S W, Meek A H (1986) Dairy calf management and mortality in Ontario Holstein herds. iii. Association of management with morbidity. *Preventive Veterinary Medicine* **4**: 139–58.

Wannall W R (1991) Animal-rights activism's dark side. *Chicago Tribune*, August 6, p. 13.

Ward K A, Nancarrow C D, Byrne C R, Shanahan C M, Murray J D, Leish Z, et al. (1990) The potential of transgenic animals for improved agricultural productivity. In Blancou J (ed) *Rev. sci. tech. Off. int. Epiz.* **9**(3): 847–64.

Wassell T R, Esslemont R J (1992) Survey of the operation of dairy herd health schemes by veterinary practices in the U.K. *Veterinary Record* (in press).

Wathes C M, Jones C D R, Webster A J F (1983) Ventilation, air hygiene and animal health. *Veterinary Record* **113**: 554–9.

Wathes C M, Miller B G, Bourne F J (1989) Cold stress and post-weaning diarrhoea in piglets inoculated orally or by aerosol. *Animal Production* **49**: 483–96.

Wathes C M, Zaidan W A R, Pearson G R, Hinton M, Todd J W (1988) Aerosol infection of calves and mice with *Salmonella typhimurium*. *Veterinary Record* **123**: 590–4.

Watts S (1990) DNA gene on target for gene therapy. *New Scientist*, nr. 1734–34.

Webster A J F (1983) Nutrition and the thermal environment. In Rook J A F, Thomas P C (eds) *Nutritional physiology of farm animals*. Longman, London, pp 639–69.

Webster A J F (1984) *Calf husbandry, health and welfare*. Collins, London.

Webster A J F (1987) *Understanding the dairy cow*. Blackwell Scientific Publications, London.

Webster A J F (1989a) Bioenergetics, bioengineering and growth. *Animal Production* **48**: 249–69.

Webster A J F (1989b) Animal housing as perceived by the animal. *Veterinary Annual* **29**: 1–8.

Webster A J F, Clarke A F, Madelin T M, Wathes C M (1987) Air hygiene in stables. 1. Effects of stable design, ventilation and management on the concentration of respirable dust. *Equine Veterinary Journal* **19**: 448–53.

Wegner R M (1983) Production performance in laying hens kept under different housing conditions. In Schmidt D (ed) *Indicators relevant to farm animal welfare*. Martinus Nijhoff, The Hague, pp 189–97.

Weiss J M (1972) Stress and disease. *Scientific American* **226**: 104–13.

Weiss G M, Topel D G, Siers D G, Magilton J H (1970) Relationships of plasma cortisol and growth hormone levels to muscle quality characteristics in normal and stress-prone swine. *Journal of Animal Science* **31**: 1018 (Abstract).

Welch R A S, Day A M, Duganzich D M, Featherstone R (1979) Induced calving, a comparison of treatment regimes. *New Zealand Veterinary Journal* **27**: 190–8.

Westerterp K R, Saris I J H M, Vanes A, Ten Hoor R (1986) Use of the doubly labelled water technique in humans during heavy sustained exercise. *Journal of Applied Physiology* **61**: 2162–7.

Widowski T M, Curtis S E, Graves C N (1989) The neutrophil: lymphocyte ratio in pigs fed cortisol. *Canadian Journal of Animal Science* **69**: 501–4.

Wiepkema P R (1987) Developmental aspect of motivated behavior in domestic animals. *Journal of Animal Science* **65**: 1220–7.

Wiepkema P R, Broom D M, Duncan I J H, van Putten G (1983) *Abnormal behaviours in farm animals*. CEC Report, Brussels.

Wiepkema P R, van Hellemond K K, Roessingh P, Romberg H (1987) Behaviour and abomasal damage in individual veal calves. *Applied Animal Behaviour Science* **18**: 257–68.

Wierenga H K (1983) The influence of the space for walking and lying on a cubicle system on the behaviour of dairy cattle. In Baxter S H, Baxter M R, McCormack J A C (eds) *Farm animal housing and welfare*. Martinus Nijhoff, The Hague, pp 171–81.

Wilkins D B (1989) Animal welfare societies in Europe. Presented to British Veterinary Association Congress, September 6–10.

Willard J G, Willard J C, Wolfral S A, Baker J P (1977) Effect of diet on caecal pH and feeding behavior of horses. *Journal of Animal Science* **45**: 87–93.

Williamson N B (1987) Evaluating herd

reproductive status. *Proceedings of the AABP Annual Congress* **19**: 117–21.

Williamson N B (1988) A health and management program for heifers. *Proceedings of the XVth World Congress on Diseases of Cattle, Palma, Mallorca*, pp 1020–37.

Wokac R M (1987) Skeletal deformations in laying hens in battery and deep litter husbandry. *Berliner und Munchener Tierarztliche Wochenschrift* **100**: 191–8.

Wood G (1990) Factory farming: the pig product. *Animal Welfare Institute Quarterly*, Fall, pp 4–5.

Wood P D P (1976) *Animal Production* **22**: 275.

Wood-Gush D G M (1988) The relevance of the knowledge of free ranging domesticated animals for animal husbandry. In van Putten G, Unshelm J, Zeeb K (eds) *International Congress of Applied Ethology of Farm Animals, Skara, Sweden*. KTBL, Darmstadt.

World Veterinary Association (1991) Policy statement on animal welfare, well-being and ethology. *World Veterinary Association Bulletin* **7**(2): 38–9.

Yaukey J (1991) Animal research is right, expert says. *Ithaca Journal*, January 9.

Yong Kang (1989) Vaccine production by recombinant DNA technology. In Babink L A, Phillips, J P, Moo-Young M (eds) *Animal biotechnology*. Pergamon, Oxford, pp 39–63.

Young E M, Anderson D B (1986) First service conception rate in dairy cows treated with dinoprost tromethamine early post partum. *Veterinary Record* **118**: 212–13.

Zappavigna P (1983) Space and equipment requirements for feeding in cattle housing. In Baxter S H, Baxter M R, MacCormack J A C (eds) *Farm animal housing and welfare*. Martinus Nijhoff, The Hague, pp 155–64.

Zayan R, Doyen J, Duncan I J H (1983) Social and space requirements for hens in battery cages. In Baxter S H, Baxter M R, McCormack J A D (eds) *Farm animal housing and welfare*. Martinus Nijhoff, The Hague, pp 67–91.

Zijpp A J van der, Sybesma W (eds) (1989) *Improving genetic disease resistance in farm animals*. Kluwer Academic Publishers, Dordrecht/Boston, London.

Legislation

European Economic Community
Directive 77/489/EEC Protection of Animals during International Transport

France
Loi no: 76-629 10 July 1976 modified by Loi no: 87-501 8 July 1987

Great Britain
Protection of Animals Act 1911 as amended

Agriculture (Miscellaneous Provisions) Act 1968

Welfare of Livestock (Intensive Units) Regulations 1978

Welfare of Livestock (Prohibited Operations) Regulations 1982 and amendment 1987

Docking of Pigs (use of Anaesthetics) Order 1974

Removal of Antlers in Velvet (Anaesthetics) Order 1980

Codes of Welfare Practice

Luxembourg
Law of 15th March 1983: covering protection of life and well-being of animals

Northern Ireland
The Welfare of Animals Act 1972

Norway
Welfare of Animals Act 1974

Transport of Live Animals Regulations 1984

Sweden
Swedish Animal Protection Act 1988

Animal Protection Ordinance 1988

West Germany
Law on Animal Protection 1986.

Brochure on Animal Protection: Federal Minister of Food, Agriculture and Forestry: issued 1986.

INDEX